Nutritional Assessment
A Laboratory Manual

Nutritional Assessment
A Laboratory Manual

ROSALIND S. GIBSON

Professor of Applied Human Nutrition

University of Guelph

New York   Oxford

OXFORD UNIVERSITY PRESS

1993

Oxford University Press

Oxford   New York   Toronto
Delhi   Bombay   Calcutta   Madras   Karachi
Kuala Lumpur   Singapore   Hong Kong   Tokyo
Nairobi   Dar es Salaam   Cape Town
Melbourne   Auckland   Madrid

and associated companies in
Berlin   Ibadan

Published by Oxford University Press, Inc.,
198 Madison Avenue, New York, New York 10016-4314

Oxford is a registered trademark of Oxford University Press

Library of Congress Cataloging-in-Publication Data
Gibson, Rosalind, S.
    Nutritional assessment : a laboratory manual / Rosalind S. Gibson.
      p.   cm.   Includes bibliographical references and index.
    ISBN 0-19-508547-7
    1. Nutrition—Evaluation—Laboratory manuals. I. Title.
  RC621.G52   1993
  613.2—dc20   93-1087

Grateful acknowledgment is made to the University of Michigan Press for
Tables II.2, 4.2, 4.9, 4.13, 4.15, 4.16, 5.1, 5.5, 5.6, 5.7, 6.1, 6.5, 6.8, 6.9, 6.10,
6.11, 6.12 and 6.13, adapted from *Anthropometric Standards for the Assessment of Growth
and Nutritional Status* by Roberto A. Frisancho. Copyright by the University of Michigan 1990.
Published by the University of Michigan Press.

9 8 7 6 5 4 3 2

Printed in the United States of America
on acid-free paper

Preface

This laboratory manual has been written to accompany my earlier text (Principles of Nutritional Assessment, Oxford University Press, New York, 1990), and is a guide to practical dietary, anthropometric, and biochemical nutritional assessment. It was written initially for my students, because of the lack of any comparable text, and in the hope of increasing awareness of the importance of rigorous methodology in nutritional assessment. I also hope the book will encourage the teaching of laboratory work in assessment. Students of nutrition, dietetics, home economics, public health, and nursing, as well as health professionals involved in nutritional assessment, should find this new manual useful.

The arrangement of the material follows that of the original text, with separate parts on dietary, anthropometric and biochemical assessment. Each part commences with an overview of the advantages, limitations and applicability of each form of nutritional assessment. The overview is then followed by detailed instructions on standardized procedures for each of the assessment methods. Although particular emphasis is placed on practical and laboratory methods of nutritional assessment, some associated text from the earlier volume provides a theoretical framework; key references are also given. Laboratory assignments have not been included as it was thought that instructors would want to devise these to suit the needs of their own students.

Three separate chapters deal with quantitative and qualitative dietary methods and the evaluation of nutrient intakes. The anthropometric part covers the assessment of growth, the fat-free mass, and body fat. Evaluation of the anthropometric measurements used is discussed at the end of each method and reference data from national surveys in Canada and the United States are included where possible.

Biochemical assessment is covered in five chapters dealing with specific groups of nutrients, and a chapter on hematology. Examples of both static and functional biochemical methods are included. The biochemical methods have been selected as appropriate for use by undergraduate students with limited practical laboratory experience. Thus the methods are not necessarily 'state of the art' but are instead proven standard laboratory procedures. Commercial kits are used for some methods to minimize preparation time and maximize accuracy and precision of the analytical results. Interpretive criteria for evaluating the biochemical measurements are also included at the end of each method, based on reference distributions compiled from national surveys; alternatively, cutoff points are given.

A glossary is given at the end of the text for the convenience of the reader. Other appendices give abbreviations, a conversion table for weights and measures, and a list of suppliers of anthropometric equipment.

I am particularly grateful to the individuals, editors, and publishers who granted permission to reproduce figures and tables. In most cases these tables have been reset and the figures redrawn; the sources have been acknowledged in the text. During the initial stages of preparation of the material, numerous undergraduate and graduate students in the Division of Applied Human Nutrition at the University of Guelph provided suggestions and corrections. Many have been incorporated into this final version of the text and I am grateful for this help. I am also indebted to Fiona Yeudell and Cristine Grunt for their assistance with the references and proofs. I would also like to thank Ingeborg Brouwer of the University of Wageningen, The Netherlands, who kindly proofread the entire text, although I am responsible for remaining defects of fact, treatment, judgment or style.

This book has been printed from computer-typeset material prepared by myself and my husband, Ian L. Gibson. Mr Philip Taylor, University of London, kindly provided advice and assistance with the typesetting.

R. S. G.
Guelph, Ontario, Canada.
February, 1993.

This book is dedicated to our daughter Isobel, and our son Simon, who introduced us to TeX and LaTeX, and who was tragically killed in a climbing accident on Guye Peak, Washington, USA, on June 17th, 1990.

Table of Contents

Nutritional Assessment
A Laboratory Manual

Part I
Dietary Assessment

Contents

Overview

There are four stages in any dietary assessment protocol designed to assess nutrient intakes. These stages are: (1) the measurement of food consumption; (2) the calculation of the nutrient content of food eaten; (3) the assessment of absorbed intakes; and (4) the evaluation of nutrient intakes in relation to recommendations.

Stage 1. Methods for assessing food consumption of individuals can be classified into two major groups—quantitative and qualitative: these are described in detail in Chapters 1 and 2; the choice of the method depends primarily on the objectives of the study; Callmer et al. (1985) describe four possible levels of objectives.

For level one, the mean intake of a group is required. This can be accomplished by measuring the food intake of each subject for one day only.

Level two involves estimating the proportion of the population 'at risk' of inadequate intake by measuring the food consumed by each subject over more than one day.

For level three, multiple replicates of daily food intake must be measured, the number of days depending upon the day-to-day variation in the intake of the nutrients of interest. With such data, intakes of individuals can be ranked within the distribution.

When data on usual food intakes of individuals are required for individual counselling or for correlation and regression analysis, an even larger number of measurement days for each individual are required. Some investigators recommend using qualitative dietary methods, such as the dietary history or semi-quantitative food frequency questionnaire, to obtain this level-four data (Hankin, 1987).

Additional factors which should be considered when selecting a method for measuring food intake include the characteristics of the subjects within the study population, the respondent burden of the method, and the available resources. Generally, the more accurate methods are associated with higher costs, greater respondent burden, and lower response rates.

Stage 2. For the conversion of food to nutrient intakes, food composition tables or nutrient databases stored on a computer are used. Nutrient intakes calculated in this way represent the maximum amount available to the body. For most nutrients, however, the amount actually absorbed and utilized by the body cells will be lower than the determined values (O'Dell, 1983).

Stage 3. In the third stage of the dietary assessment protocol, an estimate of the bioavailability of the nutrients is made, often derived from the proportion of plant- to animal-based foods in the diet.

Stage 4. The fourth stage involves evaluating the adequacy of the nutrient intakes, by comparison with tables of recommended nutrient intakes. This stage is discussed in detail in Chapter 3.

References

Callmer E, Haraldsdottir J, Løker E B, Seppänen R, Solvoll K (1985). Selecting a method for a dietary survey. Närings-forskning 2: 43–52.

Hankin J H (1987). Dietary methods for estimating vitamin A and carotene intakes in epidemiologic studies of cancer. Journal of Canadian Dietetic Association 48: 219–224.

O'Dell B L (1983). Bioavailability of trace elements. Federation Proceedings 42: 1714–1715.

Chapter 1
Quantitative dietary assessment

Contents

Introduction

Quantitative dietary assessment methods consist of recalls or food records designed to measure the quantity of individual foods consumed over a one-day period. These methods are described in detail in Sections 1.1 and 1.2. By increasing the number of measurement days, quantitative estimates of recent food intake, or—for longer time periods—habitual food intake of individuals can be obtained. The number of measurement days, their selection and spacing, all depend on the objectives of the study, the diversity of food intake, and the day-to-day variation in intake of the nutrients of interest. Assessment of habitual intake is particularly critical when relationships between diet and biological parameters are assessed (Anderson, 1986).

Both systematic and random errors may occur during the measurement of food intake; the major sources of error are summarized in Table 1.1 (van Staveren and Burema, 1985). The direction and extent of these errors vary with the method used and the population and nutrients studied. Random errors affect the precision of the methods; such errors can be reduced by increasing the number of measurement days, but cannot be entirely eliminated. In contrast, systematic measurement errors cannot be minimized by extending the number of measurement days; these errors are important, as they can introduce a significant bias into the results which cannot be removed by subsequent statistical analysis.

Both types of measurement errors can be minimized by incorporating appropriate quality control procedures during each stage of the measurement process. For example, respondent and interviewer biases can be minimized by training the interviewers, and by developing standard interviewing techniques and questionnaires. Errors arising from respondent memory lapses can be reduced by probing questions and/or by using visual aids such

Sources of Error	24-hr Recall	Estimated Record	Weighed Record
Omitting foods	●	○	○
Adding foods	●	-	-
Estimating food weights	●	●	-
Estimating frequency	-	-	-
Day-to-day variation	●	●	●
Changes in diet	-	○	●
Coding errors	●	●	●

Table 1.1: Sources of error in quantitative dietary assessment techniques. ● error is likely; ○ error is possible; - error is unlikely. Modified from Staveren W A van, Burema J. Food consumption surveys: frustrations and expectations. Närings-forskning 2: 38–42, 1985.

as food models. To improve the accuracy of estimating portion sizes for recall methods, graduated food models can be used.

After the food consumption data have been collected, nutrient intakes can be calculated by hand using a food composition table or by computer if a computer-stored nutrient database is available; this procedure is discussed in Section 1.3. When a computer is used for this calculation, the recalls or records must first be coded; to minimize coding errors, 'coding rules' should be established to deal with incomplete or ambiguous descriptions of the foods (Anderson, 1986).

The recognition of the various potential sources of error in food composition values is important, as these errors affect the calculation of nutrient intakes whether food composition tables or nutrient databases are used. The errors may be a result of true random variability in the nutrient content of a food, or alternatively, the errors may be systematic and difficult to detect.

References

Anderson S A (1986). Guidelines for Use of Dietary Intake Data. Life Sciences Research Office, Federation of American Societies for Experimental Biology, Bethesda, Maryland.

Staveren W A van, Burema J (1985).   Food consumption surveys: frustrations and expectations. Näringsforskning 2: 38–42.

1.1 The twenty-four-hour recall

Principle

The purpose of the twenty-four-hour recall is to provide information on the respondent's exact food intake during the previous twenty-four-hour period or preceding day. Such information can be used to characterize the mean intake of a group. If habitual intakes of individuals are required, however, multiple replicate twenty-four-hour recalls must be used.

The twenty-four-hour recall is conducted in four stages using a standardized protocol. In the first stage, a complete list of all foods and beverages consumed during the previous twenty-four-hour period or preceding day is obtained. In the second stage, detailed descriptions of all the foods and beverages consumed, including cooking methods and brand names (if possible) are recorded, together with the time and place of consumption. In the third stage, estimates of the amounts of all foods and beverages consumed are obtained. Finally, in the fourth stage, the recall is reviewed to ensure that all items have been recorded correctly.

The advantages of the twenty-four-hour recall method include low respondent burden, high compliance, low cost, ease and speed of use, use of a standardized interview, an element of surprise (so that the respondent is less likely to modify his or her eating habits), and its suitability for illiterate respondents. Disadvantages include its reliance on memory, making it an unsatisfactory method for the elderly and for young children. Errors in the estimation of portion sizes of foods also occur, but can be reduced by using food models of various types to assist the respondent. Graduated food models are preferred because their use tends to prevent 'directed' responses, a phenomenon observed when simulated plastic food models representing 'average' portion sizes are used (Samuelson, 1970). The flat slope syndrome may be a problem in the twenty-four-hour recall method (Gersovitz et al., 1978): in this syndrome, individuals appear to overestimate low intakes and underestimate high intakes— sometimes referred to as "talking a good diet". Subjects completing single twenty-four-hour recalls

are likely to omit foods which are infrequently consumed.

When conducting the interview, both interpersonal and technical skills are important: for example, the interview must always be conducted with an open and pleasant manner, with the aim of being friendly, diplomatic, empathetic, and determined, as appropriate.

If possible, the interview should be conducted somewhere quiet. The interviewer should start by establishing a rapport with the respondent, who should be told that questions will cover all the food and beverages consumed during the preceding day with emphasis on the pattern of eating. Stress that all responses will be confidential and emphasise the importance of providing the correct information. Avoid asking questions about specific meals (e.g. breakfast, lunch, supper) or about snacks. Avoid showing any signs of surprise, approval, or disapproval of the subject's eating pattern (i.e. be non-judgemental at all times). Respondents should not be told in advance that a twenty-four-hour recall will be conducted on a particular day's food intake to avoid any changes in the food intake of the subject.

The success of the twenty-four-hour recall depends on the subject's memory, the ability of the respondent to convey accurate estimates of portion sizes consumed, the degree of motivation of the respondent, and the skill and persistence of the interviewer (Acheson et al., 1980).

Stage 1: Recall of foods and drinks consumed

The recall interview should commence with the first food and/or drink consumed in the morning. The interviewer should use neutral questions such as:

> *I would like you to tell me what you had to eat or drink after you woke up yesterday morning. What was the time? Did you eat that food at home? What did you have next and when was that?*

Proceed through the day, repeating these questions as necessary, and record each food or drink consumed in the appropriate column of the twenty-four-hour recall form (Table 1.2)

Stage 2: Description of foods and drinks consumed

During this stage, the interviewer should go over each of the responses made by the respondent, probing for more specific descriptions of all the foods and drinks consumed, including cooking methods and (if possible) brand names. These details are recorded in the third and fourth columns of the form (Table 1.2). Information on the place and time of eating should also be obtained and recorded in the first two columns. For homemade composite dishes, the amount of each raw ingredient used in the recipe should be recorded, the number of serving sizes for the recipe, and the amount of the composite dish consumed by the subject.

Guidelines for appropriate prompts for specific food items are given below:

- meat:
  - kind of meat
  - description of cut
  - raw or cooked weight
  - method of cooking
  - lean or lean + fat
  - bone in or not (waste factor)

- fish/sea food:
  - kind of fish/sea food
  - raw or cooked weight
  - method of cooking
  - bones/skin/shell (waste factor)

- poultry:
  - kind of poultry
  - parts or pieces eaten (e.g. breast, thigh)
  - raw or cooked weight
  - method of cooking
  - white or dark meat
  - meat + skin or meat only
  - bones (waste factor)

- fats:
  - kind of fat
  - brand name (if possible)

- milk products:
  - kind of dairy product
  - brand name (if possible)
  - percentage fat (as butter fat or milk fat)

- cheese:
  - type (Edam, Swiss, cream, etc.)
  - percentage fat (if possible)

- bread/rolls:
  - type of grain (rye, whole-wheat, etc.)
  - homemade/bought
  - size: standard or unusual
  - toasted or not
  - topping/condiments

- baked goods:
  - type of product
  - whether iced or not
  - homemade or commercial
  - type of filling

- cereal/pasta/rice:
  - type of grain
  - brand name
  - raw or cooked weight
  - enriched or not
  - record cereal + milk (if dry quantity unknown)

- vegetables:
  - fresh/frozen/canned
  - peeled/unpeeled
  - method of cooking
  - topping (butter, etc.)

- fruits:
  - fresh/frozen/canned
  - peeled/unpeeled
  - type of liquid (heavy, light)
  - sweetened/unsweetened

- beverages/soup:
  - volumetric or fluid ounces
  - size of can or bottle
  - fresh/frozen/canned/bottled
  - fruit juice: sweetened/unsweetened
  - added vitamins/minerals (e.g. Vit. C)
  - coffee: brewed, instant, decaffeinated, regular
  - soups: homemade/canned
  - soups: dilutant (milk/water)

- take-out foods:
  - restaurant name
  - food/beverage name
  - size of portion (small, medium, large)
  - condiments added

- candies, etc.:
  - brand name
  - size, price, or amount

- mixed dishes:
  - product name
  - homemade or commercial

Stage 3: Estimation of amounts

- Quantities can be recorded by the interviewer as volumes—milliliters, pints, cups, etc.; or as weights—grams, pounds, ounces, etc. Then convert all amounts to the equivalent number of grams.
- Use graduated food models (Fig. 1.1), such as those developed by Nutrition Canada (Health and Welfare Canada, 1973), to assist the respondent in estimating amounts. Display only appropriate models and emphasize that they are only a guide.
- Household cups, glasses, bowls and spoons, familiar to the respondent, can also be used to estimate amounts. If used, these should be calibrated.
- A ruler can be useful for estimating the thickness of slices of meat, cheese, and cake.
- Use counts for eggs and slices of bread.

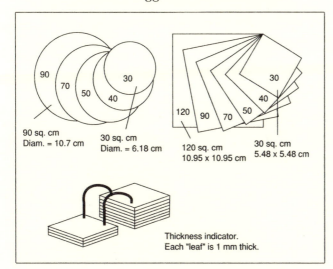

Fig. 1.1: Models for use in the estimation of portion size developed by Health and Welfare Canada (1973).

Stage 4: Review of interview data

At the end of the interview, it is important that the interviewer reviews the recall to ensure that all the items have been recorded correctly. This can be accomplished using a statement such as the following:

> *I will read back to you what I have recorded to make sure that I have not made any mistakes.*

Finally the respondent should be asked about the use of vitamin and mineral supplements, protein or diet drinks and also asked in a non-threatening manner about any alcohol consumed, e.g.

> *Did you have any alcoholic drinks during the day?*

Enquire about anything consumed in the middle of the night. As a final check, the interviewer should scan the recall in case any food groups have been omitted and should politely enquire about any missing items (e.g. meat or milk). The interviewer should then ask the subject whether the day of the recall represented a 'normal' day. At the end of the interview, the interviewer should thank the respondent for his or her time and co-operation.

References

Acheson K J, Campbell I T, Edholm O G, Miller D S, Stock M J (1980). The measurement of food and energy intake in man—an evaluation of some techniques. American Journal of Clinical Nutrition 33: 1147–1154.

Gersovitz M, Madden J P, Smiciklas-Wright H (1978). Validity of the twenty-four-hour dietary recall and seven-day record for group comparisons. Journal of the American Dietetic Association 73: 48–55.

Health and Welfare Canada (1973). Nutrition Canada National Survey. Health and Welfare, Ottawa.

Samuelson G (1970). An epidemiological study of child health and nutrition in a northern Swedish county. 2. Methodological study of the recall technique. Nutrition and Metabolism 12: 321–340.

1.2   The three-day food record

Principle

The purpose of the three-day food record is to provide a quantitative assessment of food intake over three days. Two weekdays and one weekend day should be included to take into account potential differences in food consumption patterns on weekdays versus weekend days.   To assess portion sizes, household measures or weighing scales should be used. Accuracy and precision are of course greater for the weighed record compared to the estimated record method, because the portion sizes are weighed. Misreading the weighing scale and/or errors in recording, however, may still occur (Cameron and van Staveren, 1988).

Respondents must be numerate and literate when a food record is used. They must also be highly motivated because the method is more time consuming than a twenty-four-hour recall, and the respondent burden is higher. Respondents may change their usual eating pattern to simplify the measuring or weighing process, or, alternatively, to impress the investigator (Burk and Pao, 1976).

Recording procedure

1. All food and beverages consumed throughout the three-day period must be recorded on the appropriate form (Table 1.2). Include all snacks, condiments and spices (e.g. pickles, catsup, sauces), tonics, alcoholic beverages, candy, etc.

2. All snacks, meals, or beverages consumed away from home must also be recorded.

3. Begin each new day on a new page of the record form. If a day uses more than one page, continue on to the next page but start the subsequent day at the top of a new page.

4. Record the day of the week and the date at the top of each page.

5. Record each item of a composite dish on a separate line. For example, a ham sandwich would be recorded as bread, ham, mayonnaise and butter, each on a separate line.

6. Record where (e.g. home, restaurant, office) and at what time, each meal, snack, or drink was consumed.

7. If vitamin or mineral supplements are used, list the amount taken each day, the brand name, and label information. If possible, the latter should be read directly from the bottle/package used by the respondent. Alternatively, the respondent can include the label with the completed record.

How to describe foods and drinks

Use a separate line for each food or food type when recording, and separate out components of composite dishes such as sandwiches, salads, or casseroles.   For all foods, include the following details:

1. Method of cooking (e.g. roasted, stewed, fried, boiled, steamed).

2. Kind of food (e.g. raw or cooked; peeled or unpeeled; white or whole wheat bread; fresh, canned, frozen, dried; 2%, whole or skim milk).

3. Brand names of all processed foods wherever applicable (e.g. Kraft Macaroni and Cheese, Campbell's soup, Kellogg's corn flakes).

4. Include all condiments (e.g. pickles, sauces, catsup, mustard).

5. Provide as much label information as possible and the brand name of any unusual or special foods consumed (e.g. sodium-reduced soup).

6. If a recipe is used to make composite products such as casseroles, baked goods, sauces, etc., record, on the back of the food record sheet, the complete recipe, giving the measured amount of each ingredient, the total number of servings for the dish, and the amount of the dish eaten by the respondent.

How to record amounts of foods and drinks

1. Record the amounts of all food and beverages in the form they are consumed. For example, do not record the weight or size of a raw pork chop: instead, record the amount of a fried pork chop.

Date		Day of the week			
Subject ID No.		Name of Subject			
Place Eaten	Time	Description of Food or Drink		Brand Name	Amount

Table 1.2: Form used to record detailed food intakes.

	Incorrect		Correct	
Group	Description	Amount	Description	Amount
Meat and Fish	Hamburger Lamb Fish	medium patty medium chop small portion	Beef hamburger Lamb chop, lean and fat Cod fried in batter	3 oz $2 \times 4 \times 1''$ $2 \times 3 \times 1''$
Fruits and vegetables	Apple Tomato	medium dish small amount	Stewed apple Fried tomato	1 cup 2 tbs.
Prepared foods	Bread Muffin Spaghetti	a few slices small portion large serving	Wholemeal bread Bran muffin Campbell's spaghetti and tomato sauce	2 slices $1 \times 2''$ 3/4 cup
Others	Small candies	handful	Smarties	6

Table 1.3: The correct and incorrect methods for describing and quantifying foods when using household measures.

2. Record the amount of all leftovers; any remaining bones from meat, apple cores, or the skin from a baked potato, etc. Subtract the amount left over from the original weight or volume for that food.

3. Remove the peel from fruit such as bananas or oranges before recording the weight eaten.

Method using household measures

- Use measuring cups for soup, casseroles, and drinks.

- Use measuring spoons for small-quantity food items e.g. for butter, sugar, coffee, jam. Record amounts in teaspoons or tablespoons. Always use level measures.

- For meat, cheese, pies, and cakes, estimate the size of the portion by measuring with a ruler, e.g. cheddar cheese: one $1''$ cube; roast beef: two slices $2'' \times 4'' \times 1/2''$ thick.

Table 1.3 shows examples of correct and incorrect methods for describing and quantifying the food items consumed using household measures.

Method using dietary scales

- Adjust the scale to zero.

- Place the serving dish or cup on the scale.

- Adjust the scale to zero.

- Place the food or beverage in a serving dish or cup.

- Read and record the weight in grams.

- Repeat this weighing procedure for the next food item.

If some food remains, weigh the leftovers and deduct the weight of these from the initial weight, thus recording only the amount eaten.

References

Burk M C, Pao E M (1976). Methodology for large-scale surveys of household and individual diets. Home Economics Research Report No. 40. Agriculture Research Service, U.S. Department of Agriculture, Washington, D.C.

Cameron M E, Staveren W A van (1988). Manual on Methodology for Food Consumption Studies. Oxford Medical Publications, Oxford University Press, Oxford.

1.3 Calculation of nutrient intakes

Principle

Nutrient intakes can be calculated from food consumption data collected by quantitative or semi-quantitative methods. Food composition values, representative of the average composition of a particular foodstuff on a year-round nation-wide basis, are used to calculate nutrient intakes. These are available in food composition tables, or in nutrient databases stored on a computer. All food composition values represent the total amount of the constituent in the food, and not the amount absorbed. The availability of most nutrients in individual food items has not been assessed, and hence when nutrient intake data are evaluated, the potential bioavailability of the nutrients from the diets must always be considered.

Food composition values can be expressed in terms of the nutrient content of the edible portion of the food per hundred grams and/or per common household measure. Data on the number of food samples used to derive the average energy or nutrient value, and a statistical parameter to describe the observed variation (i.e. the standard deviation, standard error, or coefficient of variation) are sometimes available.

It is important to have information on the source of the food composition values used. Most frequently, they are compiled from a variety of sources such as the food industry, published research, contract research, and government research laboratories. Very few food composition tables are based exclusively on analyses of locally grown foods: indeed, for some countries, all the values for local foods are taken from tables of other countries (Périssé, 1982).

Both random and systematic errors may occur in food composition data, depending on the food item and the nutrient. The sources of error include:

- Inadequate sampling protocols resulting in data for unrepresentative food samples being included in the food composition tables and/or nutrient databases;
- the use of inappropriate analytical methods for the analysis of the nutrients for the food composition data;
- errors in the analytical methods used in the analysis of the nutrients for the food composition data;
- a lack of standardized conversion factors for calculating energy and protein content of foods included in the food composition tables and/or nutrient databases;
- inconsistencies in terminology used to express certain nutrients;
- incorrect description of individual food items and/or source of nutrient values in food composition tables;
- inconsistencies resulting from genetic, environmental, food preparation, and processing factors.

These errors generate additional uncertainty in calculated nutrient intakes.

Nutrient intakes can be calculated using food composition tables; alternatively, intakes can be calculated using a computer program and a nutrient database. These two procedures are described below.

Calculation of nutrient intakes using food composition tables

1. Select the food composition tables appropriate for the country of interest. For Canada, the tables entitled 'Nutrient Values for some Common Foods' (Health and Welfare Canada, 1988) should be used. For the United States, the revised USDA Handbooks No. 8 (Consumer and Food Economic Institute, 1976–1992) are appropriate. In the United Kingdom, McCance and Widdowson's 'Composition of Foods' (Holland et al., 1991) is the most important source of food composition data; supplemental information to these tables is also available for fruits and nuts, and for vegetable dishes (Holland et al., 1992a, 1992b).

2. Record each type of food or beverage listed during the recall or food record in column 1 of Table 1.4.

3. Calculate the sum of the edible portion sizes of each food or beverage item consumed during the period of study. Record the sum in grams or household measures in column 2 of Table 1.4.

4. Convert this total sum into a decimal fraction of the amount given in the food composition tables for that particular food item.

5. Record this decimal fraction in column 3 of Table 1.4.

6. Multiply the nutrient values for each food item in the food composition table by the corresponding decimal fraction in column 3, and enter these adjusted values in the appropriate nutrient columns in Table 1.4.

7. After entering all the nutrient values for each food item listed, calculate the totals for energy and for each of the nutrients investigated. Record the totals in the last line of Table 1.4.

Computer calculation of nutrient intakes

Before selecting a computer program for the calculation of nutrient intakes, the source of the accompanying nutrient database,[1] its completeness—both in terms of the range of foods listed and in the availability of nutrient values for individual foods—must be determined. In addition, the validity of the computer program for calculating nutrient intakes must also be assessed. Both these factors can be checked using the diagnostic tool developed by Hoover and Perloff (1981).

The first stage in the use of a nutrient database involves coding the food intake data obtained from the twenty-four-hour recall or the three-day record into a defined machine readable form. This procedure is generally done manually and usually involves assigning a numerical code to the subject, day, meal, food, and amount. The food identification code can define the food group, major and minor food subgroup, and finally the individual food. The code may also provide information on preserving or processing techniques, storage conditions, etc. The coding is not arbitrary, and will be defined either in the documentation which accompanies the program or in an appropriate food code handbook (Arab, 1988).

The second stage involves the use of a software package to calculate the nutrient intakes. In detail, the following steps can be identified:

1. Assign a food identification code to each food and beverage item recorded in Table 1.4, using an appropriate food code handbook. Note: If the food or beverage consumed is not listed in the food code handbook, substitute a food which most closely resembles the item consumed. If necessary, the substitution can involve two or more items so as to more closely resemble the item consumed; for example, the addition of an ingredient such as honey to breakfast cereal can be used when an unlisted honey-coated breakfast cereal was eaten.

2. Code the day, meal, and amount of each edible portion of food consumed. For the amount code, depending on the computer program, use either a decimal fraction of the amount given in the nutrient database for that particular food item, or the actual amount consumed expressed in grams.

3. Enter the coded food consumption data into the computer system. This may be done on-line or off-line, depending on the software package used.

4. Check the input data for transcription errors. Incorrect food codes can be rapidly identified if check digits[2] are included in the food code. Weight errors are more readily detected if the computer program flags those subjects whose daily intakes of energy and selected nutrients, foods, or portion sizes falls outside the 2 SD limits for the data set; if such an situation occurs, checks should be made for weight errors in the coded data for the reported subjects.

5. Carry out spot checks on subsamples of the stored data against the original data forms.

6. Select an appropriate software package to calculate the energy and nutrient intakes from the food intake data. A software package that can provide the following output is recommended:

---

[1] The majority of suitable computer programs are supplied with an accompanying nutrient database

[2] Check digits provide a simple method of improving the integrity of data by incorporating some redundancy into the encoding of the data; a program which is capable of dealing with check digits will be able to report when an impossible code has been entered.

Date Subject ID No.	Day of the week Name of Subject															
Food or Beverage	Amount in grams or household measures	Fraction	Energy (KJ)	Protein (g)	Total fat (g)	Calcium (mg)	Iron (mg)	Zinc (mg)	Vitamin D (ug)	Vitamin A (RE)	Thiamin (mg)	Riboflavin (mg)	Niacin (NE)	Vitamin C (mg)	Dietary fiber (g)
Totals															

Table 1.4: Form for the hand calculation of nutrient intakes.

- total nutrients per meal
- total nutrients for each day
- average daily nutrient intake per day
- average daily nutrient intake per major food group and food subgroup
- average daily intake (in grams) of major food groups and food subgroups
- average frequency of consumption of major food groups and food subgroups

References

Arab L (1988). Analyses, presentation, and interpretation of results. In: Cameron M E, Staveren W A van (eds), Manual on Methodology for Food Consumption Studies. Oxford University Press, pp. 145–169.

Consumer and Food Economic Institute (1976–1992). Composition of foods—raw, processed, and prepared. Agriculture Handbook 8, Nos. 1–21, US Government Printing Office, Washington, D.C.

Health and Welfare Canada. Nutrient Value of some Common Foods. Health Services and Promotion Branch and Health Protection Branch, Health and Welfare Canada, Ottawa, 1988.

Holland B, Welch A A, Unwin I D, Buss D H, Paul A A, Southgate D A T (1991). McCance and Widdowson's The Composition of Foods. Fifth revised and extended edition. The Royal Society of Chemistry and Ministry of Agriculture, Fisheries and Food, Cambridge, UK.

Holland B, Unwin I D, Buss D H (1992a). Fruit and Nuts. The First Supplement to the Fifth Edition of McCance and Widdowson's The Composition of Foods. Royal Society of Chemistry and Ministry of Agriculture, Fisheries and Food, Cambridge, UK.

Holland B, Welch A A, Buss D H (1992b). Vegetable Dishes. The Second Supplement to the Fifth Edition of McCance and Widdowson's The Composition of Foods. Royal Society of Chemistry and Ministry of Agriculture, Fisheries and Food, Cambridge, UK.

Hoover L W, Perloff B P (1981). Model for Review of Nutrient Data Base System Capabilities. University of Missouri, Columbia, Missouri.

Périssé J (1982). The heterogeneity of food composition tables. In: Hautvast J G A J, Klaver W (eds) The Diet Factor in Epidemiological Research. Euronut Report 1, Wageningen, pp. 100–105.

Chapter 2
Qualitative dietary assessment

Contents

Introduction

Qualitative dietary assessment methods include the food frequency questionnaire and the dietary history. Both obtain retrospective information on the patterns of food use during a longer, less precisely defined time period than are associated with the methods of quantitative assessment, and are most frequently used to assess habitual intake of foods or specific classes of foods. With modification, they can provide data on habitual nutrient intakes.

A food frequency questionnaire consists of a list of foods and an associated set of frequency-of-use response categories. The list of foods may be extensive enough to enable estimates of total food intake, and hence dietary diversity, to be made. Alternatively, the list may focus on specific groups of foods or particular food items. The questionnaire may also quantify the usual portion sizes consumed for each food item.

The dietary history method, first developed by Burke in 1947, attempts to estimate the usual food intakes of individuals over a relatively long period of time (Burke, 1947). It is an interview method and should be carried out by a nutritionist trained in interviewing techniques.

Variation in dietary intakes within one individual (within- or intra-subject variation) cannot be estimated using either of these methods. Hence, the effect of intra-subject variation cannot be taken into account during the interpretation of dietary data collected by qualitative methods. This is a disadvantage if data on habitual intakes are required for correlation with biochemical or clinical parameters. When intra-subject variation in a dietary component is large in relation to variation among subjects (between or inter-subject variation), the effect is to mask significant correlations (Liu et al., 1978). The theoretical reduction in the absolute value of the correlation coefficient can be calculated provided that the intra-subject variation can be measured using analysis of variance. This approach is only possible, however, when a quantitative food consumption method is used which measures food intake for at least two separate days on each individual.

References

Burke B S (1947). The dietary history as a tool in research. Journal of the American Dietetic Association 23: 1041–1046.

Lui K, Stamler J, Dyer A, McKeever J, McKeever P (1978). Statistical methods to assess and minimize the role of intra-individual variability in obscuring relationship between dietary lipids and serum cholesterol. Journal of Chronic Diseases 31: 399–418.

2.1 The semi-quantitative food frequency questionnaire

Principle

A food frequency questionnaire is designed to obtain qualitative or semi-quantitative descriptive information about usual food consumption patterns. This is accomplished by assessing the frequency with which certain food items or food groups are consumed during a specified time period (e.g. daily, weekly, monthly or yearly).

The questionnaire has two main components: (a) a list of foods and (b) a set of frequency-of-use response categories. The list of foods may focus on specific foods or groups of foods, or on foods consumed periodically in association with special events or seasons. Alternatively, the food list may be extensive, to enable estimates of total food intake—and hence dietary diversity—to be made (Anderson, 1986). If the questionnaire is modified to quantify the usual portion sizes consumed for each food item, then semi-quantitative food frequency data can be obtained. Usual portion sizes can be estimated by means of photographs or pictures of standard-size servings, or by using food models (Jain et al., 1982). The data for a food frequency questionnaire may be obtained by a standardized interview or self-administered questionnaire.

The advantages of a food frequency questionnaire include a high response rate and a low respondent burden. The method is also speedy, relatively inexpensive, and assesses usual food intake. The questionnaire can be administered by non-professionals or can be self-administered, and generates standardized results (Howarth, 1990).

The three-part questionnaire shown is a semi-quantitative food frequency questionnaire modified from Block et al. (1986). The food list consists of 98 food items (Tables 2.2, 2.3, and 2.4). The respondent is requested to indicate the use of each food item as the number of times per day, week, month, or year, and to indicate the usual portion size as small, medium, or large. The medium portion sizes (Table 2.1) are specified, and were obtained from USDA Foods Commonly Eaten by Individuals (Pao et al., 1982) and Nutrition Canada Food Consumption Portion Data (Sabry, 1981), using, respectively, the median portion consumed per eating occasion for females aged 19–34 years, and the mean portion consumed for females aged 20–29 years. Small and large portion sizes were based on the 25th and 75th percentiles for food portions from the USDA data and ±1 SD for food portions from the Nutrition Canada data respectively. Comparable data for males and for other age groups are available from the same sources.

Procedure

1. Complete the three-part semi-quantitative food frequency questionnaire (Tables 2.2 – 2.4) using graduated food models to estimate the portion sizes (Fig. 1.1).

2. Five categories for the frequency of food use are available: daily (D), weekly (W), monthly (M), yearly (Y), rarely/never (N). Select the most appropriate category for the frequency of consumption of each of the food items chosen, and record the number of times each food item is consumed in the appropriate box.

3. A choice of three portion sizes is available: small (S), medium (M), and large (L). Indicate the usual portion size consumed for each food item in the appropriate box.

4. Convert all the frequency-of-use categories to a daily basis with once per day equal to one. Assume there are 30 days per month. For example: tomato juice consumed four times per month is equivalent to 4/30 per day, ≈ 0.13 per day. Apples consumed five times per week are equivalent to 5/7 per day, ≈ 0.71 per day. For seasonal fruits and vegetables, use the yearly category. For example, peaches consumed fifteen times over the summer is equivalent to 15/365 per day, ≈ 0.04 per day.

5. Multiply frequency per day by the usual portion size (in grams) to provide weight consumed in grams per day.

6. Refer to Section 1.3 to calculate nutrient intakes from the semi-quantitative food frequency questionnaire using food composition tables or a computer.

	Percentiles (g)		
	25th	**50th**	**75th**
Fruits			
Apples	138	138	138
Bananas	95	119	119
Peaches (canned or frozen)	125	128	250
Peaches (fresh)	152	152	152
Cantaloupe	80	136	272
Watermelon		300	
Strawberries (fresh)	57	75	149
Oranges	145	145	145
Orange juice	125	187	249
Grapefruit (fresh)	134	134	165
Grapefruit juice	185	188	250
Tang or other fruit drinks	190	250	313
Any other fruit including			
berries or fruit cocktail	123	128	255
Vegetables			
String beans or green beans	68	70	135
Peas	56	85	85
Beans (baked or pintos or			
kidney or lima)	95	185	190
Corn	77	83	123
Mixed vegetables	94	94	182
Winter and baked squash	108	108	215
Tomato juice	151	182	243
Tomatoes (raw)	34	62	91
Broccoli	78	93	155
Cauliflower or brussel sprouts		100	
Spinach (raw)	10	28	55
Spinach (cooked)	95	103	180
Cole slaw or cabbage or			
sauerkraut	30	60	60
Carrots raw or cooked	35	62	70
Green salad	65	93	140
French fries and fried			
potatoes (1-2 inch strips)	35	57	70
Sweet potatoes or yams	103	114	200
Other potatoes including			
boiled or baked or mashed	92	122	184
Rice	88	175	175
Eggs, Meat, and Fish			
Hamburger or meatloaf	74	113	169
Beef (steaks or roasts)	84	112	168
Beef stew	245	245	490
Pot pie with veg	227	227	250
Organ meats (liver etc)	84	112	150
Pork (incl. chops or roasts)	20	56	92
Chicken, fried	84	112	168
Chicken, baked or broiled	84	112	168
Turkey, baked or broiled	84	112	168
Shellfish or shrimp or lobster	24	43	68
Tuna fish	40	80	96
Other fish (haddock etc)	84	112	168
Eggs (large)	50	64	104
Bacon (med sliced)	16	16	24
Sausage (links)	26	45	57
Weiners (small)	44	66	88
Ham or luncheon meats	43	67	112

	Percentiles (g)		
	25th	**50th**	**75th**
Mixed dishes and Soups			
Spagetti or lasagna or other			
pasta with tomato sauce	250	375	500
Pizza (slices)	94	152	227
Mixed dishes with cheese			
(macaroni and cheese)	100	200	240
Vegetable soup or veg beef or			
minestrone or tomato soup	240	245	360
Creamed soup	240	245	360
Breads, Snacks, and Spreads			
White bread or rolls	25	44	50
Dark bread or rolls	25	34	50
Crackers	12	15	28
Muffins *	33	62	91
High fiber cereals	28	43	84
Other cold cereals	15	20	23
Cooked cereals	123	240	245
Sugar added to cereal			
Salty snacks (chips etc.)	9	18	27
Peanuts	19	36	72
Peanut butter	16	16	32
Butter	5	7	14
Margarine	5	9	14
Salad dressing or mayonnaise	5	14	15
Gravies *	18	71	124
Pancakes	54	81	128
Sweets			
Ice cream	67	133	133
Sweet rolls or doughnuts	42	43	84
Cookies	14	25	40
Cake	41	66	100
Pies (8 pieces/pie)	93	118	135
Pudding *	42	99	146
Chocolate candy	18	32	48
Liquorice *		23	
Other candy i.e. hard		10	
Jelly or Jam or Syrup	6	18	19
Dairy Products			
Whole milk	31	183	244
2% Milk	123	245	245
Skim milk	123	245	245
Cottage cheese	75	113	113
Other cheese or spreads	28	28	57
Flavoured yogurt	123	227	245
Beverages and other foods			
Coffee (decaffeinated)	240	240	240
Coffee (not decaffeinated)	240	240	480
Tea	240	240	360
Non-dairy creamer in coffee or tea	2	2	4
Milk in coffee or tea			
Cream in coffee or tea (creamers)			
Sugar in coffee or tea			
Artificial sweetner in coffee or tea *			
Wine	116	174	232
Beer (12 oz/bottle)	360	360	720
Whiskey or vodka or rum	42	56	56
Brewer's yeast *	3	19	35
Wheat germ	28	43	84
Bran	25	25	30

Table 2.1: Small, medium, and large portion sizes (g) for foods commonly consumed by individuals. Data given are for females 19–34 years of age (Pao et al., 1982); and the mean portion (*) consumed by females 20–29 years of age (Sabry, 1981).

	Weight (g)	Medium Amount	Frequency					Portion			Frequency per day	Grams per day
			D	W	M	Y	N	S	M	L		
Fruits												
Apples	138	medium										
Bananas	119	small										
Peaches (canned or frozen)	128	1/2 cup										
Peaches (fresh)	152	medium										
Cantaloupe	136	one-sixth										
Watermelon	300	slice										
Strawberries (fresh)	75	2/3 cup										
Oranges	145	medium										
Orange juice	187	3/4 cup										
Grapefruit (fresh)	134	1/2 med.										
Grapefruit juice	188	6 oz										
Tang or other fruit drink	250	9 oz										
Any other fruit including												
berries or fruit cocktail	128	2/3 cup										
Vegetables												
String beans or green beans	70	2/3 cup										
Peas	85	1/2 cup										
Beans (baked or pintos or												
kidney or lima)	185	3/4 cup										
Corn	83	1/2 cup										
Mixed vegetables	94	2/3 cup										
Winter and baked squash	108	3/4 cup										
Tomato juice	182	5 oz										
Tomatoes (raw)	62	3 slices										
Broccoli	93	2/3 cup										
Cauliflower or brussel sprouts	100	1/2 cup										
Spinach (raw)	28	2/3 cup										
Spinach (cooked)	103	2/3 cup										
Cole slaw or cabbage or												
sauerkraut	60	1/2 cup										
Carrots raw or cooked	62	1/2 cup										
Green salad	93	1 cup										
French fries and fried												
potatoes (1-2 inch strips)	57	eighteen										
Sweet potatoes or yams	114	medium										
Other potatoes including												
boiled or baked or mashed	122	medium										
Rice	175	3/4 cup										
Eggs, Meat, and Fish												
Hamburger or meatloaf	113	3 oz										
Beef (steaks or roasts)	112	4 oz										
Beef stew	245	4/3 cup										
Pot pie with veg	227	1 (8 oz)										
Organ meats (liver etc)	112	4 oz										
Pork (including chops or roasts)	56	med. chop										

Table 2.2: Food frequency questionnaire (Part 1)

	Weight (g)	Medium Amount	Frequency					Portion			Frequency per day	Grams per day
			D	W	M	Y	N	S	M	L		
Eggs, Meat, and Fish (cont.)												
Chicken, fried	112	(1 leg or two										
		drum sticks										
		or 1/2 breast)										
Chicken baked or broiled	112	4 slices										
Turkey baked or broiled	112	4 slices										
Shellfish or shrimp or lobster	43	2.5 oz										
Tuna fish	80	2.5 oz										
Other fish (haddock etc)	112	5 oz										
Eggs (large)	64	one										
Bacon (med sliced)	16	2 slices										
Sausage (links)	45	2 links										
Weiners (small)	66	two										
Ham or luncheon meats	67	3 oz										
Mixed dishes and Soups												
Spagetti or lasagna or other												
pasta with tomato sauce	375	1 cup										
Pizza (slices)	152	2 slices										
Mixed dishes with cheese												
(macaroni and cheese)	200	1 cup										
Vegetable soup or vegetable-beef												
or minestrone or tomato soup	245	5/4 cup										
Creamed soup	245	5/4 cup										
Breads, Snacks, and Spreads												
White bread or rolls	44	3/2 slices										
Dark bread or rolls	34	2 slices										
Crackers	15	5										
Muffins *	62	medium										
High fiber cereals	43	2/3 cup										
Other cold cereals	20	1 cup										
Cooked cereals	240	5/4 cup										
Sugar added to cereal		1 tsp										
Salty snacks (chips etc.)	18	1 cup										
Peanuts	36	1/3 cup										
Peanut butter	16	1 tbsp										
Butter	7	2 tsp										
Margarine	9	2 tsp										
Salad dressing or mayonnaise	14	1 tbsp										
Gravies *	71	1/4 cup										
Pancakes	81	3 medium										
Sweets												
Ice cream	133	3/4 cup										
Sweet rolls or doughnuts	43	one										
Cookies	25	three										
Cake	66	1 slice										

Table 2.3: Food frequency questionnaire (Part 2)

	Weight (g)	Medium Amount	Frequency					Portion			Frequency per day	Grams per day
			D	W	M	Y	N	S	M	L		
Sweets (cont.)												
Pies (8 pieces/pie)	118	1/8 pie										
Pudding *	99	1/3 cup										
Chocolate candy	32	1/8 cup										
Liquorice *	23	1 pc										
Other candy i.e. hard	10	two										
Jelly or Jam or Syrup	18	1 tbsp										
Dairy Products												
Whole milk	183	5 oz										
2% Milk	245	6 oz										
Skim milk	245	5 oz										
Cottage cheese	113	1/2 cup										
Other cheese and spreads	28	2 cubes										
Flavored yogurt	227	3/4 cup										
Beverages and other foods												
Coffee (decaffeinated)	240	1 cup										
Coffee (not decaffeinated)	240	1 cup										
Tea	240	1 cup										
Non-dairy creamer in coffee or tea		2 tsp										
Milk in coffee or tea		1 tbsp										
Cream in coffee or tea (creamers)		1 tbsp										
Sugar in coffee or tea		1 tsp										
Artificial sweetner in coffee or tea *		0.5 tsp										
Wine	174	5 oz										
Beer (12 oz bottle)	360	1 bot										
Whiskey or vodka or rum	56	1.5 oz										
Brewer's yeast *	19	0.5 oz										
Wheat germ	43	2/3 cup										
Bran	25	1/3 cup										

Table 2.4: Food frequency questionnaire (Part 3)

References

Anderson S A (1986). Guidelines for Use of Dietary Intake Data. Life Sciences Research Office, Federation of American Societies for Experimental Biology, Bethesda, Maryland.

Block G, Hartman A M, Dresser C M, Carroll M D, Gannon J, Gardner L (1986). A data-based approach to diet questionnaire design and testing. American Journal of Epidemiology 124: 453–469.

Howarth C C (1990). Food frequency questionnaires: a review. Australian Journal of Nutrition and Dietetics 47: 71–76.

Jain M G, Harrison L, Howe G R, Miller A M (1982). Evaluation of a self-administered dietary questionnaire for use in a cohort study. American Journal of Clinical Nutrition 36: 931–935.

Pao E M, Fleming K H, Guenther P, Mickle S (1982). Foods commonly eaten by individuals. Amount per day and per eating occasion. Home Economics Research Report No. 44.

Sabry J H (1981). Nutrition Canada Food Consumption Portion Data. Department of Family Studies, University of Guelph, Guelph, Ontario.

2.2 The dietary history

Principle

The purpose of a dietary history is to obtain retrospective information on the usual food intake and meal pattern of individuals over varying periods of time. The time periods covered often include the previous month, six months, or (sometimes) the previous year. The maximum time period which can be used has not been established, although measurements of food intake over a one-year period are probably unrealistic if seasonal variations in food intake occur (Callmer et al., 1985). A dietary history is usually conducted by a nutritionist during a personal interview which may be 1.5–2 hours in length.

The dietary history technique was developed by Burke in 1947 as an interview method consisting initially of three components: (a) a twenty-four-hour recall of actual intake, as well as the collection of general information on the overall eating pattern of the respondent both at mealtimes and between meals; (b) a questionnaire on the frequency of consumption of specific food items, which was used to verify and clarify the information on the kinds and amounts of foods given as the usual intake in the first component; (c) a three-day food record using household measures. The latter component was used as a cross-check, and was found to be the least helpful. Consequently, it is often omitted.

Advantages of the dietary history include its ability to provide information on habitual dietary intake and its relatively low respondent burden compared to that of a food record. As a result, compliance using this method is generally high. A major disadvantage of the dietary history, however, is its reliance on the respondent's memory and ability to estimate portion sizes correctly, making it unsuitable for children less than 14 years of age and for the elderly. The method is also unsuitable for those subjects who have erratic meal patterns: it tends to underestimate any irregularities in food intake and meal patterns because of its emphasis on regular eating patterns (Cameron and van Staveren, 1988).

Numerous modifications of the dietary history method exist. The example given below is modified from that developed by van Staveren et al. (1985) and is designed to assess usual food intake and meal patterns over the previous one month period.

Procedure

1. Question the respondent about a typical day's eating pattern, commencing with the foods consumed during the first meal of a typical weekday during the previous month. Record the responses on a copy of Table 1.2 and then proceed to deal with subsequent meals and snacks consecutively.

2. Question the respondent about a typical eating pattern for a Saturday, again commencing with the foods consumed during the first meal; proceed through each of the meals and snacks consecutively, recording the results on the form.

3. Question the respondent about a typical eating pattern for a Sunday; proceed through each of the meals and snacks consecutively, starting with the first, and record the results as above.

4. To estimate the usual portion sizes of each food item consumed, weigh the portion size of each food item said to be most frequently consumed by the respondent; use dietary scales for this procedure. Alternatively, estimate portion sizes using the respondent's household utensils, which should be calibrated by the investigator.

5. Calculate a weighted daily average intake of each food item consumed using the formula:

$$\text{Avg. intake} = \frac{((5 \times \text{workday}) + \text{Saturday} + \text{Sunday})}{7}$$

6. Use the methods outlined in Section 1.3 to calculate nutrient intakes from the dietary history, either using food composition tables or a computer.

References

Burke B S (1947). The dietary history as a tool in research. Journal of the American Dietetic Association 23: 1041–1046.

Callmer E, Haraldsdottir J, Løker E B, Seppänen R, Solvoll K (1985). Selecting a method for a dietary survey. Närings-forskning 2: 43–52.

Cameron M E, Staveren W A van (1988). Manual on Methodology for Food Consumption Studies. Oxford University Press, Oxford.

Staveren W A van, Boer J O de, Burema J (1985). Validity and reproducibility of dietary history method estimating the usual food intake during one month. American Journal of Clinical Nutrition 42: 554–559.

Chapter 3
Evaluation of nutrient intake data

Contents

Introduction

Most of the methods for evaluating nutrient intakes involve comparison with tables of recommended nutrient intakes. Recommended nutrient intakes are set for a particular group of healthy individuals with specified characteristics, consuming a typical dietary pattern of the country. They refer to the average recommended intake for a nutrient consumed over a reasonable period of time and do not take into account possible interactions involving nutrients and other dietary components (International Union of Nutritional Sciences, 1983). The values for the recommended nutrient intakes for the same nutrient vary among countries.

Methods used to evaluate nutrient intakes of individuals include a nutrient adequacy ratio (NAR), an index of nutritional quality (INQ), a standard deviation score or Z score, and comparison of individual intakes with corresponding recommended nutrient intakes. In the latter approach, the percentage of individuals with intakes below the recommended nutrient intake, or an arbitrary proportion of the recommended nutrient intake, is calculated. More recently, a probability approach has been developed in an attempt to assess more reliably the risk of nutrient inadequacy for an individual, or, for a population, an estimate of the prevalence of inadequate intakes (Beaton, 1988). Such an approach is preferable for identifying and targeting nutrition and food intervention programs at the more vulnerable groups.

All the methods provide an estimate of the risk of a population and/or individual to nutrient inadequacy. None of the methods identify actual individuals in the population who have a specific nutrient deficiency. This can only be achieved if biochemical and clinical assessments are also carried out with the dietary investigation. Dietary data alone provide an estimate of the *risk* for nutrient inadequacies. The reliability of this risk estimate depends on the method used for the evaluation.

References

Beaton GH (1988). Twelfth Boyd Orr Memorial Lecture. Nutrient Requirements and Population Data. Proceedings of the Nutrition Society 47: 63–78.

International Union of Nutritional Sciences (1983). Recommended Dietary Intakes around the World. A Report by Committee 1/5 of the International Union of Nutritional Sciences (1982). Nutrition Abstracts and Reviews 53: 1075–1118.

3.1 Nutrient adequacy ratio

Principle

The nutrient adequacy ratio (NAR) represents an index of adequacy for a nutrient based on the corresponding U.S. Recommended Daily Allowance (RDA) for that nutrient (Food and Nutrition Board, 1989). The nutrients selected for the calculation of NAR's vary (Guthrie and Scheer, 1981; Krebs-Smith et al., 1987). Calculation of the average for the NAR values yields a mean adequacy ratio (MAR) for each subject, which provides an index of the overall quality of the diet. All the nutrients included in the MAR are assigned equal importance using this approach. Furthermore, the MAR does not identify which specific nutrients are inadequate in the diet or provide a means of evaluating the proportion of energy derived from protein, fat, and carbohydrate (Crocetti and Guthrie, 1981).

Procedure

1. Calculate the NAR for protein, calcium, iron, zinc, vitamins A, C, thiamin, and riboflavin as follows:

$$NAR = \frac{\text{Subject's daily intake of a nutrient}}{\text{RDA of that nutrient}}$$

2. Truncate the NAR values at 1.0 to prevent intakes in excess of the RDA for any nutrient from increasing the index. In this way, any false impressions of nutritional adequacy can be avoided.

3. Average the NAR values for the selected nutrients to yield a mean adequacy ratio (MAR) for each subject:

$$MAR = \frac{\text{Sum of the NARs for x nutrients}}{x}$$

References

Crocetti AF, Guthrie HA (1981). Food consumption patterns and nutritional quality of U.S. diets: A preliminary report. Food Technology 35 (9): 40–49.

Food and Nutrition Board, National Research Council—National Academy of Sciences (1989). Recommended Dietary Allowances. Tenth edition. National Academy of Sciences, Washington, D.C.

Guthrie HA, Scheer JC (1981). Validity of a dietary score for assessing nutrient adequacy. Journal of the American Dietetic Association 78: 240–245.

Krebs-Smith SM, Smiciklas-Wright H, Guthrie HA, Krebs-Smith J (1987). The effects of variety in food choices on dietary quality. Journal of the American Dietetic Association 87: 897–903.

3.2 Index of nutritional quality

Principle

This method, developed at Utah State University by Hansen (1973), was designed to evaluate the adequacy of meals and diets of individuals and can therefore be used for individual counselling. The index of nutritional quality (INQ) for each nutrient represents the quality of a nutrient in a food, meal, or diet relative to the recommended nutrient intake.

An INQ value greater than 1.0 for any nutrient indicates that an amount of a particular food or a combination of foods that would satisfy the total energy requirement would also provide a sufficient amount of the nutrient. An INQ less than 1.0 indicates that for that nutrient, an excess of a particular food or groups of foods must be consumed to meet the recommended nutrient intake. Thus the capacity of an individual's diet to provide both energy and nutrient needs can be evaluated.

Procedure

Calculate the INQ for protein, calcium, iron, zinc, vitamins A, C, thiamin and riboflavin using the reference values given in Table 3.1 and the equation given below:

$$INQ = \frac{\text{Amount of nutrient in 1000 kcal of food}}{\text{Allowance of the nutrient per 1000 kcal}}$$

The reference values for the nutrient allowances per 1000 kcal (with the exception of carbohydrate, sugar, fat and cholesterol) are based on the 1980 United States Recommended Dietary Allowances (Food and Nutrition Board, 1980). These single-value nutrient allowances were designed to meet and in some cases exceed the needs of all age groups and physiological states in the population when the energy needs of each group were met.

To meet nutritional needs, composite diets must have INQ values of 1.0 or more for all vitamins, minerals, and protein. For sodium and cholesterol, INQ should not greatly exceed 1.0 because moderate intakes of these nutrients are recommended. In some instances, the INQ value may be misleading. Whole milk, for example, has an INQ value for calcium which is lower (INQ = 4.0) than that of skim milk (INQ = 7.8), despite a similar calcium content per gram of fluid milk.

Nutrient	Allowance per 1000 kcal
Protein (g)	25
Fat (g)	39
Carbohydrate (g)	137.5
Sugar, added (g)	25
Calcium (mg)	450
Iron (mg)	8
Magnesium (mg)	150
Zinc (mg)	8
Potassium (mg)	1875
Sodium (mg)	1100
Vitamin A (IU)	2000
Thiamin (mg)	0.5
Riboflavin (mg)	0.6
Vitamin B-6 (mg)	1
Vitamin B-12 (μg)	1.5
Vitamin C (mg)	30
Folacin (μg)	200
Cholesterol (mg)	175

Table 3.1: Single-value nutrient allowances per 1000 kcal for heterogeneous populations one year of age and older. From Hansen RG, Wyse BW. Expression of nutrient allowances per 1,000 kilocalories. © The American Dietetic Association. Reproduced by permission from Journal of the American Dietetic Association, Vol. 76: 223–227, 1980.

References

Food and Nutrition Board, Committee on Dietary Allowances (1980). Recommended Dietary Allowances, Ninth edition. National Academy of Sciences, Washington, D.C.

Food and Nutrition Board, National Research Council—National Academy of Sciences (1989). Recommended Dietary Allowances. Tenth edition. National Academy of Sciences, Washington, D.C.

Hansen RG (1973). An index of food quality. Nutrition Reviews 31: 1–7.

Hansen RG, Wyse BW (1980). Expression of nutrient allowances per 1,000 kilocalories. Journal of American Dietetic Association 76: 223–227.

3.3 Comparison with recommended nutrient intakes

Principle

This method compares, for a specific country, a subjects's nutrient intake with the corresponding recommended nutrient intake of an individual of the same age, sex, and physiological state. Estimates of recommended nutrient intakes are derived from measurements of nutrient requirements on individuals of the same age and sex. These measurements generate a distribution of requirements because of individual variability for a specific nutrient, valid for a specific age and sex group. Data are available for the distribution of nutrient requirements for energy, protein, iron, and calcium; data for other nutrients are limited. The requirements are generally considered to follow a Gaussian distribution. The mean of this distribution represents the average requirement for that particular group of individuals, and the standard deviation is a measure of the variability in the requirement. When the standard deviation is unknown, it is assumed to be 15% of the mean. Recent committees in Canada and the United States have generally set the recommended nutrient intake at the average requirement (for a particular age and sex category) plus two standard deviations (Beaton, 1985). This means that the recommended nutrient intakes exceeds the needs of all but 2% to 3% of individuals in the population (Fig. 3.1). This conservative approach, taking into account inter-subject variability in nutrient requirements, has been adopted because most of the health risks are associated with inadequate rather than excess intakes of nutrients.

Recommended intakes for energy are based on estimates of the average energy requirement for a group of comparable individuals, and not on the average requirement plus two standard deviations. This approach has been adopted because excessive energy intake is injurious to health.

When tables of recommended intakes for a particular country are not available, the FAO and/or the WHO requirements are often used (FAO/WHO, 1970; WHO, 1973; Passmore et al., 1974; FAO/WHO/UNU, 1985; FAO/WHO, 1988). Individuals should not be classified as 'deficient' or 'inadequate' in any nutrient just because

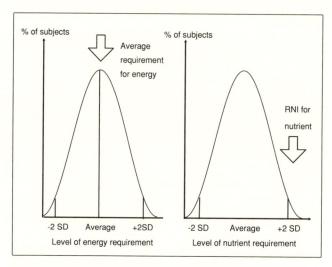

Fig. 3.1: Comparison of the average requirement for energy and the recommended intake of a nutrient. It is assumed that in both cases individual requirements are normally distributed about the mean. From Health and Welfare Canada (1983). Reproduced with permission of the Minister of Supply and Services Canada.

the short-term nutrient intake appears to fall below the recommended intake. Nevertheless, the more the habitual intake of an individual falls below the recommended intake and the longer the duration of the low intake, the greater the risk of nutrient deficiency for that individual.

Procedure

1. Select the appropriate recommended nutrient intake value for age, sex, and physiological state from the Canadian (Tables 3.2 and 3.3), the United States (Table 3.4), or the United Kingdom (Table 3.5) tables of recommended intakes for energy and the following nutrients: protein, calcium, iron, zinc, vitamin C, vitamin A, thiamin, riboflavin, niacin, and vitamin D.

2. Calculate the nutrient intakes obtained from the three-day food record and food frequency questionnaire as percentages of the corresponding recommendation. Note that a nutrient intake below the recommended level does not necessarily mean that the intake is inadequate to meet requirements. The recommended levels for the nutrient requirements

(except for energy) exceed the actual requirements of most individuals because they are generally set at the mean requirement plus two standard deviations.

3. Observe whether the intake for any nutrient falls below 66% of the corresponding recommendation.

References

Beaton GH (1985). Uses and limits of the use of the Recommended Dietary Allowances for evaluating dietary intake data. American Journal of Clinical Nutrition 41: 155–164.

Department of Health and Social Security (1981). Recommended Daily Amounts of Food Energy and Nutrients for Groups of People in the United Kingdom. Second impression. Report by the Committee on Medical Aspects of Food Policy. Report on Health and Social Subjects No. 15. Her Majesty's Stationery Office, London.

FAO/WHO/UNU (Food and Agriculture Organization / World Health Organization / United Nations University) (1985). Energy and protein Requirements. WHO Technical Report Series No. 724. World Health Organization, Geneva.

FAO/WHO (Food and Agriculture Organization / World Health Organization) (1970). Requirements of Ascorbic Acid, Vitamin D, Vitamin B-12, Folate and Iron. Report of a Joint FAO/WHO Expert Group. WHO Technical Report Series No. 452. FAO Nutrition Meetings Report Series No. 47. World Health Organization, Geneva.

FAO/WHO (Food and Agriculture Organization / World Health Organization) (1988). Requirements of Vitamin A, Iron, Folate and Vitamin B-12. Report of a Joint FAO/WHO Expert Consultation, FAO Food and Nutrition Series No. 23, Rome.

Food and Nutrition Board, Commission on Life Sciences, National Research Council (1989). Recommended Dietary Allowances. National Academy Press.

Health and Welfare (1990). Nutrition Recommendations. The Report of the Scientific Review Committee. Health and Welfare, Ottawa.

Passmore R, Nicol BM, Rao MN (1974). Handbook on Human Nutritional Requirements. World Health Organization Monograph Series No. 61, World Health Organization, Geneva.

WHO (World Health Organization) (1973). Trace Elements in Human Nutrition. WHO Technical Report Series No. 532. World Health Organization, Geneva.

Age	Sex	Weight (kg)	Protein (g)[c]	Minerals						Fat-soluble Vitamins			Water-soluble Vitamins		
				Ca (mg)	P (mg)	Mg (mg)	Fe (mg)	I (µg)	Zn (mg)	Vit. A (RE)[a]	Vit. D (µg)	Vit. E (mg)	Vit. C (mg)	Folate (µg)	Vit. B-12 (µg)
Months															
0–4	Both	6.0	12[b]	250[c]	150	20	0.3[d]	30	2[d]	400	10.0	3	20	25	0.3
5–12	Both	9.0	12	400	200	32	7	40	3	400	10.0	3	20	40	0.4
Years															
1	Both	11	13	500	300	40	6	55	4	400	10.0	3	20	40	0.5
2–3	Both	14	16	550	350	50	6	65	4	400	5.0	4	20	50	0.6
4–6	Both	18	19	600	400	65	8	85	5	500	5.0	5	25	70	0.8
7–9	M	25	26	700	500	100	8	110	7	700	2.5	7	25	90	1.0
7–9	F	25	26	700	500	100	8	95	7	700	2.5	6	25	90	1.0
10–12	M	34	34	900	700	130	8	125	9	800	2.5	8	25	120	1.0
10–12	F	36	36	1100	800	135	8	110	9	800	2.5	7	25	130	1.0
13–15	M	50	49	1100	900	185	10	160	12	900	2.5	9	30	175	1.0
13–15	F	48	46	1000	850	180	13	160	9	800	2.5	7	30	170	1.0
16–18	M	62	58	900	1000	230	10	160	12	1000	2.5	10	40[e]	220	1.0
16–18	F	53	47	700	850	200	12	160	9	800	2.5	7	30[e]	190	1.0
19–24	M	71	61	800	1000	240	9	160	12	1000	2.5	10	40[e]	220	1.0
19–24	F	58	50	700	850	200	13	160	9	800	2.5	7	30[e]	180	1.0
25–49	M	74	64	800	1000	250	9	160	12	1000	2.5	9	40[e]	230	1.0
25–49	F	59	51	700	850	200	13[g]	160	9	800	2.5	6	30[e]	185	1.0
50–74	M	73	63	800	1000	250	9	160	12	1000	5.0	7	40[e]	230	1.0
50–74	F	63	54	800	850	210	8	160	9	800	5.0	6	30[e]	195	1.0
75+	M	69	59	800	1000	230	9	160	12	1000	5.0	6	40[e]	215	1.0
75+	F	64	55	800	850	210	8	160	9	800	5.0	5	30[e]	200	1.0
Pregnancy (additional)															
1st Trimester			5	500	200	15	0	25	6	0	2.5	2	0	200	1.0
2nd Trimester			20	500	200	45	5	25	6	0	2.5	2	10	200	1.0
3rd Trimester			24	500	200	45	10	25	6	0	2.5	2	10	200	1.0
Lactation (additional)			20	500	200	65	0	50	6	400	2.5	3	25	100	0.5

Table 3.2: Recommended[a,b] nutrient intakes for Canadians based on age and body weight expressed as daily rates. [a] Retinol equivalents. [b] Protein is assumed to be from breast milk and must be adjusted for infant formula. [c] Infant formula with high phosphorus should contain 375 mg calcium. [d] Breast milk is assumed to be the source of the mineral. [e] Smokers should increase vitamin C by 50%. From Health and Welfare Canada (1990). Reproduced with permission of the Minister of Supply and Services Canada.

Age	Sex	Energy (kcal)	Thiamin (mg)	Riboflavin (mg)	Niacin (NE)[b]	n-3PUFA[a] (g)	n-6PUFA (g)
Months							
0–4	Both	600	0.3	0.3	4	0.5	3
5–12	Both	900	0.4	0.5	7	0.5	3
Years							
1	Both	1100	0.5	0.6	8	0.6	4
2–3	Both	1300	0.6	0.7	9	0.7	4
4–6	Both	1800	0.7	0.9	13	1.0	6
7–9	M	2200	0.9	1.1	16	1.2	7
	F	1900	0.8	1.0	14	1.0	6
10–12	M	2500	1.0	1.3	18	1.4	8
	F	2200	0.9	1.1	16	1.2	7
13–15	M	2800	1.1	1.4	20	1.5	9
	F	2200	0.9	1.1	16	1.2	7
16–18	M	3200	1.3	1.6	23	1.8	11
	F	2100	0.8	1.1	15	1.2	7
19–24	M	3000	1.2	1.5	22	1.6	10
	F	2100	0.8	1.1	15	1.2	7[c]
25–49	M	2700	1.1	1.4	19	1.5	9
	F	1900	0.8	1.0	14[c]	1.1[c]	7[c]
50–74	M	2300	0.9	1.2	16	1.3	8
	F	1800	0.8[c]	1.0[c]	14[c]	1.1[c]	7[c]
75+	M	2000	0.8	1.0	14	1.1	7
	F[d]	1700	0.8[c]	1.0[c]	14[c]	1.1[c]	7[c]
Pregnancy (additional)							
1st Trimester		100	0.1	0.1	0.1	0.05	0.3
2nd Trimester		300	0.1	0.3	0.2	0.16	0.9
3rd Trimester		300	0.1	0.3	0.2	0.16	0.9
Lactation (additional)		450	0.2	0.4	0.3	0.25	1.5

Table 3.3: Summary of examples of recommended nutrients based on energy expressed as daily rates. [a] PUFA, polyunsaturated fatty acids. [b] Niacin equivalents. [c] level below which intake should not fall. [d] Assumes moderate physical activity. From Health and Welfare Canada (1990). Reproduced with permission of the Minister of Supply and Services Canada.

Age yr	Wt[b] kg	Ht[b] cm	Pro-tein g	Minerals							Fat-soluble Vits.				Water-soluble Vitamins						
				Ca mg	P mg	Mg mg	Fe mg	Zn mg	I µg	Se µg	Vit. A[c] µg RE	Vit. D[d] µg	Vit. E[e] mg	Vit. K µg	Vit. C mg	Thia-min mg	Ribo flavin mg	Nia-cin[f] NE	Vit. B-6 mg	Fola-cin[g] µg	Vit. B-12 µg
Infants																					
0–0.5	6	60	13	400	300	40	6	5	40	10	375	7.5	3	5	30	0.3	0.4	5	0.3	25	0.3
0.5–1.0	9	71	14	600	500	60	10	5	50	15	375	10	4	10	35	0.4	0.5	6	0.6	35	0.5
Children																					
1–3	13	90	16	800	800	80	10	10	70	20	400	10	6	15	40	0.7	0.8	9	1.0	50	0.7
4–6	20	112	24	800	800	120	10	10	90	20	500	10	7	20	45	0.9	1.1	12	1.1	75	1.0
7–10	28	132	28	800	800	170	10	10	120	30	700	10	7	30	45	1.0	1.2	13	1.4	100	1.4
Males																					
11–14	45	157	45	1200	1200	270	12	15	150	40	1000	10	10	45	50	1.3	1.5	17	1.7	150	2.0
15–18	66	176	59	1200	1200	400	12	15	150	50	1000	10	10	65	60	1.5	1.8	20	2.0	200	2.0
19–24	72	177	58	1200	1200	350	10	15	150	70	1000	10	10	70	60	1.5	1.7	19	2.0	200	2.0
25–50	79	176	63	800	800	350	10	15	150	70	1000	5	10	80	60	1.5	1.7	19	2.0	200	2.0
51+	77	173	63	800	800	350	10	15	150	70	1000	5	10	80	60	1.2	1.4	15	2.0	200	2.0
Females																					
11–14	46	157	46	1200	1200	280	15	12	150	45	800	10	8	45	50	1.1	1.3	15	1.4	150	2.0
15–18	55	163	44	1200	1200	300	15	12	150	50	800	10	8	55	60	1.1	1.3	15	1.5	180	2.0
19–24	58	164	46	1200	1200	280	15	12	150	55	800	10	8	60	60	1.1	1.3	15	1.6	180	2.0
25–50	63	163	50	800	800	280	15	12	150	55	800	5	8	65	60	1.1	1.3	15	1.6	180	2.0
51+	65	160	50	800	800	280	10	12	150	55	800	5	10	65	60	1.0	1.2	13	1.6	180	2.0
Pregnant			60	1200	1200	320	30	15	175	65	800	10	12	65	70	1.5	1.6	17	2.2	400	2.2
Lactating (1st 6 mo.)			65	1200	1200	355	15	19	200	75	1300	10	12	65	95	1.6	1.8	20	2.1	280	2.6
Lactating (2nd 6 mo.)			62	1200	1200	340	15	16	200	75	1200	10	11	65	90	1.6	1.7	20	2.1	260	2.6

Table 3.4: Recommended Dietary Allowances, Revised 1989. Designed for the maintenance of good nutrition of practically all healthy people in the U.S.A. [a] The allowances, expressed as average daily intakes over time, are intended to provide for individual variations among most normal persons as they live in the United States under usual environmental stresses. Diets should be based on a variety of common foods in order to provide other nutrients for which human requirements have been less well defined. [b] Weights and heights of Reference Adults are actual medians for the U.S. population of the designated age, as reported by NHANES II. The median weights and heights of those under 19 years of age were taken from Hamill et al.,(1979). The use of these figures does not imply that the height-to-weight ratios are ideal. [c] Retinol equivalents. 1 retinol equivalent = 1 µg retinol or 6 µg β-carotene. See original reference for calculation of vitamin A activity of diets as retinol equivalents. [d] As cholecalciferol. 10 µg cholecalciferol = 400 IU of vitamin D. [e] α-Tocopherol equivalents. 1 mg *d*-α-tocopherol = 1 α-TE. See original reference for variation in allowances and calculation of vitamin E activity of the diets as α-tocopherol equivalents. [f] 1 NE (niacin equivalent) is equal to 1 mg of niacin or 60 mg of dietary tryptophan. From: Food and Nutrition Board, Commission on Life Sciences, National Research Council (1989). Recommended Dietary Allowances. Reproduced with permission of the National Academy Press, Washington, D.C.

Age[a] (yrs)	Activity level	Energy[b] (MJ)	(kcal)	Protein[c] (g)	Calcium (g)	Iron (mg)	Thiamin (mg)	Riboflavin (mg)	Nicotinic acid equiv. (mg)[f]	Vit. C (mg)	Vit. A (µg)[g]	Vit. D (µg)[h]
Boys												
1		5.0	1200	30	600	7	0.5	0.6	7	20	300	10
2		5.75	1400	35	600	7	0.6	0.7	8	20	300	10
3–4		6.5	1560	39	600	8	0.6	0.8	9	20	300	10
5–6		7.25	1740	43	600	10	0.7	0.9	10	20	300	–
7–8		8.25	1980	49	600	10	0.8	1.0	11	20	400	–
9–11		9.5	2280	57	700	12	0.9	1.2	14	25	575	–
12–14		11.0	2640	66	700	12	1.1	1.4	16	25	725	–
15–17		12.0	2880	72	600	12	1.2	1.7	19	30	750	–
Girls												
1		4.5	1100	27	600	7	0.4	0.6	7	20	300	10
2		5.55	1300	32	600	7	0.5	0.7	8	20	300	10
3–4		6.25	1500	37	600	8	0.6	0.8	9	20	300	10
5–6		7.0	1680	42	600	10	0.7	0.9	10	20	300	–
7–8		8.0	1900	47	600	10	0.8	1.0	11	20	400	–
9–11		8.5	2050	51	700	12[d]	0.8	1.2	14	25	575	–
12–14		9.0	2150	53	700	12[d]	0.9	1.4	16	25	725	–
15–17		9.0	2150	53	600	12[d]	0.9	1.7	19	30	750	–
Men												
18–34	Sedentary	10.5	2510	63	500	10	1.0	1.6	18	30	750	–
	Moderately active	12.0	2900	72	500	10	1.2	1.6	18	30	750	–
	Very active	14.0	3350	84	500	10	1.3	1.6	18	30	750	–
35–64	Sedentary	10.0	2400	60	500	10	1.0	1.6	18	30	750	–
	Moderately active	11.5	2750	69	500	10	1.1	1.6	18	30	750	–
	Very active	14.0	3350	84	500	10	1.3	1.6	18	30	750	–
65–74	Sedentary	10.0	2400	60	500	10	1.0	1.6	18	30	750	–
75+	Sedentary	9.0	2150	54	500	10	0.9	1.6	18	30	750	–
Women												
18–54	Most occupations	9.0	2150	54	500	12[d]	0.9	1.3	15	30	750	–
	Very active	10.5	2500	62	500	12[d]	1.0	1.3	15	30	750	–
55–74	Sedentary	8.0	1900	47	500	10	0.8	1.3	15	30	750	–
75+	Sedentary	7.0	1680	42	500	10	0.7	1.3	15	30	750	–
	Pregnancy	10.0	2400	60	1200[e]	13	1.0	1.6	18	60	750	10
	Lactation	11.5	2750	69	1200	15	1.1	1.8	21	60	1200	10

Table 3.5: Recommended daily amounts of food energy, protein, calcium and iron for population groups in the United Kingdom. [a] Since the recommendations are average amounts, the figures for each age range represent the amounts recommended at the middle of the range. Within each age range, younger children will need less, and older children more than the amount recommended. [b] Megajoules (10^6 joules). Calculated from the relation 1 kilocalorie = 4.184 kilojoules, i.e., 1 MJ = 240 kilocalories. [c] Recommended amounts have been calculated as 10% of the recommendations for energy. [d] This intake may not be sufficient for 10% of girls and women with large menstrual losses. [e] For the third trimester only. [f] 1 nicotinic acid equivalent = 1 mg available nicotinic acid or 60 mg tryptophan. [g] 1 retinol equivalent = 1 µg retinol or 6 µg β-carotene or 12 µg other biologically active carotenoids. [h] No dietary sources may be necessary for children and adults who are sufficiently exposed to sunlight, but during the winter children and adolescents should receive 10 µg (400 IU) daily by supplementation. Adults with inadequate exposure to sunlight, for example those who are housebound, may also need a supplement of 10 µg daily. From Department of Health and Social Security (1981). Recommended Intakes of Nutrients for the United Kingdom. Second Impression. Reproduced with the permission of the Controller of Her Majesty's Stationery Office.

3.4 Standard deviation score or Z score

Principle

The standard deviation or Z score is a measure of an individual's nutrient intake in relation to the distribution of corresponding nutrient intakes of the group (Sanjur, 1982). It does not evaluate nutrient intakes in relation to the recommended nutrient intakes.

Procedure

The standard deviation score is calculated as follows:

$$\frac{\text{Subject's nutrient intake} - \text{mean value for group}}{\text{SD value for that nutrient for the group}}$$

A person with an intake one standard deviation above the group mean has a standard deviation score or Z score of $+1.0$. This method of evaluating individual intakes is particularly useful in longitudinal studies for monitoring nutrient intakes of individuals relative to the group.

Reference

Sanjur D (1982). Social and Cultural Perspectives in Nutrition. Prentice-Hall Inc., Englewood Cliffs, New Jersey.

3.5 Probability approach to evaluating nutrient intakes

Principle

The probability approach attempts to assess more reliably the risk of nutrient inadequacy both for an individual and a population. For individuals, the method estimates the relative probability that the nutrient intake does not meet the individual's actual requirement. It is essential to note that this procedure does not identify with certainty which individuals are 'at risk' because of the absence of information about the actual requirements of each individual (Beaton, 1988). For a group, the method described below predicts the number of individuals within the group with nutrient intakes below their own requirements and hence provides an estimate of the proportion of the population at risk, or the prevalence of inadequate intakes, for specific nutrients (Anderson et al., 1982).

The absence of reliable estimates of the mean nutrient requirements and their variability for many nutrients, and the limitations of food composition data for certain nutrients, limit the general applicability of the probability approach to estimate the prevalence of inadequacy for every nutrient at the present time. Nevertheless, the United States Subcommittee on Dietary Evaluation (NRC, 1986) recommended the adoption of the probability approach to estimate the prevalence of inadequate intakes of most nutrients in future national nutrition surveys, with the exception of vitamin C, vitamin A, folate, and energy.

Procedure

Nutrient intake data derived from the three-day food records for each member of a group should be used.

1. Select a nutrient of interest (e.g. calcium).

2. Classify the individual intakes of calcium of each member of the group into the six classes defined in Table 3.6, row A. Each class is defined by the recommended nutrient intake for the nutrient and the associated standard deviation units.

3. Calculate the number of individuals with intakes of calcium within each class.

4. Multiply this number by the appropriate probability for each class (Table 3.6, row C) to give the estimated number of individuals in each of the six classes likely to have intakes of calcium below their own requirements.

5. Sum these estimated numbers to give the total number of individuals in the group who are at risk for inadequate intakes for calcium.

6. Express the sum as a percentage of the total number of subjects in the group. This is the percentage of the group who are predicted to have intakes for calcium below their own requirements and represents a probability estimate for the population as a whole as long as the group is a representative sample of that population.

7. Steps 2–6 can be repeated for the following nutrients: protein, iron, zinc, thiamin, riboflavin, and niacin.

It may be useful to construct a table to compare, for any nutrient, the following approaches to evaluating nutrient intakes: mean intake of the group as

	Class 1	Class 2	Class 3	Class 4	Class 5	Class 6
A	$< -2\,SD$ of R.N.I.	$-2\,SD$ to $-1\,SD$	$-1\,SD$ to mean	mean to $+1\,SD$	$+1\,SD$ to $+2\,SD$	$> +2\,SD$ of R.N.I.
B	$<54\%$	54% to 65.5%	65.5% to 77%	77% to 88.5%	88.5% to 100%	$>100\%$
C	1.0	0.93	0.69	0.31	0.07	0.0

Table 3.6: Assignment of 'risk' or probability statements to six classes of observed intakes expressed as proportions of the Canadian Recommended Nutrient Intake. Assumptions in this model are: requirements are normally distributed with the coefficient of variation = 15%; the recommended intake is set at the average requirement $+2\,SD$. Row 'A' shows the individual's intake in terms of the distribution of requirements; 'B' gives the intake in terms of the percentage of the RNI; 'C' indicates the probability that the individual's intake does not meet the requirement. Modified after Beaton (1985). © Am. J. Clin. Nutr. American Society for Clinical Nutrition.

a percentage of the RNI; percentage of the group below the RNI; percentage of the group below two-thirds RNI; probability estimate of inadequacy as a percentage.

References

Anderson GH, Peterson RD, Beaton GH (1982). Estimating nutrient deficiencies in a population from dietary records: the use of probability analyses. Nutrition Research 2: 409–415.

Beaton GH (1985). Uses and limits of the use of the Recommended Dietary Allowances for evaluating dietary intake data. American Journal of Clinical Nutrition 41: 155–164.

Beaton GH (1988). Twelfth Boyd Orr Memorial Lecture. Nutrient Requirements and Population Data. Proceedings of the Nutrition Society 47: 63–78.

NRC (National Research Council) (1986). Nutrient Adequacy. Assessment using Food Consumption Surveys. Subcommittee on Criteria for Dietary Evaluation, Coordinating Committee on Evaluation of Food Consumption Surveys. Food and Nutrition Board, Commission on Life Sciences. National Academy Press, Washington, D.C.

Part II
Anthropometric Assessment

Contents

Overview

The term 'nutritional anthropometry' has been defined by Jelliffe (1966) as:

measurements of the variations of the physical dimensions and the gross composition of the human body at different age levels and degrees of nutrition.

Anthropometric measurements are widely used in the assessment of nutritional status, particularly when a chronic imbalance between intakes of protein and energy occurs. Such disturbances modify the patterns of physical growth and the relative proportions of body tissues such as fat, muscle, and total body water.

Anthropometric measurements are of two types: growth and body composition measurements. Details of these measurement techniques are given in the following chapters. Body composition measurements can be further subdivided into measurements of body fat and fat-free mass, the two major compartments of total body mass. To assist in the interpretation of these measurements, anthropometric indices are derived. These are constructed from two or more raw anthropometric measurements. They can be simple numerical ratios such as weight$/$(height)^2, or combinations such as weight for age, weight for height, skinfold thicknesses at various sites, and/or limb circumferences (WHO, 1986). Selection of the most appropriate anthropometric index depends on the study objectives, the prevalence of malnutrition, as well as the validity, precision, sensitivity, specificity, and

Measurement	Common Error	Proposed Solution
All	Inadequate instrument Restless child Reading Recording	Select method appropriate to resources Postpone measurement, involve parent in procedure, use culturally appropriate procedures Training and refresher exercises stressing accuracy, with intermittent supervision by supervisor Record results immediately after measurement is taken and then have the results checked by second person
Length	Incorrect method for age Footwear or headwear not removed Head not in correct plane Child not straight along board and/or feet not parallel with movable board Board not firmly against heels	Use only when subject is < 2 years old Remove as local culture permits or make allowances Correct position of child before measuring Have assistant and child's parent present; don't take the measurement while the child is struggling; settle child correct pressure should be practised
Height	Incorrect method for age Footwear or headwear not removed Head not in correct plane, subject not straight, knees bent, or feet not flat on floor Board not firmly against head	Use only when subject is ≥ 2 years old Remove as local culture permits or make allowances Correct technique with practice and regular retraining. Provide adequate assistance. Calm non-co-operative children Move head board to compress hair
Weight	Room cold, no privacy Scale not calibrated to zero Subject wearing heavy clothing Subject moving or anxious as a result of prior incident	Use appropriate clinic facilities Re-calibrate after every subject Remove or make allowances for clothing Wait until subject is calm or remove cause of anxiety (e.g. scale too high)
Arm circ.	Subject not standing in correct position Tape too thick, stretched, or creased Wrong arm Mid-arm point incorrectly marked Arm not hanging loosely by side during measurement, examiner not comfortable or level with subject, tape around arm not at midpoint: too tight (causing skin contour indentation), too loose	Position subject correctly Use correct instrument Use left arm Measure midpoint carefully Correct techniques with training, supervision, and regular refresher courses. Take into account any cultural problems, such as wearing of arm band
Head circ.	Occipital protuberance / supraorbital landmarks poorly defined Hair crushed inadequately, ears under tape, or tension and position poorly maintained at time of reading Headwear not removed	Position tape correctly Correct technique with training regular refresher courses. Remove as local culture permits
Triceps skinfold	Wrong arm Mid-arm point or posterior plane incorrectly measured or marked Arm not loose by side during measurement Finger-thumb pinch or caliper placement too deep (muscle) or too superficial (skin) Caliper jaws not at marked site Reading done too early, pinch not maintained, caliper handle not fully released. Examiner not comfortable or level with subject	Use left arm Measure midpoint carefully Reposition and relax arm Correct technique with training etc. Reposition calipers Correct technique with training etc. Ensure examiner is level with subject for measurement

Table II.1: Common errors and possible solutions when measuring mid-upper-arm circumference, head circumference, and triceps skinfold. Modified from Zerfas AJ (1979). In: Jelliffe DB, Jelliffe EFP (eds). Human Nutrition. A Comprehensive Treatise, Volume 2. Nutrition and Growth. Plenum Press.

predictive value of the index. Definitions for these terms are given in the glossary.

Anthropometric indices are of increasing importance in nutritional assessment because the measurement procedures have several advantages:

- The procedures use simple, safe, noninvasive techniques which can be used at the bedside and are applicable to large sample sizes (Heymsfield and Casper, 1987).
- Equipment required is inexpensive, portable, and durable and can be made or purchased locally.
- Relatively unskilled personnel can perform measurement procedures.
- The methods are precise and accurate, provided that standardized techniques are used.
- Information is generated on past long-term nutritional history, which cannot be obtained with equal confidence using other techniques.
- The procedures can assist in the identification of mild to moderate malnutrition, as well as severe states of malnutrition.
- The methods may be used to evaluate changes in nutritional status over time and from one generation to the next, a phenomenon known as the secular trend.
- Screening tests, to identify individuals at high risk to malnutrition, can be devised.

Despite these advantages, nutritional anthropometry has several limitations. For example, it is a relatively insensitive method, and it cannot detect disturbances in nutritional status over short time periods or distinguish between specific nutrient deficiencies (e.g. zinc and protein). Certain nonnutritional factors (such as disease, genetics, diurnal variation, and reduced energy expenditure) can reduce the specificity and sensitivity of anthropometric measurements.

Errors occur in nutritional anthropometry which may affect the precision, accuracy, and validity of the measurements/indices. The errors can be attributed to three major effects: measurement errors, alterations in the composition and physical properties of certain tissues, and use of invalid assumptions in the derivation of body composition from anthropometric measurements (Heymsfield and Casper, 1987). Sources of error may be random or systematic and may include

examiner error resulting from inadequate training, instrument error, and measurement difficulties (Himes, 1987). Some common sources of measurement errors in anthropometry are shown in Table II.1. Some of these measurement errors can be minimized by training personnel to use instruments that are precise and correctly calibrated, and standardized, validated measurement techniques.

Alterations in the composition and/or physical properties of certain tissues may occur in both healthy and diseased subjects, resulting in inaccuracies in certain anthropometric measurements/indices. Even in healthy individuals, body weight may be affected by variations in tissue hydration with the menstrual cycle (Heymsfield and Casper, 1987), whereas skinfolds may be influenced by alterations in compressibility with age and site of the measurements (Himes et al., 1979). Generally, anthropometric measurements are not corrected to account for these effects. Errors also arise when the prediction equations, developed for healthy lean subjects, are applied to patients with certain diseases in which increases in the total body water and alterations in the distribution of body fat occur.

Invalid assumptions may lead to erroneous estimates of body composition when derived from anthropometric measurements, especially in protein-energy malnutrition, certain disease states, or obesity. For instance, use of skinfold thickness measurements to estimate total body fat assumes that: (a) the thickness of the subcutaneous adipose tissue reflects a constant proportion of the total body fat, and (b) the sites selected represent the average thickness of the subcutaneous adipose tissue. In fact, the relationship between subcutaneous and internal fat is nonlinear, and varies with body weight, age, and disease state. Very lean subjects have a smaller proportion of body fat deposited subcutaneously than obese subjects (Allen et al., 1956), and in malnourished persons there is probably a shift of fat storage from subcutaneous to deep visceral sites. Variations in the distribution of subcutaneous fat also occur with sex, race, and age (Robson et al., 1971; Durnin and Womersley, 1974).

The selection of appropriate reference data to allow comparison of the distributions of the anthropometric indices of the study group with those of an apparently healthy population, and to establish 'risk' categories or cutoff points, is a difficult problem. There is lack of agreement regarding the use of local versus international reference data. Some investigators advocate the use of local reference data derived from ethnically similar but privileged groups living in the same country, to minimize genetic influences (Goldstein and Tanner, 1980); others suggest that the advantages of one universal standard drawn from a well-defined and accurately sampled population outweigh the problems of genetic influence (Habicht et al., 1974; Graitcer and Gentry, 1981). The World Health Organization (WHO, 1983) has recommended the use of the United States National Center for Health Statistics (NCHS) growth percentiles (Hamill et al., 1979) as an international reference for comparisons of health and nutritional status among countries.

Several systems are available for estimating the prevalence of malnutrition in the study population or identifying individuals 'at risk' to malnutrition. All utilize at least one anthropometric index and one or more reference limits drawn from the frequency distribution of the appropriate reference data, or cutoff points. Reference limits can be based on percentiles for designating individuals as 'at risk' to malnutrition. Often below the 3rd or 5th percentiles or above the 97th or 95th percentiles are used, depending on the reference data used.

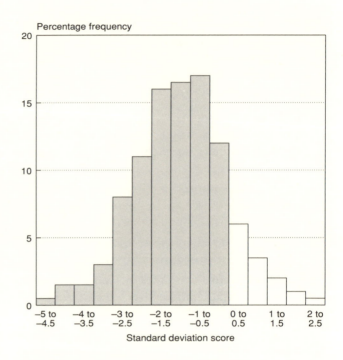

Fig. II.2: Frequency distribution of SD scores of height for age for 1395 children measured during the Sahel nutrition studies and who were aged 12 to 23.9 months. From: Measuring Change in Nutritional Status: Guidelines for assessing the nutritional impact of supplementary feeding programmes for vulnerable groups. Geneva, World Health Organization, 1983: page 26, Figure 4, with permission.

A percentile refers to the position of the measurement value in relation to all (or 100%) of the measurements for the reference population, ranked in order of magnitude. Fig. II.1 is a cumulative frequency distribution of the heights of boys aged thirteen years, illustrating the use of percentiles. In this figure, a height of 152 cm represents the 50th percentile. This means that 50% of the boys have a height at or below this value, and 50% at or above this value. Similarly, 10% of the boys have a height at or below the 10th percentile which, in Fig. II.1, falls at 141.8 cm. For data with a Gaussian distribution (e.g. height for age), the 50th percentile corresponds to both the mean and the median; for skewed data (e.g. weight for age) the 50th percentile corresponds to the median.

For population studies, the number and the percentage of individuals falling within specified percentiles of the reference data can be tabulated or presented as a histogram (Fig. II.2) (WHO, 1983). This procedure is recommended for the evaluation of anthropometric measurements from relatively well-nourished populations

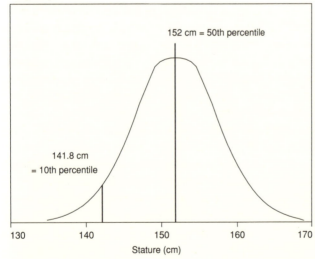

Fig. II.1: Frequency distribution for stature in 13-year old boys.

Below Mean		Above Mean	
Percentile	Z-score	Percentile	Z-score
0–5	less than −1.645	50–55	0.000 to 0.126
5–10	−1.645 to −1.282	55–60	0.126 to 0.253
10–15	−1.282 to −1.036	60–65	0.253 to 0.385
15–20	−1.036 to −0.842	65–70	0.385 to 0.524
20–25	−0.842 to −0.675	70–75	0.524 to 0.675
25–30	−0.675 to −0.524	75–80	0.675 to 0.842
30–35	−0.524 to −0.385	80–85	0.842 to 1.036
35–40	−0.385 to −0.253	85–90	1.036 to 1.282
40–45	−0.253 to −0.126	90–95	1.282 to 1.645
45–50	−0.126 to 0.000	95–100	greater than 1.645

Table II.2: Equivalents of percentile and Z-scores in a normal distribution. Modified from Frisancho (1990), Table III.1

from industrialized countries, as no errors are introduced if the data have a skewed distribution. Weight for age, weight for height, and many circumferential and skinfold indices have skewed distributions.

Percentiles are not recommended for evaluating anthropometric indices from less developed areas when reference data from industrialized countries, such as the NCHS data (Hamill et al., 1979), are used. In these circumstances, many of the study population may have indices below the extreme percentile of the reference population (i.e. below the 5th percentile). As a result it may be very difficult to accurately classify large numbers of individuals in the study population (Waterlow et al., 1977).

As an alternative, standard deviation scores or Z scores should be used (Waterlow et al., 1977). The method measures the deviation of the anthropometric measurement from the reference median in terms of standard deviations or Z scores. Standard deviation scores can be defined beyond the limits of the original reference data. Consequently, individuals with indices well below the extreme percentiles of the original reference data can be classified accurately. The number and proportion of subjects within a specified range of standard deviation scores for each age and sex group can be presented graphically (Fig. II.2), or as a table, as noted for percentiles.

The SD score, is calculated using the following formula, a modified version of the standard statistical Z-score transformation:

$$\frac{\text{Individual's value} - \text{median value of reference population}}{\text{Standard deviation value of reference population}}$$

The score is a measure of an individual's value with respect to the distribution of the reference population and is calculated for each subject within the sample. The standard deviation values for the NCHS reference population are recommended for use in calculating SD scores and are published by WHO (1983). These reference standard deviations have been calculated by transforming the original NCHS reference data. Specific details of this process are given in Dibley et al. (1987). As the distributions of weight for age and weight for height are not symmetrical, standard deviations below and above the median differ and hence were calculated separately. In contrast, the distribution for height for age is symmetrical, so that a single set of age-specific standard deviations was calculated.

Reference limits can also be based on SD scores, in which case, often scores of below −2.0 are designated as indicating risk of severe protein-energy malnutrition whereas scores above +2.0 are taken to indicate risk of obesity. Table II.2 illustrates the relationship between percentiles and standard deviation score values in a normal distribution (Frisancho, 1990).

Reference limits are comparable across all indices and at all ages, when based on the same standard deviation score values (e.g. −2.0 SD). For example, a reference limit of −2.0 SD represents the same degree of malnutrition, irrespective of the anthropometric index used (e.g. weight-for-age or weight-for-height) or the age of the child (Waterlow et al., 1977).

Cutoff points may also be expressed as standard deviation scores or percentiles and, in some cases, as a percentage of the reference median. They differ from reference limits, however, because they are based on functional impairment and/or clinical signs of deficiency, and occasionally mortality risk. They are generally established by reviewing anthropometric characteristics of individuals with clinically moderate and/or severe malnutrition or who subsequently die. For example, height-for-age below the 5th percentile is often referred to as a 'cutoff point' rather than a reference limit, because children with indices below this value are stunted.

The use of percentiles and standard deviation scores to classify individuals is preferable to calculating the index value of the subject as a percentage of the reference median. Although this latter approach continues to be widely used, it does not take into account the distribution of the data within the reference set or the variability in the relative width of the distributions of the weight-for-age, weight-for-height, and height-for-age indices (Waterlow et al., 1977). Such variability inhibits the universal use of a constant percentage of the reference median (e.g. 70%) across all ages and for all growth indices. For example, 60% of median weight for age represents a more severe state of malnutrition for younger compared to older children. Moreover, when the index weight for height is used, 60% of the median is inappropriate; such a deficit at any age is incompatible with life (Dibley et al., 1987).

In the following chapters on anthropometry, data from two reference populations are given: data from U.S. surveys conducted by the National Center for Health Statistics (NCHS) and from the Nutrition Canada Survey (Nutrition Canada, 1980). The NCHS reference growth data has been recommended by the World Health Organization as an international standard for comparisons of health and nutritional status of children among countries.

References

Dibley M J, Goldsby J B, Staehling N W, Trowbridge F L (1987). Development of normalized curves for the international growth reference: historical and technical considerations. American Journal of Clinical Nutrition 46: 736–748.

Frisancho A R (1990). Anthropometric Standards for the Assessment of Growth and Nutritional Status. The University of Michigan Press, Ann Arbor.

Goldstein H, Tanner J M (1980). Ecological considerations in the creation and the use of child growth standards. Lancet 1: 582–585.

Graitcer P L, Gentry E M (1981). Measuring children: one reference for all. Lancet 2: 297–299.

Habicht J P, Martorell R, Yarbrough C, Malina R M, Klein R E (1974). Height and weight standards for preschool children. How relevant are ethnic differences in growth potential? Lancet I: 611–615.

Hamill P V V, Drizd T A, Johnson C L, Reed R B, Roche A F, Moore W M (1979). Physical growth: National Center for Health Statistics Percentiles. American Journal of Clinical Nutrition 32: 607–629.

Heymsfield S B, Casper K (1987). Anthropometric assessment of the adult hospitalized patient. Journal of Parenteral and Enteral Nutrition 11: 36S–41S.

Himes J H (1987). Purposeful assessment of nutritional status. In: Johnston F E (ed) Nutritional Anthropology. Alan R. Liss Inc., New York, pp. 85–99.

Himes J H, Roche A F, Siervogel R M (1979). Compressibility of skinfolds and measurements of subcutaneous fat. American Journal of Clinical Nutrition 32: 1734–1740.

Jelliffe D B (1966). The Assessment of the Nutritional Status of the Community. WHO Monograph No. 53. World Health Organization, Geneva.

Lohman T G, Roche A F, Martorell R (eds) (1988). Anthropometric Standardization Manual. Human Kinetics Books, Champagne, Illinois.

Nutrition Canada (1980). Anthropometry Report: Height, Weight and Body Dimensions. Bureau of Nutritional Sciences, Health Protection Branch, Health and Welfare, Ottawa.

Robson J R F, Bazin M, Soderstrom R (1971). Ethnic differences in skin-fold thickness. American Journal of Clinical Nutrition 24: 864–868.

Waterlow J C, Buzina R, Keller W, Lane J M, Nichaman M Z, Tanner J M (1977). The presentation and use of height and weight data for comparing the nutritional status of groups of children under the age of 10 years. Bulletin of the World Health Organization 55: 489–498.

WHO (World Health Organization) (1983). Measuring Change in Nutritional Status. Guidelines for Assessing the Nutritional Impact of Supplementary Feeding Programmes for Vulnerable Groups. World Health Organization, Geneva.

WHO (World Health Organization) (1986). Use and interpretation of anthropometric indicators of nutritional status. Bulletin of the World Health Organization 64: 929–941.

Zerfas A J (1979). Anthropometric field methods: general. In: Jelliffe D B, Jelliffe E F P (eds) Human Nutrition. A Comprehensive Treatise. Volume 2. Nutrition and Growth. Plenum Press, New York, pp. 339–364.

Chapter 4
Assessment of growth

Contents

Introduction

The most widely used anthropometric measurements of growth are those of stature (height or length) and body weight. These measurements can be made quickly and easily, and, with care and training, accurately. Head circumference measurements are often taken in association with stature. Details of the standardized procedures for these growth measurements are summarized below and are given in detail in Lohman et al. (1988).

Growth indices can be derived from raw measurements. They can be simple numerical ratios such as weight/(height)^2, or combinations such as head circumference for age, or weight for stature. Such combinations should not be written as head circumference/age, weight/stature to avoid confusion with the numerical ratios. Some growth indices have been recommended by the World Health Organization (WHO, 1983) as primary measures of past (e.g. height for age) or current (e.g. weight for height) nutritional status in children. Together, they can distinguish between linear growth failure (stunting) and wasting. In hospital patients, anthropometric growth indices are used primarily to identify protein-energy malnutrition and obesity, and to monitor changes following a nutrition intervention program.

The World Health Organization has recommended the National Center for Health Statistics (NCHS) reference growth data as an international standard, allowing comparisons of health and nutritional status of children among countries. The NCHS sample was cross-sectional, data collection procedures were well-standardized and fully documented, and the population examined appear to have attained their full growth potential. In contrast, in less industrialized countries, well-nourished children are often few, and sometimes unrepresentative; as a result, appropriate 'local' reference data are rare.

References

Lohman T G, Roche A F, Martorell R (eds) (1988). Anthropometric Standardization Manual. Human Kinetics Books, Champagne, Illinois.

WHO (World Health Organization) (1983). Measuring Change in Nutritional Status. Guidelines for assessing the nutritional impact of supplementary feeding programmes for vulnerable groups. World Health Organization, Geneva.

4.1 Head circumference

Principle

Chronic malnutrition during the first few months of life, or intra-uterine growth retardation, may impair brain development and result in an abnormally low head circumference (Winick, 1969). Consequently, measurement of head circumference is important because it is closely related to brain size. When assessed in relation to age, head circumference can be used as an index of protein-energy nutritional status during the first two years of life. Beyond two years, growth in head circumference is so slow that its measurement is no longer useful. Head circumference is often used with other measurements to detect pathological conditions associated with an unusually large (macrocephalic) or small (microcephalic) head. Certain non-nutritional factors, including disease and pathological conditions, genetic variation, and cultural practices (such as binding of the head during infancy) may also influence head circumference.

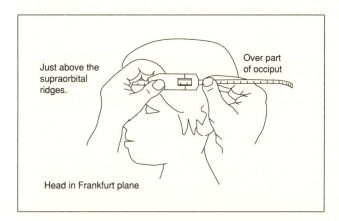

Fig. 4.1: Measurement of head circumference

Procedure for infants and young children

For the measurement of head circumference, a narrow, flexible, and nonstretch tape made of fiberglass or steel about 0.6 cm wide should be used.

1. Stand the subject with the left side facing the measurer, with arms relaxed and legs apart.

2. The subject must look straight ahead so the line of vision is perpendicular to the body and the plane of the head is horizontal (i.e. in the Frankfurt plane). To check the subject's head is in the Frankfurt plane, an imaginary line which passes through the external auditory meatus (the small flap of skin on the forward edge of the ear) and across the top of the lower bone of the eye socket immediately under the eye must be horizontal.

3. Place the tape just above the supraorbital ridges covering the most prominent part of the frontal bulge, and over the part of the occiput which gives the maximum circumference (Fig. 4.1). Care must be taken to ensure that the tape is at the same level on each side of the head and pulled tightly to compress the hair (Weiner and Lourie, 1969; Lohman et al., 1988).

4. Measurements are made to the nearest millimeter.

5. Calculate the percentage of the median with the reference data cited below, using the appropriate age, sex, and median head circumference.

$$\% \text{ Median} = \frac{100 \times \text{observed head circ.}}{\text{median head circ. for age and sex}}$$

6. Determine in which percentile range the subject's head circumference falls using the reference data cited below.

Evaluation

Tables of percentiles for head circumference for Canadian children from birth up to and including age five years were calculated from the Nutrition Canada data (Nutrition Canada, 1980). Percentiles for head circumference for US children from birth to thirty-six months, compiled by the National Center for Health Statistics (Johnson et al., 1978), are given in Table 4.1.

References

Johnson T R, Moore W M, Jeffries J E (eds) (1978). Children are different: Developmental Physiology. Ross Laboratories, Columbus, Ohio.

Age (months)	Percentiles of head circumference (cm) by age							Percentiles of head circumference (cm) by age						
	5	10	25	50	75	90	95	5	10	25	50	75	90	95
	Male subjects							Female subjects						
Birth	32.6	33.0	33.9	34.8	35.6	36.6	37.2	32.1	32.9	33.5	34.3	34.8	35.5	35.9
1	34.9	35.4	36.2	37.2	38.1	39.0	39.6	34.2	34.8	35.6	36.4	37.1	37.8	38.3
3	38.4	38.9	39.7	40.6	41.7	42.5	43.1	37.3	37.8	38.7	39.5	40.4	41.2	41.7
6	41.5	42.0	42.8	43.8	44.7	45.6	46.2	40.3	40.9	41.6	42.4	43.3	44.1	44.6
9	43.5	44.0	44.8	45.8	46.6	47.5	48.1	42.3	42.8	43.5	44.3	45.1	46.0	46.4
12	44.8	45.3	46.1	47.0	47.9	48.8	49.3	43.5	44.1	44.8	45.6	46.4	47.2	47.6
18	46.3	46.7	47.4	48.4	49.3	50.1	50.6	45.0	45.6	46.3	47.1	47.9	48.6	49.1
24	47.3	47.7	48.3	49.2	50.2	51.0	51.4	46.1	46.5	47.3	48.1	48.8	49.6	50.1
30	48.0	48.4	49.1	49.9	51.0	51.7	52.2	47.0	47.3	48.0	48.8	49.4	50.3	50.8
36	48.6	49.0	49.7	50.5	51.5	52.3	52.8	47.6	47.9	48.5	49.3	50.0	50.8	51.4

Table 4.1: Percentiles of head circumference (cm) by age for males and females from birth to thirty-six months, compiled by the NCHS. From Johnson et al. (1978).

Lohman T G, Roche A F, Martorell R (eds) (1988). Anthropometric Standardization Manual. Human Kinetics Books, Champagne, Illinois.

Nutrition Canada (1980). Anthropometry Report: Height, Weight and Body Dimensions. Bureau of Nutritional Sciences, Health Protection Branch, Health and Welfare, Ottawa.

Weiner J S, Lourie J A (1969). Human Biology: A Guide to Field Methods: International Biological Programme Handbook. IBP No. 9. Blackwell Scientific Publications, Oxford-Edinburgh.

Winick M (1969). Malnutrition and brain development. Journal of Pediatrics 74: 667–679.

4.2 Weight in infants, children, and adults

Principle

Body weight represents the sum of protein, fat, water, and bone mineral mass, and does not provide any information on relative changes in these four chemical compartments. In normal adults, there is a tendency to increased fat deposition with age, concomitant with a reduction in muscle protein. Such changes are not evident in body weight measurements and can only be evaluated by determining body fat and/or fat-free mass. In persons with edema or ascites, an increase in total body water occurs, which may mask any body weight deficit resulting from losses of fat and/or muscle. Massive tumour growth may also mask losses of fat and muscle tissue which may occur during severe undernutrition. Conversely, in obese subjects, loss of muscle may be masked by residual fat (Heymsfield and Casper, 1987).

Several indices can be constructed from the measurement of body weight. For example, weight for age, an acute index of malnutrition, is widely used to assess protein-energy malnutrition and overnutrition, especially in infancy when the measurement of length is difficult. A major limitation of weight for age as an index of protein-energy malnutrition, however, is that it does not take into account height differences: as a result, children with a low weight for age are not necessarily wasted. They may be genetically short, or their low weight for age may be associated with nutritional growth failure or 'stunting', a condition characterized by low height for age but a weight appropriate for their short stature. Consequently, the prevalence of malnutrition in small children may be overestimated if only weight for age is used.

To interpret a single measurement of weight in relation to the reference data, the exact age of the child must be known. In some countries, local calendars of special events can be constructed to assist in identifying the birth date of a child. In areas where the ages of the children are uncertain, weight for height should be used instead of weight for age. Weight for height is a sensitive index of current nutritional status and is relatively independent of age between one and ten years. For ages less than one year, however, older infants at a given height tend to be heavier, so that age groupings with a narrower range should be used. Weight for height also appears to be relatively independent of ethnic group, particularly for children aged one to five years (Waterlow et al., 1977). In contrast to weight for age, weight for height differentiates between nutritional stunting, when weight may be appropriate for height, and wasting, when weight is very low for height as a result of deficits in both tissue and fat mass. The highest prevalence of wasting occurs during the postweaning period (i.e. from 12 to 23 months) (WHO, 1986). Weight for height is also useful in evaluating the benefits of intervention programs, as this index is more sensitive to changes in nutritional status than height for age. The index is also frequently used in the nutritional assessment of hospital patients, to identify wasting.

Unfortunately, edema and obesity may significantly complicate the interpretation of weight-for-height measurements. A further disadvantage is that it classifies children with poor linear growth as 'normal'. Consequently, it is preferable to use a combination of weight for height, and height for age (Section 4.3).

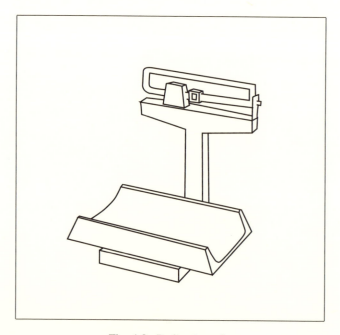

Fig. 4.2: Pediatric scale

Procedures for infants and children

A pediatric scale (Fig. 4.2) should be used where possible, with a scale pan large enough to support the weight of the child.

1. Cover the pan with a blanket or towel.

2. Zero the scale and calibrate with standard weights.

3. Place the infant on the pan scale so the weight is well distributed equally over the the pan.

4. Once the infant is lying quietly, record the weight to the nearest 10 g.

5. Calculate the percentage of the median with the reference data given in Table 4.2 or 4.7, using the appropriate age, sex, and median weight.

$$\% \text{ Median} = \frac{100 \times \text{observed weight}}{\text{median weight for age and sex}}$$

6. Determine in which percentile range the subject's weight falls using the same reference data.

In the field, a suspended spring balance and a weighing sling may be used (Fig. 4.3). After slipping the subject into the sling, the weight is recorded as soon as the indicator on the scale has stabilized.

If there is no alternative, the mother and subject can be weighed together, and then the mother alone, using a beam balance. The subject's weight can then be calculated by subtraction. This

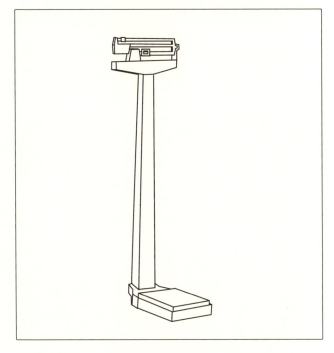

Fig. 4.4: Beam balance

method should only be used as a last resort as the precision of the measurement of the weight of the infant will be much reduced.

Procedure for older children and adults

Use a beam balance with nondetachable weights for the measurement of weight in older children and adults who can stand without support (Fig. 4.4). The balance should be calibrated regularly and whenever it is moved to another location. Measurements should preferably be made after the bladder has been emptied, and before a meal. Unfortunately, beam balances tend to be heavy and bulky, and therefore unsuitable for field use. In such cases, spring balance scales, although less accurate and reliable, are often used.

1. Place the balance on a hard flat surface.

2. Zero the scale and calibrate with standard weights.

3. Ask the subject to stand unassisted, in the center of the platform, and to look straight ahead, standing relaxed but still, preferably in the nude. If this is not possible, the subject should wear light underclothing and/or a paper examination gown. The weight of these garments should be recorded for later subtraction; standard corrections for clothing should not be used.

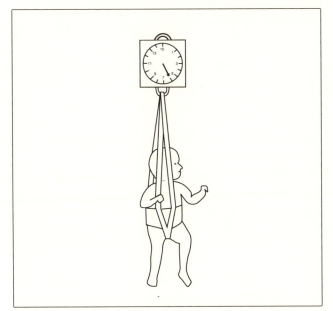

Fig. 4.3: Measurement of weight using a spring balance

Age (yr)	Percentiles of weight (kg) by age							Percentiles of weight (kg) by age						
	5	10	25	50	75	90	95	5	10	25	50	75	90	95
	Male subjects							Female subjects						
1.0–1.9	9.6	10.0	10.7	11.6	12.6	13.7	14.4	8.7	9.2	9.9	10.8	11.8	12.8	13.4
2.0–2.9	11.1	11.6	12.5	13.6	14.6	15.8	16.6	10.8	11.2	12.0	12.8	13.9	15.1	15.9
3.0–3.9	12.8	13.4	14.4	15.5	16.8	18.1	19.4	11.8	12.6	13.6	14.7	16.2	17.6	18.6
4.0–4.9	14.1	15.0	16.1	17.5	19.0	20.6	21.5	13.7	14.3	15.5	16.8	18.4	20.1	21.3
5.0–5.9	16.0	16.7	17.8	19.6	21.4	23.5	25.4	15.3	16.2	17.3	19.0	21.0	23.6	25.3
6.0–6.9	17.5	18.8	20.2	21.9	24.0	27.7	30.0	17.0	17.7	19.4	21.3	23.7	26.5	28.9
7.0–7.9	19.0	20.4	22.2	24.7	27.2	29.9	33.1	19.2	19.8	21.9	23.8	26.5	29.9	32.7
8.0–8.9	21.5	22.7	24.5	26.8	29.7	33.6	37.3	20.9	21.9	24.0	26.9	30.4	35.1	39.9
9.0–9.9	23.6	24.7	27.1	30.3	33.6	40.3	43.2	23.7	24.8	26.8	30.7	34.7	41.7	46.5
10.0–10.9	26.2	27.7	30.2	33.8	38.6	45.6	53.1	25.6	27.0	29.6	33.9	39.2	46.5	52.4
11.0–11.9	28.3	30.0	33.4	37.6	43.3	52.3	58.6	29.1	30.5	34.3	39.8	46.3	56.9	61.9
12.0–12.9	30.8	32.8	36.6	42.2	49.0	59.0	66.9	32.5	34.3	39.1	45.9	53.0	61.2	66.7
13.0–13.9	34.6	37.1	41.6	48.5	56.1	65.2	69.6	37.2	39.3	44.3	49.6	55.7	66.8	76.2
14.0–14.9	41.3	44.0	49.2	55.3	63.0	70.1	76.9	40.3	42.9	47.3	52.7	60.0	69.5	75.6
15.0–15.9	44.7	48.6	54.2	60.0	66.2	74.4	81.3	43.4	45.3	48.6	54.2	60.3	69.5	79.4
16.0–16.9	51.7	54.2	59.0	64.8	72.9	81.6	89.0	43.4	46.1	50.8	55.7	62.8	73.1	80.8
17.0–17.9	51.1	54.1	59.3	65.7	72.5	83.3	91.4	43.2	46.4	51.9	57.4	63.3	74.7	86.0
18.0–24.9	56.4	59.8	64.8	71.4	80.5	91.5	99.9	45.6	48.4	52.6	58.3	65.4	76.1	84.3
25.0–29.9	58.7	61.8	68.1	76.0	84.8	95.1	103.4	46.6	49.0	53.4	59.4	68.4	81.6	90.8
30.0–34.9	59.8	63.3	69.8	78.4	87.4	96.8	103.0	47.5	50.1	54.9	61.5	72.2	86.5	97.9
35.0–39.9	58.4	62.9	72.2	79.8	87.8	96.7	102.8	48.6	51.7	56.4	63.3	73.7	88.1	98.2
40.0–44.9	60.7	64.3	71.9	79.6	89.4	98.8	104.8	49.2	51.8	57.0	64.0	75.1	89.8	99.1
45.0–49.9	60.0	64.0	71.4	79.7	89.2	97.2	103.6	47.8	51.4	57.1	64.9	75.9	87.4	98.4
50.0–54.9	58.7	63.3	70.0	78.0	87.4	99.3	103.6	48.8	51.9	58.1	65.8	75.8	88.4	97.1
55.0–59.9	58.2	63.0	70.2	78.5	86.8	97.1	103.5	48.6	52.2	58.2	66.3	77.2	89.4	98.5
60.0–64.9	57.9	61.8	68.8	76.8	84.9	92.5	100.0	48.5	51.7	58.1	66.0	75.8	86.0	94.1
65.0–69.9	55.1	58.5	66.4	74.5	83.2	91.8	97.2	47.8	51.4	57.7	65.7	74.8	86.1	93.9
70.0–74.9	53.9	57.5	65.2	73.0	81.3	90.4	95.9	46.5	50.1	57.0	64.5	74.4	83.3	88.8

Table 4.2: Percentiles of weight (kg) by age for males and females of one to seventy-four years. Data are from the U.S. NHANES I (1971–74) and NHANES II (1976–80) surveys and were compiled by Frisancho (1990).

4. Record any signs of visible edema, if present.

5. Record the body weight to the nearest 0.1 kg.

6. Calculate the percentage of the median with the reference data cited below, using the appropriate age, sex, and median weight.

$$\% \text{ Median} = \frac{100 \times \text{observed weight}}{\text{median weight for age and sex}}$$

7. Determine in which percentile range the subject's weight falls using the same reference data.

Electronic scales that are both accurate and light in weight are now available, but are expensive. Usually, such scales can be connected to a portable computer, allowing the recording of the weights to be automated, and recording errors to be eliminated.

Evaluation

Weight percentiles by age for U.S. males and females aged one to seventy-four years, compiled by Frisancho (1990) from the NHANES I (1971–74) and the NHANES II (1976–80) surveys conducted by the National Center for Health Statistics are given in Table 4.2. Measurements were made on 7,125 blacks and 35,931 whites, and 718 of other ethnic groups, using standardized techniques.

Weight percentiles by height and age for U.S. adults aged eighteen to seventy-four years, derived from the NHANES I survey (1971–1974) and compiled by Abraham et al. (1979), are given in Tables 4.3 and 4.4. Height-weight tables are presented for men and women, with mean weight values (in kilograms) for each inch (or centimeter) of height ranging from 62 to 74 inches for men, and 57 to 68 inches for women, aged 18 to 74 and

18 to 24, 25 to 34, 35 to 44, 45 to 54, 55 to 64, and 65 to 74 years.

Percentiles for weight by frame size and height for U.S. adults aged twenty-five to fifty-four years and fifty-five to seventy-four years old are given in Tables 4.5 and 4.6 (Frisancho, 1984). These are also from the cross-sectional data collected by the NHANES I (1971–1974) and NHANES II (1976–1980) surveys, conducted by NCHS. The frame size categories—small, medium, and large— correspond to below the 15th, between the 15th and 85th, and above the 85th sex-and age-specific percentiles of elbow breadth.

Percentiles for weight (kg) of Canadians by age and sex for children and adults are given in Table 4.7. Data are from the Nutrition Canada (1980) Anthropometry Report.

The Metropolitan Life Insurance (MLI) height-weight table for adults by frame size is shown in Table 4.8. The table is based on the 1979 Build Study and is derived from measurements on life insurance policyholders aged from twenty-five to fifty-nine during the years from 1950 to 1971. The applicability of this table to the general population, especially the elderly, is questionable. The weight ranges given in the tables are those for which people should have the greatest longevity. They do not refer to weights that minimize illness or incidence of diseases. Weight is related to three frame sizes, small, medium, and large, based on elbow breadth. Categories of frame size were developed from the elbow breadth measurements such that 50% of the population falls within the medium frame and 25% each fall within the small

and large frames (Metropolitan Height and Weight Tables, 1983). The range of weights given fall below the average weights of the NCHS reference data.

References

Abraham S, Johnson C L, Najjar M F (1979). Weight by height and age for adults 18–74 years, U.S. 1971–74, vital and health statistics. Series 11, No. 211, Department of Health, Education, and Welfare. Washington, D.C: U.S. Government Printing Office.

Frisancho A R (1984). New standards of weight and body composition by frame size and height for assessment of nutritional status of adults and the elderly. American Journal of Clinical Nutrition 40: 808–819.

Frisancho A R (1990). Anthropometric Standards for the Assessment of Growth and Nutritional Status. The University of Michigan Press, Ann Arbor.

Heymsfield S B, Casper K (1987). Anthropometric assessment of the adult hospitalized patient. Journal of Parenteral and Enteral Nutrition 11: 36S–41S.

Metropolitan Height and Weight Tables (1983). Statistical Bulletin, Metropolitan Life Insurance Company, New York 64: 1–9.

Nutrition Canada (1980). Anthropometry Report: Height, Weight and Body Dimensions. Bureau of Nutritional Sciences, Health Protection Branch, Health and Welfare, Ottawa.

Waterlow J C, Buzina R, Keller W, Lane J M, Nichaman M Z, Tanner J M (1977). The presentation and use of height and weight data for comparing the nutritional status of groups of children under the age of 10 years. Bulletin of the World Health Organization 55: 489–498.

WHO (World Health Organization Working Group) (1986). Use and interpretation of anthropometric indicators of nutritional status. Bulletin of the World Health Organization 64: 929–941.

Height		Males (18–24 yr)						Height		Females (18–24 yr)					
in	cm	5	10	20	50	80	90	95	in	cm	5	10	20	50	80	90	95
62	157.5	38.5	43.1	48.5	58.9	69.4	74.8	79.4	57	144.8	30.8	35.4	40.8	51.7	62.6	68.0	72.6
63	160.0	40.8	45.3	50.8	61.2	71.6	77.1	81.6	58	147.3	32.2	36.7	42.2	53.1	63.9	69.4	73.9
64	162.6	43.1	47.6	53.1	63.5	73.9	79.4	83.9	59	149.9	33.6	38.1	43.5	54.4	65.3	70.7	75.3
65	165.1	45.4	49.9	55.3	65.8	76.2	81.6	86.2	60	152.4	34.9	39.5	44.9	55.8	66.7	72.1	76.6
66	167.6	47.6	52.2	57.6	68.0	78.5	83.9	88.4	61	154.9	36.3	40.8	46.3	57.1	68.0	73.5	78.0
67	170.2	49.4	54.0	59.4	69.8	80.3	85.7	90.2	62	157.5	37.6	42.2	47.6	58.5	69.4	74.8	79.4
68	172.7	51.7	56.2	61.7	72.1	82.5	88.0	92.5	63	160.0	39.0	43.5	49.0	59.9	70.7	76.2	80.7
69	175.3	54.0	58.5	63.9	74.4	84.8	90.2	94.8	64	162.6	40.4	40.8	50.3	61.2	72.1	77.6	82.1
70	177.8	55.8	60.3	65.8	76.2	86.6	92.1	96.6	65	165.1	41.7	46.3	51.7	62.6	73.5	78.9	83.4
71	180.3	58.0	62.6	68.0	78.5	88.9	94.3	98.9	66	167.6	43.1	48.1	53.1	63.9	74.8	80.3	84.8
72	182.9	60.3	64.9	70.3	80.7	91.2	96.6	101.1	67	170.2	44.4	49.0	54.4	65.3	76.2	81.6	86.2
73	185.4	62.6	67.1	72.6	83.0	93.4	98.9	103.4	68	172.7	45.8	50.3	55.8	66.7	77.6	83.0	87.5
74	188.0	64.9	69.4	74.8	85.3	95.7	101.1	105.7									

Height		Males (25–34 yr)						Height		Females (25–34 yr)					
in	cm	5	10	20	50	80	90	95	in	cm	5	10	20	50	80	90	95
62	157.5	41.3	46.3	52.2	63.9	75.7	81.6	86.6	57	144.8	29.5	34.9	41.3	53.5	65.8	72.1	77.6
63	160.0	43.1	48.1	54.0	65.7	77.5	83.4	88.4	58	147.3	30.8	36.3	42.6	54.9	67.1	73.5	78.9
64	162.6	45.4	50.3	56.2	68.0	79.8	85.7	90.7	59	149.9	32.7	38.1	44.4	56.7	68.9	75.3	80.7
65	165.1	48.1	53.1	59.0	70.7	82.5	88.4	93.4	60	152.4	34.0	39.5	45.8	58.0	70.3	76.6	82.1
66	167.6	49.9	54.9	60.8	72.6	84.4	90.2	95.2	61	154.9	35.8	41.3	47.6	59.9	72.1	79.4	83.9
67	170.2	52.1	57.1	63.0	74.8	86.6	92.5	97.5	62	157.5	37.6	43.1	49.4	61.7	73.9	80.3	85.7
68	172.7	54.4	59.4	65.3	77.1	88.9	94.8	99.8	63	160.0	39.0	44.4	50.8	63.0	75.3	81.6	87.1
69	175.3	56.2	61.2	67.1	78.9	90.7	96.6	101.6	64	162.6	40.4	45.8	52.2	64.4	76.6	83.0	88.4
70	177.8	58.5	63.5	69.4	81.2	93.0	98.9	103.9	65	165.1	42.2	47.6	54.0	66.2	78.5	84.8	90.2
71	180.3	60.8	65.8	71.7	83.4	95.2	101.1	106.1	66	167.6	44.0	49.4	55.8	68.0	80.3	86.6	92.1
72	182.9	63.0	68.0	73.9	85.7	97.5	103.4	108.4	67	170.2	45.4	50.8	57.1	69.4	81.6	88.0	93.4
73	185.4	65.3	70.3	76.2	88.0	99.8	105.7	110.7	68	172.7	47.2	52.6	59.0	71.2	83.4	89.8	95.2
74	188.0	67.6	72.6	78.5	90.2	102.0	107.9	112.9									

Height		Males (35–44 yr)						Height		Females (35–44 yr)					
in	cm	5	10	20	50	80	90	95	in	cm	5	10	20	50	80	90	95
62	157.5	44.4	49.0	54.4	64.8	75.3	80.7	85.3	57	144.8	30.4	36.3	43.5	56.7	69.8	77.1	83.0
63	160.0	46.7	51.2	56.7	67.1	77.5	83.0	87.5	58	147.3	32.2	38.1	45.4	58.5	71.7	78.9	84.8
64	162.6	49.0	53.5	58.9	69.4	79.8	85.3	89.8	59	149.9	34.0	39.9	47.2	60.3	73.5	80.7	86.6
65	165.1	51.2	55.8	61.2	71.7	82.1	87.5	92.1	60	152.4	35.8	41.7	49.0	62.1	75.3	82.5	88.4
66	167.6	53.5	58.0	63.5	73.9	84.4	89.8	94.3	61	154.9	37.6	43.5	50.8	63.9	77.1	84.4	90.2
67	170.2	56.2	60.8	66.2	76.6	87.1	92.5	97.1	62	157.5	39.0	44.9	52.2	65.3	78.5	85.7	91.6
68	172.7	58.5	63.0	68.5	78.9	89.3	94.8	99.3	63	160.0	40.8	46.7	54.0	67.1	80.3	87.5	93.4
69	175.3	60.8	65.3	70.7	81.2	91.6	97.1	101.6	64	162.6	42.6	48.5	55.8	68.9	82.1	89.3	95.2
70	177.8	63.0	67.6	73.0	83.4	93.9	96.1	103.9	65	165.1	44.4	50.3	57.6	70.7	83.9	91.2	97.1
71	180.3	65.8	70.3	75.7	86.2	96.6	102.0	106.6	66	167.6	45.8	51.7	59.0	72.1	85.3	92.5	98.4
72	182.9	67.6	72.1	77.6	88.0	98.4	103.9	108.4	67	170.2	47.6	71.7	60.8	73.9	87.1	94.3	100.2
73	185.4	70.3	74.8	80.3	90.7	101.1	106.6	111.1	68	172.7	49.4	55.3	62.6	75.7	88.9	96.1	102.0
74	188.0	72.6	77.1	82.5	93.0	103.4	108.8	113.4									

Table 4.3: Weight percentiles by height and age data for U.S. adults aged eighteen to forty-four years, derived from the NHANES I survey (1971–1974) and compiled by Abraham et al. (1979).

Height		Males (45–54 yr)							Height		Females (45–54 yr)						
in	cm	5	10	20	50	80	90	95	in	cm	5	10	20	50	80	90	95
62	157.5	45.4	50.3	55.8	66.7	77.6	83.0	88.0	57	144.8	33.1	39.0	45.8	58.5	71.2	78.0	83.9
63	160.0	47.6	52.6	58.0	68.9	79.8	85.3	90.2	58	147.3	34.9	40.8	47.6	60.3	73.0	79.8	85.7
64	162.6	49.4	54.4	59.9	70.7	81.6	87.1	92.1	59	149.9	36.3	42.2	49.0	61.7	74.4	81.2	87.1
65	165.1	51.2	56.2	61.7	72.6	83.4	88.9	93.9	60	152.4	38.1	44.0	50.8	63.5	76.2	83.0	88.9
66	167.6	53.1	58.0	63.5	74.4	85.3	90.7	95.7	61	154.9	39.5	45.4	52.2	64.9	77.6	84.4	90.2
67	170.2	55.3	60.3	65.8	76.6	87.5	93.0	98.0	62	157.5	41.3	47.2	54.0	66.7	79.4	86.2	92.1
68	172.7	57.1	62.1	67.6	78.5	89.3	94.8	99.8	63	160.0	42.6	48.5	55.3	68.0	80.7	87.5	93.4
69	175.3	59.0	63.9	69.4	80.3	91.2	96.6	101.6	64	162.6	44.4	49.9	57.1	69.8	82.5	89.3	95.2
70	177.8	61.2	66.2	71.7	82.5	93.4	98.9	103.9	65	165.1	46.3	52.2	59.0	71.7	84.4	91.2	97.1
71	180.3	63.5	68.5	73.9	84.8	95.7	101.1	106.1	66	167.6	47.6	53.5	60.3	73.0	85.7	92.5	98.4
72	182.9	65.3	70.3	75.7	86.6	97.5	102.9	107.9	67	170.2	49.4	55.3	62.1	74.8	87.5	94.3	100.2
73	185.4	67.6	72.6	78.6	88.9	99.8	105.2	110.2	68	172.7	50.8	56.7	63.5	76.2	88.9	95.7	101.6
74	188.0	69.4	74.4	79.8	90.7	101.6	107.0	112.0									

Height		Males (55–64 yr)							Height		Females (55–64 yr)						
in	cm	5	10	20	50	80	90	95	in	cm	5	10	20	50	80	90	95
62	157.5	43.5	48.1	54.0	64.9	75.7	81.6	86.2	57	144.8	34.9	40.4	47.2	59.9	72.6	79.4	84.8
63	160.0	45.4	49.9	55.8	66.7	77.6	83.4	88.0	58	147.3	36.7	42.2	49.0	61.7	74.4	81.2	86.6
64	162.6	48.1	52.6	58.5	69.4	80.3	86.2	90.7	59	149.9	38.5	44.0	50.8	63.5	76.2	83.0	88.4
65	165.1	50.3	54.9	60.8	71.7	82.5	88.4	93.0	60	152.4	39.9	45.4	52.2	64.9	77.6	84.4	89.8
66	167.6	52.6	57.1	63.0	73.9	84.8	90.7	95.2	61	154.9	41.7	47.2	54.0	66.7	79.4	86.2	91.6
67	170.2	54.9	59.4	65.3	76.2	87.1	93.0	97.5	62	157.5	43.1	48.5	55.3	68.0	80.7	87.5	93.0
68	172.7	57.1	61.7	67.6	78.5	89.3	95.2	99.8	63	160.0	44.4	49.9	56.7	69.4	82.1	88.9	94.3
69	175.3	59.4	63.9	69.8	80.7	91.6	97.5	102.0	64	162.6	46.3	51.7	58.5	71.2	83.9	90.7	96.1
70	177.8	61.7	66.2	72.1	83.0	93.9	99.8	104.3	65	165.1	47.6	53.1	59.9	72.6	85.3	92.1	97.5
71	180.3	64.4	68.9	74.8	85.7	96.6	102.5	107.0	66	167.6	49.4	54.9	61.7	74.4	87.1	93.9	99.3
72	182.9	66.2	70.7	76.6	87.5	98.4	104.3	108.8	67	170.2	50.8	56.2	63.0	75.7	88.4	95.2	100.7
73	185.4	68.0	72.6	78.5	89.3	100.2	106.1	110.7	68	172.7	52.6	58.0	64.9	77.6	90.2	97.1	102.5
74	188.0	70.7	75.3	81.2	92.1	102.9	108.8	113.4									

Height		Males (55–64 yr)							Height		Females (55–64 yr)						
in	cm	5	10	20	50	80	90	95	in	cm	5	10	20	50	80	90	95
62	157.5	45.3	49.9	54.9	64.8	74.8	79.8	84.4	57	144.8	37.2	42.2	48.1	59.0	69.8	75.7	80.7
63	160.0	47.2	51.7	56.7	66.7	76.6	81.6	86.2	58	147.3	39.0	44.0	49.9	60.8	71.7	77.6	82.5
64	162.6	49.0	53.5	58.5	68.5	78.5	83.4	88.0	59	149.9	40.4	45.4	51.2	62.1	73.0	78.9	83.9
65	165.1	51.2	55.8	60.8	70.7	80.7	85.7	90.2	60	152.4	41.7	46.7	52.6	63.5	74.4	80.3	85.3
66	167.6	53.1	57.6	62.6	72.6	82.5	87.5	92.1	61	154.9	43.5	43.5	54.4	65.3	76.2	82.1	87.1
67	170.2	54.9	59.4	64.4	74.4	84.4	89.3	93.9	62	157.5	44.9	49.9	55.8	66.7	77.6	83.4	88.4
68	172.7	57.1	61.7	66.7	76.6	86.6	91.6	96.1	63	160.0	46.7	51.7	57.6	68.5	79.4	85.3	90.2
69	175.3	59.0	63.5	68.5	78.5	88.4	93.4	98.0	64	162.6	48.1	53.1	59.0	69.8	80.7	86.6	91.6
70	177.8	60.8	65.3	70.3	80.3	90.2	95.2	99.8	65	165.1	49.9	54.9	60.8	71.7	82.5	88.4	93.4
71	180.3	63.0	67.6	72.6	82.5	92.5	97.5	102.0	66	167.6	51.2	56.2	62.1	73.0	83.9	89.8	94.8
72	182.9	64.9	69.4	74.4	84.4	94.3	99.3	103.0	67	170.2	53.1	58.0	63.9	74.8	85.7	91.6	96.6
73	185.4	66.7	71.2	76.2	86.2	96.1	101.1	105.7	68	172.7	54.9	59.9	65.8	76.6	87.5	93.4	98.4
74	188.0	68.5	73.0	78.0	88.0	98.0	102.9	107.5									

Table 4.4: Weight percentiles by height and age data for U.S. adults aged forty-five to seventy-four years, derived from the NHANES I survey (1971–1974) and compiled by Abraham et al. (1979).

Height in	cm	Male subjects 25–54 yr old (small frame) 5	10	20	50	80	90	95	Height in	cm	Female subjects 25–54 yr old (small frame) 5	10	20	50	80	90	95
62	157	46	50	52	64	71	74	77	58	147	37	43	43	52	58	62	66
63	160	48	51	53	61	70	75	79	59	150	42	43	44	53	63	69	72
64	163	49	53	55	66	76	76	80	60	152	42	44	45	53	63	65	70
65	165	52	53	58	66	77	81	84	61	155	44	46	47	54	64	66	72
66	168	56	57	59	67	78	83	84	62	157	44	47	48	55	63	64	70
67	170	56	60	62	71	82	83	88	63	160	46	48	49	55	65	68	79
68	173	56	59	62	71	79	82	85	64	163	49	50	51	57	67	68	74
69	175	57	62	65	74	84	87	88	65	165	50	52	53	60	70	72	80
70	178	59	62	67	75	87	86	90	66	168	46	49	54	58	65	71	74
71	180	60	64	70	76	79	88	91	67	170	47	50	52	59	70	72	76
72	183	62	65	67	74	87	89	93	68	173	48	51	53	62	71	73	77
73	185	63	67	69	79	89	91	94	69	175	49	52	54	63	72	74	78
74	188	65	68	71	80	90	92	96	70	178	50	53	55	64	73	75	79

Height in	cm	Male subjects 25–54 yr old (medium frame) 5	10	20	50	80	90	95	Height in	cm	Female subjects 25–54 yr old (medium frame) 5	10	20	50	80	90	95
62	157	51	55	58	68	81	83	87	58	147	41	46	50	63	77	75	79
63	160	52	56	59	71	82	85	89	59	150	47	50	52	66	76	79	85
64	163	54	60	61	71	83	84	90	60	152	47	50	52	60	77	79	85
65	165	59	62	65	74	87	90	94	61	155	47	49	51	61	73	78	86
66	168	58	61	65	75	85	87	93	62	157	49	50	52	61	73	77	83
67	170	62	66	68	77	89	93	100	63	160	49	51	53	62	77	80	88
68	173	60	64	66	78	89	92	97	64	163	50	52	54	62	76	82	87
69	175	63	66	68	78	90	93	97	65	165	52	54	55	63	75	80	89
70	178	64	66	70	81	90	93	97	66	168	52	54	55	63	75	78	83
71	180	62	68	70	81	92	96	100	67	170	54	56	57	65	79	82	88
72	183	68	71	74	84	97	100	104	68	173	58	59	60	67	77	85	87
73	185	70	72	75	85	100	101	104	69	175	49	58	60	68	79	82	87
74	188	68	76	77	88	100	100	104	70	178	50	54	57	70	80	83	87

Height in	cm	Male subjects 25–54 yr old (large frame) 5	10	20	50	80	90	95	Height in	cm	Female subjects 25–54 yr old (large frame) 5	10	20	50	80	90	95
62	157	57	62	66	82	99	103	108	58	147	56	63	67	86	105	110	117
63	160	58	63	67	83	100	104	109	59	150	56	62	67	78	105	109	116
64	163	59	64	68	84	101	105	110	60	152	55	62	66	87	104	109	116
65	165	60	65	69	79	102	106	111	61	155	54	64	66	81	105	117	115
66	168	60	65	75	84	103	106	112	62	157	59	61	65	81	103	107	113
67	170	62	70	71	84	102	111	113	63	160	58	63	67	83	105	109	119
68	173	63	74	76	86	101	104	114	64	163	59	62	63	79	102	104	112
69	175	68	71	74	89	103	105	114	65	165	59	61	63	81	103	109	114
70	178	68	72	74	87	106	112	114	66	168	55	58	62	75	95	100	107
71	180	73	78	82	91	113	116	123	67	170	58	60	65	80	100	108	114
72	183	73	76	78	91	109	112	121	68	173	51	66	66	76	104	105	111
73	185	72	77	79	93	106	107	116	69	175	50	57	68	79	105	104	111
74	188	69	74	82	92	105	115	120	70	178	50	56	61	76	99	104	110

Table 4.5: Percentiles for weight by frame size and height for U.S. adults aged twenty-five to fifty-four years old. Data are from the NHANES I (1971–1974) and NHANES II (1976–1980) surveys. From Frisancho (1984). © Am. J. Clin. Nutr. American Society for Clinical Nutrition.

Height		Male subjects 55–74 yr old (small frame)							Height		Female subjects 55–74 yr old (small frame)						
in	cm	5	10	20	50	80	90	95	in	cm	5	10	20	50	80	90	95
62	157	45	49	56	61	68	73	77	58	147	39	46	48	54	63	65	71
63	160	47	49	51	62	71	71	79	59	150	41	45	48	55	66	68	74
64	163	47	50	54	63	72	74	80	60	152	43	45	47	54	67	70	73
65	165	48	54	59	70	80	90	90	61	155	43	43	45	56	65	70	71
66	168	51	55	59	68	77	80	84	62	157	47	49	52	58	67	69	73
67	170	55	60	61	69	79	81	88	63	160	42	45	49	58	67	68	74
68	173	54	54	58	70	79	81	86	64	163	43	47	49	60	68	70	75
69	175	56	59	63	75	81	84	88	65	165	43	47	49	60	69	72	75
70	178	57	61	63	76	83	86	89	66	168	44	48	50	68	70	72	76
71	180	59	62	65	69	85	87	91	67	170	45	48	51	61	71	73	77
72	183	60	64	66	76	86	89	92	68	173	45	49	51	61	71	74	77
73	185	62	65	69	78	88	90	94	69	175	46	49	52	62	72	74	78
74	188	63	67	69	77	89	92	95	70	178	47	50	52	63	73	75	79

Height		Male subjects 55–74 yr old (medium frame)							Height		Female subjects 55–74 yr old (medium frame)						
in	cm	5	10	20	50	80	90	95	in	cm	5	10	20	50	80	90	95
62	157	50	54	59	68	77	81	85	58	147	40	44	49	57	72	82	85
63	160	51	57	60	70	80	82	87	59	150	47	49	52	62	74	78	86
64	163	55	59	62	71	82	83	91	60	152	47	50	52	65	76	79	86
65	165	56	60	64	72	83	86	89	61	155	49	51	54	64	78	81	86
66	168	57	62	66	74	83	84	89	62	157	49	53	54	64	78	82	88
67	170	59	64	66	78	87	89	94	63	160	52	54	55	65	79	83	89
68	173	62	66	68	78	88	89	101	64	163	51	54	57	66	78	81	87
69	175	62	66	68	77	90	93	99	65	165	54	56	59	67	78	84	88
70	178	62	68	71	80	90	95	101	66	168	54	57	57	66	79	85	88
71	180	68	70	72	84	94	97	101	67	170	51	59	61	72	82	85	89
72	183	66	65	69	81	96	97	101	68	173	52	56	59	70	83	86	90
73	185	68	72	79	88	93	99	103	69	175	53	57	60	72	84	87	91
74	188	69	73	76	95	98	101	104	70	178	54	58	61	73	85	88	92

Height		Male subjects 55–74 yr old (large frame)							Height		Female subjects 55–74 yr old (large frame)						
in	cm	5	10	20	50	80	90	95	in	cm	5	10	20	50	80	90	95
62	157	54	59	63	77	91	95	100	58	147	53	59	63	92	95	99	104
63	160	55	60	64	80	92	96	101	59	150	54	59	63	78	95	99	105
64	163	57	62	65	77	94	97	102	60	152	54	65	69	78	87	88	105
65	165	58	63	73	79	89	98	103	61	155	64	68	69	79	94	95	106
66	168	59	67	73	80	101	102	105	62	157	59	61	63	82	93	101	111
67	170	65	71	73	85	103	108	112	63	160	61	65	67	80	100	102	118
68	173	67	71	73	83	95	98	111	64	163	60	65	67	77	97	102	119
69	175	65	70	74	84	96	98	105	65	165	60	66	69	80	98	102	111
70	178	68	73	77	87	102	104	117	66	168	57	60	63	82	98	105	109
71	180	65	70	70	84	102	109	111	67	170	58	64	68	80	105	104	109
72	183	67	76	81	90	108	112	112	68	173	58	64	68	79	100	104	110
73	185	68	73	76	88	105	108	113	69	175	59	65	69	85	101	105	110
74	188	69	74	78	89	106	109	114	70	178	60	65	69	85	101	105	111

Table 4.6: Percentiles for weight by frame size and height for U.S. adults aged fifty-five to seventy-four years old. Data are from the NHANES I (1971–1974) and NHANES II (1976–1980) surveys. From Frisancho (1984). © Am. J. Clin. Nutr. American Society for Clinical Nutrition.

Age (years)	Male subjects							Female subjects						
	5	10	25	50	75	90	95	5	10	25	50	75	90	95
0.0–0.5	4.4	4.8	6.2	7.2	8.2	9.7	10.9	4.1	4.3	5.8	6.5	7.1	8.6	11.0
0.5–1.0	7.6	7.8	8.7	9.9	10.6	11.8	12.3	7.3	7.7	8.5	9.1	10.1	11.0	11.7
1.0–1.5	8.5	9.3	9.6	10.3	11.3	12.6	13.5	8.7	9.0	10.0	10.4	11.0	11.9	12.0
1.5–2.0	10.6	11.0	11.6	12.2	13.2	13.9	15.1	9.4	9.4	10.7	11.8	12.4	13.0	13.0
2.0–2.5	11.0	11.3	11.9	12.7	13.2	14.0	14.2	10.4	11.1	11.6	11.9	12.9	13.2	14.4
3	12.8	13.2	13.8	14.5	15.8	17.0	17.8	10.7	11.1	12.0	13.8	15.8	16.2	17.4
4	13.5	14.4	15.2	16.8	18.2	19.7	22.5	13.9	14.4	15.2	16.2	17.4	18.4	19.7
5	14.9	15.2	17.2	18.5	21.1	22.9	23.8	15.0	15.8	16.3	17.3	19.8	22.3	22.5
6	17.1	17.5	18.7	20.2	22.5	24.5	25.3	16.5	17.7	19.4	20.1	22.3	23.9	26.4
7	18.5	18.8	20.7	21.9	24.4	26.0	27.3	16.8	17.0	18.5	20.0	23.5	26.4	27.1
8	20.4	21.4	23.3	24.9	27.5	32.5	35.8	18.8	19.8	22.9	24.8	29.0	30.8	31.1
9	19.1	19.8	23.8	28.3	35.5	39.8	43.0	21.4	23.2	25.5	28.0	30.2	35.5	37.1
10	25.6	26.4	27.3	30.4	33.3	39.5	44.9	24.1	24.5	27.8	31.0	38.7	44.1	44.2
11	27.2	27.6	30.4	33.0	38.0	45.1	45.1	26.8	28.7	31.2	36.2	40.8	48.7	55.7
12	29.7	31.2	33.0	37.6	44.2	51.1	54.8	27.0	31.2	34.7	40.3	44.9	54.1	59.5
13	32.1	33.0	36.9	43.8	49.5	53.8	58.6	34.1	36.0	40.4	45.1	52.7	60.1	62.8
14	34.7	37.4	42.4	46.2	54.8	58.7	63.2	33.5	36.5	41.4	47.0	51.7	59.5	64.1
15	41.2	42.9	48.9	54.7	58.8	63.4	67.5	41.0	42.7	47.8	50.8	53.8	62.8	67.2
16	43.9	48.4	51.6	59.2	69.0	81.2	81.2	43.7	46.7	49.7	52.5	57.0	65.6	71.4
17	46.5	49.6	56.2	60.6	74.8	80.9	82.2	42.0	43.5	49.0	52.0	56.1	63.2	65.6
18	48.3	48.3	58.0	62.4	69.0	77.6	80.1	38.3	41.7	48.5	55.9	60.0	68.3	74.2
19	53.5	56.0	59.6	69.3	75.6	78.8	97.5	45.4	47.8	49.0	52.0	56.6	65.6	67.6
20–29	56.2	57.7	62.0	71.5	78.7	91.9	102.1	42.0	46.0	50.9	58.2	65.8	73.2	82.1
30–39	54.0	59.8	65.4	74.6	81.6	88.8	96.6	44.8	47.4	52.0	58.1	63.1	72.3	83.9
40–49	57.3	60.4	67.3	74.4	83.3	90.3	92.3	46.2	47.6	53.8	59.9	68.9	77.2	82.6
50–59	55.3	59.0	65.1	74.2	82.2	88.0	93.8	47.3	50.4	56.4	63.4	72.7	84.0	90.3
60–69	49.7	57.9	63.6	72.5	82.1	88.1	92.1	44.4	55.1	57.3	62.9	72.4	79.3	86.5
70+	52.4	56.6	60.6	68.7	77.6	84.7	89.1	43.7	48.3	58.0	63.8	72.0	76.3	79.9

Table 4.7: Percentiles for weight (kg) of Canadians by age. Data are from Nutrition Canada (1980) Anthropometry Report—Height, Weight and Body Dimensions. Bureau of Nutritional Sciences, Health Protection Branch, Health and Welfare, Ottawa. Reproduced with permission of the Minister of Supply and Services Canada.

Height (cm)	'Ideal' Weights (kg) for Females			'Ideal' Weights (kg) for Males		
	Small Frame	Medium Frame	Large Frame	Small Frame	Medium Frame	Large Frame
148	46.4–50.6	49.6–55.1	53.7–59.8			
149	46.6–51.0	50.0–55.5	54.1–60.3			
150	46.7–51.3	50.3–55.9	54.4–60.9			
151	46.9–51.7	50.7–56.4	54.8–61.4			
152	47.1–52.1	51.1–57.0	55.2–61.9			
153	47.4–52.5	51.5–57.5	55.6–62.4			
154	47.8–53.0	51.9–58.0	56.2–63.0			
155	48.1–53.6	52.2–58.6	56.8–63.6			
156	48.5–54.1	52.7–59.1	57.3–64.1			
157	48.8–54.6	53.2–59.6	57.8–64.6			
158	49.3–55.2	53.8–60.2	58.4–65.3	58.3–61.0	59.6–64.2	62.8–68.3
159	49.8–55.7	54.3–60.7	58.9–66.0	58.6–61.3	59.9–64.5	63.1–68.8
160	50.3–56.2	54.9–61.2	59.4–66.7	59.0–61.7	60.3–64.9	63.5–69.4
161	50.8–56.7	55.4–61.7	59.9–67.4	59.3–62.0	60.6–65.2	63.8–69.9
162	51.4–57.3	55.9–62.3	60.5–68.1	59.7–62.4	61.0–65.6	64.2–70.5
163	51.9–57.8	56.4–62.8	61.0–68.8	60.0–62.7	61.3–66.0	64.5–71.1
164	52.5–58.4	57.0–63.4	61.5–69.5	60.4–63.1	61.7–66.5	64.9–71.8
165	53.0–58.9	57.5–63.9	62.0–70.2	60.8–63.5	62.1–67.0	65.3–72.5
166	53.6–59.5	58.1–64.5	62.6–70.9	61.1–63.8	62.4–67.6	65.6–73.2
167	54.1–60.0	58.7–65.0	63.2–71.7	61.5–64.2	62.8–68.2	66.0–74.0
168	54.6–60.5	59.2–65.5	63.7–72.4	61.8–64.6	63.2–68.7	66.4–74.7
169	55.2–61.1	59.7–66.1	64.3–73.1	62.2–65.2	63.8–69.3	67.0–75.4
170	55.7–61.6	60.2–66.6	64.8–73.8	62.5–65.7	64.3–69.8	67.5–76.1
171	56.2–62.1	60.7–67.1	65.3–74.5	62.9–66.2	64.8–70.3	68.0–76.8
172	56.8–62.6	61.3–67.6	65.8–75.2	63.2–66.7	65.4–70.8	68.5–77.5
173	57.3–63.2	61.8–68.2	66.4–75.9	63.6–67.3	65.9–71.4	69.1–78.2
174	57.8–63.7	62.3–68.7	66.9–76.4	63.9–67.8	66.4–71.9	69.6–78.9
175	58.3–64.2	62.8–69.2	67.4–76.9	64.3–68.3	66.9–72.4	70.1–79.6
176	58.9–64.8	63.4–69.8	68.0–77.5	64.7–68.9	67.5–73.0	70.7–80.3
177	59.5–65.4	64.0–70.4	68.5–78.1	65.0–69.5	68.1–73.5	71.3–81.0
178	60.0–65.9	64.5–70.9	69.0–78.6	65.4–70.0	68.6–74.0	71.8–81.8
179	60.5–66.4	65.1–71.4	69.6–79.1	65.7–70.5	69.2–74.6	72.3–82.5
180	61.0–66.9	65.6–71.9	70.1–79.6	66.1–71.0	69.7–75.1	72.8–83.3
181	61.6–67.5	66.1–72.5	70.7–80.2	66.6–71.6	70.2–75.8	73.4–84.0
182	62.1–68.0	66.6–73.0	71.2–80.7	67.1–72.1	70.7–76.5	73.9–84.7
183				67.7–72.7	71.3–77.2	74.5–85.4
184				68.2–73.4	71.8–77.9	75.2–86.1
185				68.7–74.1	72.4–78.6	75.9–86.8
186				69.2–74.8	73.0–79.3	76.6–87.6
187				69.8–75.5	73.7–80.0	77.3–88.5
188				70.3–76.2	74.4–80.7	78.0–89.4
189				70.9–76.9	74.9–81.5	78.7–90.3
190				71.4–77.6	75.4–82.2	79.4–91.2
191				72.1–78.4	76.1–83.0	80.3–92.1
192				72.8–79.1	76.8–83.9	81.2–93.0
193				73.5–79.8	77.6–84.8	82.1–93.9

Table 4.8: 'Ideal' weights for U.S. adults according to frame size at ages twenty-five to fifty-nine years based on lowest mortality. Weight in kilograms in indoor clothing weighing 1.4 kg (male) and 2.3 kg (female). Heights include 2.5-cm heels. Data from the 1979 Build Study, Society of Actuaries and Association of Life Insurance Medical Directors of America, 1980. From Metropolitan Height and Weight Tables (1983). Courtesy Statistical Bulletin, Metropolitan Life Insurance Company.

4.3 Recumbent length and stature

Principle

Recumbent length and stature in relation to age, are used as indices of chronic nutritional status of children and adults. They are particularly valuable in children as indices of 'stunting' of a child's full growth potential. Stunting is a slowing of skeletal growth and of stature, defined by Waterlow (1978) as "the end result of a reduced rate of linear growth". The condition results from extended periods of inadequate food intake and increased morbidity and is generally found in countries where economic conditions are poor. The prevalence of stunting, unlike wasting, is highest during the second or third year of life. The influence of possible genetic and ethnic differences must also be considered when evaluating recumbent length and stature for age. When weight is combined with recumbent length and stature, it provides a sensitive index of current nutritional status which is relatively independent of age between one and ten years.

Procedures for infants and children

For infants, and children less than two years of age, recumbent length should be measured with a measuring board. Two examiners are required to correctly position the subject and to ensure accurate and reliable measurements of length.

1. Place the subject, face upward, with the head at the fixed end of the board and the body parallel to its long axis (Fig. 4.5). The shoulders should rest against the surface of the board.

2. Apply gentle traction to bring the crown of the child's head into contact with the fixed headboard and simultaneously position the head so that it is in the the Frankfurt plane (examiner 1).

3. Hold the subject's feet, without shoes, toes pointing directly upward, while keeping the subject's knees straight (Fig. 4.5), and bring the movable footboard to rest against the heels (examiner 2).

4. Record the length to the nearest millimeter.

5. Calculate the percentage of the median with the reference data cited below, using the appropriate age, sex, and length.

$$\% \text{ Median} = \frac{100 \times \text{observed length}}{\text{median length for age}}$$

6. Determine in which percentile range the subject's length falls, using the same reference data.

If the subject is restless, only the left leg should be positioned for the measurement. For field use, a portable infant length measuring scale can be used. This device is assembled from four separate plastic sections which lock together to form head and foot plates, with a strong, two-meter metal tape insert.

Procedures for older children and adults

Children over two years of age and adults are generally measured in the standing position using a stadiometer or portable anthropometer. A plastic instrument called the Accustat stadiometer is also available, which is less expensive than the conventional stadiometer for measuring stature (Roche et al., 1988). Alternatively, some form of right-angle headboard and a measuring rod or nonstretchable tape fixed to a vertical surface can be used. In the field, vertical surfaces are not always available. In such circumstances,

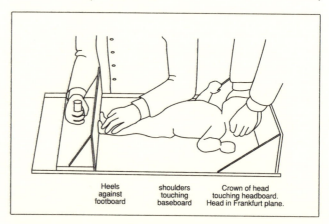

Fig. 4.5: Measurement of recumbent length. Modified from Robbins GE, Trowbridge FL. In: Nutrition Assessment: A Comprehensive Guide for Planning Intervention by M.D. Simko, C. Cowell, and J.A. Gilbride, p.75, with permission of Aspen Publishers, Inc., © 1984.

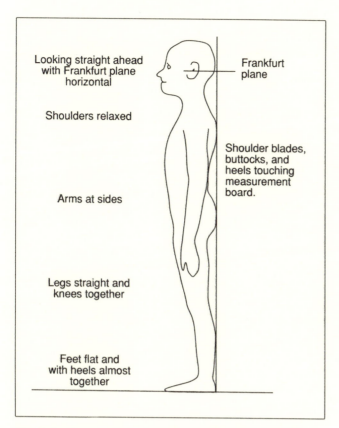

Looking straight ahead with Frankfurt plane horizontal

Frankfurt plane

Shoulders relaxed

Shoulder blades, buttocks, and heels touching measurement board.

Arms at sides

Legs straight and knees together

Feet flat and with heels almost together

Fig. 4.6: Positioning of subject for height measurement. Horizontal line is the Frankfurt plane, which should be in a horizontal position when height is measured. Modified from Robbins GE, Trowbridge FL. In: Nutrition Assessment: A Comprehensive Guide for Planning Intervention by M.D. Simko, C. Cowell, and J.A. Gilbride, p.77, with permission of Aspen Publishers, Inc., © 1984.

modified tape measures such as the Microtoise, which measure up to two meters, can be used (Cameron, 1986). Platform scales with movable measuring rods are not suitable. Clothing should be minimal when measuring height so that posture can be clearly seen. Shoes and socks should not be worn.

1. Ask the subject to stand straight with the head in the Frankfurt plane (Fig. 4.6), feet together, knees straight, and heels, buttocks, and shoulder blades in contact with the vertical surface of the stadiometer, anthropometer, or wall.

2. Make sure that the subject's arms are hanging loosely at the sides with palms facing the thighs; the head is not necessarily in contact with the vertical surface. For younger subjects, it may be necessary to hold the heels to ensure they do not leave the ground.

3. Ask the subject to take a deep breath and stand tall to aid the straightening of the spine. Shoulders should be relaxed.

4. Lower the movable headboard until it touches the crown of the head.

5. Take the height measurement at maximum inspiration, with the examiner's eyes level with the headboard to avoid parallax errors.

6. Record the time of day and the height to the nearest millimeter. If the reading falls between two values, the lower reading is always recorded. Successive measurements should agree within five millimeters (Lohman et al., 1988).

7. Calculate the percentage of the median with the NHANES (Table 4.9) or Canadian (Table 4.10) reference data cited below, using the appropriate age, sex, and height

$$\% \text{ Median} = \frac{100 \times \text{observed height}}{\text{median height for age}}$$

8. Determine in which percentile range the subject's length falls, using the same reference data.

The time at which the measurement is made should be noted because diurnal variations in height occur. In cases where large amounts of adipose tissue prevent the heels, buttocks, and shoulders from simultaneously touching the wall, subjects should simply be asked to stand erect (Chumlea et al., 1984).

When the Microtoise tape is used, it is first placed on the floor. The tape is then pulled out to its fullest extent, released, and the end fixed with a nail to a door or doorway. An anthropometrist should then position the subject's head correctly in the Frankfurt plane, before the tape is lowered by a second person until the headboard touches the crown of the head. A direct reading of height to the nearest millimeter is obtained.

Evaluation

Height percentiles by age for U.S. males and females aged one to seventy-four years, compiled by Frisancho (1990) from the NHANES I (1971–74) and the NHANES II (1976–80) surveys conducted by the NCHS. are given in Table 4.9. Percentiles for stature (cm) of Canadians by age are given in Table 4.10. Data are from Nutrition

Age (yr)	Percentiles of stature (cm) by age							Percentiles of stature (cm) by age						
	5	10	25	50	75	90	95	5	10	25	50	75	90	95
	Male subjects							Female subjects						
1.0–1.9	75.5	76.7	79.3	82.1	85.6	88.0	89.8	73.2	74.7	77.4	80.5	83.6	86.8	88.6
2.0–2.9	84.9	86.3	88.4	91.4	94.4	96.9	98.0	83.1	84.9	86.8	90.1	93.0	95.7	97.4
3.0–3.9	91.6	93.7	96.1	98.7	102.0	104.9	107.0	90.3	92.1	94.8	97.5	100.6	103.4	105.0
4.0–4.9	98.1	99.5	102.7	106.1	109.3	112.3	114.1	97.0	98.5	101.6	104.9	108.3	111.2	113.6
5.0–5.9	103.9	105.9	109.3	112.7	115.7	119.2	121.2	103.1	105.3	108.6	111.9	115.4	119.0	120.6
6.0–6.9	109.4	112.0	115.7	119.4	122.8	126.0	127.7	109.9	111.4	114.2	118.5	122.2	125.2	127.6
7.0–7.9	115.6	118.2	121.5	125.4	128.5	131.6	133.5	115.3	117.0	120.3	124.3	128.4	131.7	134.5
8.0–8.9	120.0	122.6	125.9	130.1	133.7	137.5	140.0	120.1	122.1	125.5	129.7	133.5	137.8	140.1
9.0–9.9	126.0	128.7	131.4	135.8	139.9	143.0	145.0	125.7	127.5	130.5	135.6	140.4	143.9	147.2
10.0–10.9	130.2	132.3	136.1	140.9	145.8	150.1	152.7	129.5	132.2	136.3	141.6	146.0	150.9	154.4
11.0–11.9	134.3	136.6	141.6	146.4	151.5	155.0	158.1	134.7	138.1	142.3	148.4	153.4	158.0	162.1
12.0–12.9	139.7	141.9	146.4	151.4	157.9	162.3	166.0	143.0	145.2	149.6	154.6	159.3	164.0	165.5
13.0–13.9	145.1	147.8	152.8	159.3	165.6	170.7	173.2	149.1	151.1	155.1	158.8	162.8	165.7	168.3
14.0–14.9	153.3	156.3	161.7	166.9	172.8	178.2	179.9	151.0	153.0	156.8	160.8	164.9	168.8	171.7
15.0–15.9	158.5	161.5	165.6	171.2	176.2	179.8	182.5	152.8	155.2	158.8	162.7	167.2	172.0	175.4
16.0–16.9	163.4	165.0	169.8	174.1	178.7	183.8	186.7	151.4	153.6	157.7	162.3	166.4	171.6	173.2
17.0–17.9	164.4	166.9	170.7	175.1	180.5	184.5	187.3	153.2	155.5	159.2	162.3	166.4	169.9	172.8
18.0–24.9	165.4	167.8	171.9	176.6	181.5	185.7	188.0	152.3	154.8	158.8	163.1	167.1	171.0	173.6
25.0–29.9	165.1	167.8	172.0	176.2	181.5	184.8	188.0	152.6	155.2	158.6	162.8	167.1	170.9	173.3
30.0–34.9	164.8	167.4	171.5	176.2	180.9	184.8	187.2	152.9	155.2	158.4	162.4	166.8	171.2	173.1
35.0–39.9	164.0	166.8	171.9	176.1	181.0	185.0	187.7	152.0	155.0	158.6	162.7	167.0	171.0	173.5
40.0–44.9	165.0	167.2	171.4	176.0	180.3	184.2	186.9	151.6	154.3	158.1	162.7	166.7	170.5	173.2
45.0–49.9	163.8	166.5	170.6	174.8	180.2	184.5	186.6	151.7	154.0	157.9	162.0	166.3	169.9	172.2
50.0–54.9	164.2	166.4	170.1	174.6	178.8	183.2	185.3	151.3	153.8	156.9	161.1	165.1	169.2	171.0
55.0–59.9	163.2	165.0	169.3	173.8	178.7	182.3	184.6	149.8	152.7	156.7	160.3	164.4	167.8	170.1
60.0–64.9	161.9	165.0	168.7	173.0	177.4	181.3	183.7	149.2	151.4	155.6	160.0	163.7	167.3	169.8
65.0–69.9	159.7	162.9	166.7	171.6	176.3	180.1	182.5	148.5	150.7	154.8	158.8	162.6	166.2	168.1
70.0–74.9	159.5	162.0	165.8	170.7	175.0	179.4	182.0	147.2	150.0	153.7	157.4	161.5	165.5	167.5

Table 4.9: Percentiles of stature (cm) by age for males and females of one to seventy-four years. Data are from the U.S. NHANES I (1971–74) and NHANES II (1976–80) surveys and were compiled by Frisancho (1990).

Canada (1980), collected between October 1970 and October 1972.

References

Cameron N (1986). The methods of auxological anthropometry. In: Falkner F, Tanner J M (eds). Human Growth. A Comprehensive Treatise. Volume 3. Methodology, Ecological, Genetic, and Nutritional Effects on Growth. Plenum Press, New York, pp. 3–46.

Chumlea W C, Roche A F, Mukherjee D (1984). Nutritional Assessment of the Elderly through Anthropometry. Ross Laboratories, Columbus, Ohio.

Frisancho A R (1990). Anthropometric Standards for the Assessment of Growth and Nutritional Status. The University of Michigan Press, Ann Arbor.

Lohman T G, Roche A F, Martorell R (eds) (1988). Anthropometric Standardization Manual. Human Kinetics Books, Champagne, Illinois.

Nutrition Canada (1980). Anthropometry Report: Height, Weight and Body Dimensions. Bureau of Nutritional Sciences, Health Protection Branch, Health and Welfare, Ottawa.

Robbins G E, Trowbridge F L (1984). Anthropometric techniques and their application. In: Simko M D, Cowell C, Gilbride J A (eds). Nutrition Assessment. Aspen Systems Corporation, Rockville, Maryland, pp. 69–92.

Roche A F, Guo S, Baumgartner R N, Falls R A (1988). The measurement of stature. American Journal of Clinical Nutrition 47: 922.

Waterlow J C (1978). Observations on the assessment of protein-energy malnutrition with special reference to stunting. Extrait Courrier 28: 455–460.

Age (years)	Male subjects							Female subjects						
	5	10	25	50	75	90	95	5	10	25	50	75	90	95
0.0–0.5	56.5	56.5	61.2	65.2	67.1	70.0	78.9	52.5	56.0	60.1	62.0	63.5	65.5	67.5
0.5–1.0	64.8	68.3	69.6	73.4	76.4	78.5	79.4	65.4	67.0	69.5	73.0	75.0	78.3	78.3
1.0–1.5	71.4	72.9	74.9	77.9	80.8	82.8	86.5	71.5	74.1	76.6	78.6	79.9	82.8	86.2
1.5–2.0	80.4	82.7	83.5	83.9	85.3	87.8	91.9	70.7	75.7	81.3	83.4	86.5	86.6	87.1
2.0–2.5	83.0	84.2	85.8	88.2	90.1	90.7	91.6	81.4	81.8	83.5	87.7	88.4	91.2	92.7
3	88.6	90.4	93.3	95.2	97.5	100.4	103.9	84.7	86.0	90.1	94.0	96.5	99.7	100.7
4	92.7	94.4	98.5	101.9	105.0	108.6	112.1	94.5	95.6	99.7	102.3	104.5	106.8	108.3
5	98.7	102.0	104.8	107.4	113.0	114.6	115.6	101.4	102.5	103.0	105.5	111.2	114.1	117.6
6	101.7	105.4	110.3	115.5	117.9	121.3	121.4	104.5	107.7	111.4	114.4	116.3	118.7	119.9
7	111.8	113.6	114.2	118.5	122.7	125.6	126.8	104.6	108.0	113.3	116.0	121.3	125.3	126.6
8	116.5	119.2	121.9	126.6	131.0	132.0	134.3	114.2	117.3	120.7	125.6	128.8	134.4	136.4
9	115.6	117.9	125.3	130.8	140.1	143.4	145.7	120.0	122.9	127.5	130.3	132.6	136.0	140.9
10	123.8	129.0	132.7	137.1	139.6	144.8	148.5	129.3	130.6	133.9	137.6	141.7	142.7	146.5
11	128.6	131.3	136.2	139.0	145.5	147.6	149.3	130.0	132.4	139.2	142.9	148.2	151.2	153.5
12	135.9	136.7	142.8	147.8	152.6	159.2	166.1	135.5	137.3	141.3	145.5	153.9	158.6	161.8
13	140.0	141.3	147.6	151.9	160.8	163.3	164.4	145.1	146.4	151.1	154.4	160.4	163.7	166.7
14	146.9	147.8	151.4	158.9	164.5	172.0	174.1	147.4	148.2	152.3	157.1	160.5	165.3	168.2
15	151.8	152.4	161.4	165.9	171.5	173.8	175.5	150.9	154.2	154.9	158.8	161.0	165.7	167.7
16	157.9	161.1	165.5	172.3	176.0	179.0	180.0	149.7	152.5	155.9	160.5	164.4	169.2	171.2
17	160.3	162.8	167.0	173.4	178.2	182.4	185.4	153.2	153.3	156.0	159.9	162.9	164.9	166.9
18	160.8	163.3	166.2	171.1	178.1	180.9	184.3	146.0	153.2	157.1	159.8	165.6	167.4	167.5
19	164.3	165.5	168.7	173.1	180.8	183.7	183.7	149.0	155.0	156.3	160.7	163.0	163.9	167.9
20–29	163.7	165.3	170.5	174.7	178.9	183.8	189.6	150.9	153.0	157.1	160.3	165.4	169.2	170.9
30–39	161.8	164.9	168.0	172.9	178.1	182.7	184.6	149.2	150.9	155.5	160.4	164.5	167.7	170.2
40–49	160.2	162.6	167.6	171.9	176.4	181.1	184.5	149.6	151.9	154.8	159.1	163.8	168.7	169.5
50–59	161.2	162.3	166.8	171.8	175.9	179.8	182.0	148.6	150.0	155.3	159.1	163.9	167.8	171.9
60–69	158.9	160.3	164.5	168.3	172.6	176.3	178.1	147.3	149.4	152.9	156.0	160.9	165.4	166.7
70+	157.0	159.9	163.0	167.6	171.0	174.2	176.9	144.0	146.3	149.9	155.2	158.7	162.5	164.1

Table 4.10: Percentiles for stature (cm) of Canadians by age. Data are from Nutrition Canada (1980). Anthropometry Report—Height, Weight and Body Dimensions. Bureau of Nutritional Sciences, Health Protection Branch, Health and Welfare, Ottawa. Reproduced with permission of the Minister of Supply and Services Canada.

4.4 Weight changes

Principle

Alterations in body weight may reflect a change in protein, water, minerals, and/or body fat content. In healthy persons, daily variations in body weight are generally small (i.e. less than $\pm 0.5\,\text{kg}$). In conditions of acute or chronic illness, however, negative energy-nitrogen balance may occur as the body uses endogenous sources of energy (including protein) as fuel for metabolic reactions. Consequently, body weight declines. In conditions of total starvation, the maximal weight loss is approximately 30% of the initial body weight, at which point death occurs. In chronic semistarvation, body weight may decrease to approximately 50% to 60% of ideal weight. When persistent positive energy balance occurs, there is an accumulation of adipose tissue, and body weight increases.

Procedure

1. Measure the actual weight of the subject using the appropriate procedures outlined in Section 4.2.
2. Record the usual weight of the subject.
3. Calculate the parameters:

$$\text{percentage usual weight} = \frac{W_A}{W_U} \times 100\%$$

$$\text{percentage weight loss} = \frac{W_U - W_A}{W_U} \times 100\%$$

$$\text{rate of change(kg/day)} = \frac{W_A - W_U}{\text{Day}_n - \text{Day}_1}$$

Where W_A and W_U represent actual and usual body weights measured in kilograms on Day_n and Day_1 respectively.

4. Evaluate the percentage weight loss using the guidelines of Blackburn et al. (1977) (Table 4.11).

Evaluation

In general, absolute body weight can only be used to assess the severity of protein-energy malnutrition in patients with relatively uncomplicated, nonedematous forms of semistarvation (Heymsfield et al., 1984). In disease conditions in which edema, ascites, dehydration, diuresis, massive tumor growth, or organomegaly occur, or in obese patients undergoing rapid weight loss, body weight is a poor measure of body energy-nitrogen reserves. In such conditions, a relative increase in total body water, for example, may mask actual weight loss associated with changes in fat and skeletal muscle. Hence, one should make additional anthropometric measurements (e.g. skinfold thickness and mid-upper-arm circumference) to ascertain where the change in body weight occurred (Heymsfield et al., 1984).

Time	Significant Weight Loss (%)	Severe Weight Loss (%)
1 week	1–2	> 2
1 month	5	> 5
3 months	7.5	> 7.5
6 months	10	> 10

Table 4.11: Evaluation of percentage weight changes. From GL Blackburn, BR Bistrain, BS Maini, HT Schlamm, MF Smith. Nutritional and metabolic assessment of the hospitalized patient. Journal of Parenteral and Enteral Nutrition 1: 11–22. © by Am. Soc. for Parenteral and Enteral Nutrition (1977).

References

Heymsfield SB, McManus CB, Seitz SB, Nixon DW, Smith Andrews J (1984). Anthropometric assessment of adult protein-energy malnutrition. In: Wright RA, Heymsfield S (eds), Nutrition Assessment. Blackwell Scientific Publications, Boston, pp. 27–82.

Blackburn GL, Bistrain BR, Maini BS, Schlamm HT, Smith MF (1977). Nutritional and metabolic assessment of the hospitalized patient. Journal of Parenteral and Enteral Nutrition 1: 11–22.

4.5 Weight/height ratios

Principle

Weight/height ratios are frequently called obesity or body mass indices. They measure body weight corrected for height, but cannot distinguish between excessive weight produced by adiposity, muscularity, or edema. Body mass indices are generally power-type indices which express weight relative to a power function of height, or height relative to some power function of weight (Billewicz et al., 1962). The numerical values of these indices depend on the units of measurement employed (e.g. meters and kilograms or inches and pounds).

Procedure

1. Calculate the power-type weight/height ratios:

   - weight/height

   - Quetelet's index: $wt/(ht)^2$ (meters and kilograms)

   - Ponderal index: $ht/\sqrt[3]{wt}$ (inches and pounds)

2. Calculate the percentage of the median for Quetelet's index with the NHANES reference data (Table 4.13), using the appropriate sex, age, and median weight.

$$\% \text{ Median} = \frac{100 \times \text{observed weight}}{\text{median weight for age and sex}}$$

3. Determine in which percentile range the subject's Quetelet's index falls, again using the NHANES reference data.

Evaluation

Obesity may be underestimated in short persons when they are assessed by the weight/height ratio (Billewicz et al., 1962), but overestimated by the Ponderal index because the latter has only a moderate correlation with weight and is also markedly biased by height (Goldbourt and Medalie, 1974). Some confusion may arise in the interpretation of the Ponderal index because it is negatively correlated with weight and so decreases with increasing obesity. For example, the risk

categories developed for Nutrition Canada (in inches and pounds) were: below 12.5—high risk for obesity; 12.5 and above—low risk for obesity (Nutrition Canada, 1980).

Many investigators consider Quetelet's index to be the best body mass index for most adult population groups, as it is the least biased by height and easily calculated (Garrow and Webster, 1985; Health and Welfare Canada, 1988a), although in children it is apparently more dependent on stature (Garn et al., 1986). Furthermore, in adults, Quetelet's index correlates with many health-related indices such as the mortality risk (Waaler, 1984). Factors such as diet, smoking, and levels of physical activity confound this latter relationship. Hence the range of acceptable values for Quetelet's index varies among countries.

Percentiles for the body mass index by age for U.S. males and females aged one to seventy-four years old are given in Table 4.13. Data are from the NHANES I (1971–1974) and NHANES II (1976–1980) surveys and were compiled by Frisancho (1990).

Health and Welfare Canada have adopted the term 'Body Mass Index' (BMI) for Quetelet's index. The classification (in meters and kilograms) used for this index by Health and Welfare Canada (1988a) is given in Table 4.12

Body Mass Index	Evaluation
Under 20	May be associated with health problems for some individuals.
20–25	'Ideal' index range associated with the lowest risk of illness for most people.
25–27	May be associated with health problems for some people.
Over 27	Associated with increased risk of health problems such as heart disease, high blood pressure, and diabetes.

Table 4.12: Classifications used for the Body Mass Index by Health and Welfare Canada (1988a).

Age (yr)	Percentiles of body mass index by age							Percentiles of body mass index by age						
	5	10	25	50	75	90	95	5	10	25	50	75	90	95
	Male subjects							Female subjects						
1.0–1.9	15.2	15.6	16.4	17.1	18.0	19.0	19.6	14.4	14.9	15.7	16.7	17.6	18.6	19.3
2.0–2.9	14.3	14.6	15.4	16.2	17.1	17.8	18.4	14.1	14.4	15.1	15.9	16.8	17.8	18.4
3.0–3.9	14.2	14.6	15.1	15.8	16.6	17.5	18.2	13.6	14.1	14.7	15.5	16.4	17.5	18.0
4.0–4.9	13.9	14.2	14.9	15.6	16.4	17.2	17.8	13.6	13.9	14.6	15.3	16.2	17.2	18.0
5.0–5.9	13.8	14.1	14.7	15.5	16.3	17.2	18.1	13.3	13.7	14.5	15.2	16.3	17.5	18.6
6.0–6.9	13.7	14.1	14.8	15.3	16.4	18.0	19.3	13.5	13.7	14.3	15.2	16.2	17.5	18.7
7.0–7.9	13.7	14.1	14.9	15.6	16.7	18.2	19.5	13.7	14.1	14.7	15.4	16.8	18.3	19.6
8.0–8.9	13.8	14.3	15.0	15.9	17.1	19.1	20.1	13.8	14.1	14.9	15.8	17.4	19.8	21.7
9.0–9.9	14.1	14.6	15.3	16.3	17.7	19.9	21.8	14.0	14.6	15.3	16.5	18.1	21.5	23.3
10.0–10.9	14.6	15.0	15.8	17.1	18.7	21.2	23.4	14.0	14.5	15.6	16.9	18.9	22.0	24.1
11.0–11.9	14.7	15.1	16.2	17.4	19.8	22.5	25.3	14.8	15.3	16.3	18.1	20.3	23.4	26.2
12.0–12.9	15.2	15.7	16.7	17.9	20.2	23.7	25.8	15.0	15.6	17.0	18.9	21.2	24.6	27.0
13.0–13.9	15.6	16.4	17.2	18.7	20.7	24.0	25.9	15.4	16.3	17.7	19.4	22.2	25.2	28.6
14.0–14.9	16.5	17.0	18.1	19.5	21.6	24.2	26.4	16.5	17.1	18.4	20.3	22.8	26.2	28.9
15.0–15.9	16.8	17.5	19.0	20.4	22.0	24.1	26.6	17.0	17.5	18.8	20.3	22.4	25.6	28.7
16.0–16.9	18.0	18.5	19.6	21.3	23.0	25.9	27.3	17.7	18.3	19.3	21.1	23.5	26.8	30.1
17.0–17.9	17.8	18.4	19.5	21.1	23.4	26.1	28.3	17.1	17.9	19.6	21.4	24.0	27.5	32.1
18.0–24.9	18.8	19.6	21.0	23.0	25.5	28.5	31.0	17.7	18.4	19.9	21.8	24.5	28.6	32.1
25.0–29.9	19.5	20.4	21.9	24.3	27.0	30.0	32.8	18.0	18.8	20.1	22.3	25.6	30.8	34.3
30.0–34.9	19.9	21.0	23.0	25.1	27.8	30.5	32.9	18.5	19.4	20.8	23.1	27.2	33.0	36.6
35.0–39.9	19.7	21.0	23.3	25.6	28.0	30.6	32.8	18.7	19.5	21.3	23.8	28.0	33.1	36.9
40.0–44.9	20.4	21.5	23.4	26.0	28.5	31.0	32.5	18.8	19.8	21.5	24.2	28.3	33.7	36.6
45.0–49.9	20.1	21.5	23.5	26.0	28.6	31.2	33.4	19.0	20.1	21.9	24.5	28.6	33.4	37.1
50.0–54.9	19.9	21.1	23.3	25.9	28.2	31.3	33.3	19.2	20.3	22.4	25.9	29.2	33.8	36.5
55.0–59.9	19.8	21.3	23.5	26.1	28.5	31.6	33.6	19.2	20.5	22.8	25.7	30.1	34.7	38.2
60.0–64.9	20.1	21.3	23.4	25.6	28.0	30.4	32.4	19.3	20.7	22.9	25.8	29.7	33.8	36.6
65.0–69.9	19.1	20.5	22.7	25.5	27.8	30.7	32.3	19.5	20.7	23.0	26.0	29.6	33.8	36.6
70.0–74.9	19.0	20.3	22.6	25.1	27.7	30.5	32.3	19.3	20.5	23.0	26.0	29.5	33.1	35.8

Table 4.13: Percentiles of body mass index (wt/ht^2) by age for males and females of one to seventy-four years. Data are from the NHANES I and NHANES II surveys and were compiled by Frisancho (1990).

In the survey of heights and weights of adults in Great Britain, values for Quetelet's index of < 20 were regarded as indicative of underweight, > 25 indicative of overweight, and > 30 as obese (Office of Population Censuses and Surveys, 1984).

Quetelet's index is not a valid index for children, for those under twenty years, for adults over sixty-five, or for pregnant and lactating women (Health and Welfare Canada, 1988b). Note that Quetelet's index should not be used as an index of body fatness in individuals with a grossly abnormal relationship between leg and trunk length.

References

BillewiczWZ, Kemsley WFF, ThomsonAM (1962). Indices of adiposity. British Journal of Preventive and Social Medicine 16: 183–188.

FrisanchoAR (1990). Anthropometric Standards for the Assessment of Growth and Nutritional Status. The University of Michigan Press, Ann Arbor.

Garn S M, Leonard W R, Hawthorne V M (1986). Three limitations of the body mass index. American Journal of Clinical Nutrition 44: 996–997.

GarrowJS, WebsterJ (1985). Quetelet's index (W/H^2) as a measure of fatness. International Journal of Obesity 9: 147–153.

Goldbourt U, MedalieJ (1974). Weight height indices. British Journal of Preventive and Social Medicine 28: 110–112.

Health and Welfare Canada (1988a). Promoting Healthy Weights: a discussion paper. Health Services and Promotion Branch, Health and Welfare, Ottawa.

Health and Welfare Canada (1988b). Canadian Guidelines for Healthy Weights. Report of an Expert Committee convened by Health Promotion Directorate, Health Services and Promotion Branch, Health and Welfare, Ottawa.

Nutrition Canada (1980). Anthropometry Report: Height, Weight and Body Dimensions. Bureau of Nutritional Sciences, Health Protection Branch, Health and Welfare, Ottawa.

Office of Population Censuses and Surveys, Social Survey Division (1984). The heights and weights of adults in Great Britain. Knight I. (ed): Report of a survey carried out on behalf of the Department of Health and Social Security covering adults aged 16–64 years. Her Majesty's Stationery Office, London.

Waaler H Th (1984). Height, weight, and mortality. The Norwegian experience. Acta Medica Scandinavica, Supplement No. 679.

4.6 Knee height

Principle

Knee height is highly correlated with stature, and may be used to estimate height in persons with severe spinal curvature or who are unable to stand. Knee height is measured with a caliper consisting of an adjustable measuring stick with a blade attached to each end at a 90° angle (Lohman et al., 1988).

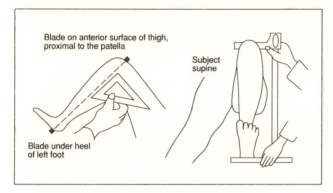

Blade on anterior surface of thigh, proximal to the patella

Subject supine

Blade under heel of left foot

Fig. 4.7: Measurement of knee height

Procedure

1. Gently bend the left leg of the subject at the knee to a 90° angle, while the subject is in the supine position.
2. Take the caliper and position one of the blades under the heel of the left foot.

3. Place the other over the anterior surface of the left thigh above the condyles of the femur and just proximal to the patella (Fig. 4.7).
4. Hold the shaft of the caliper parallel to the shaft of the tibia and apply gentle pressure to the blades of the caliper.
5. Make at least two successive measurements which should agree within five millimeters (Chumlea et al., 1985).
6. Use the appropriate formula or a nomogram (Fig. 4.8) to estimate stature in males (MS) and females (FS) from knee height (KH) (Chumlea et al., 1984).

$$MS = (2.02 \times KH\,(cm)) - (0.04 \times age\,(yr)) + 64.19$$
$$FS = (1.83 \times KH\,(cm)) - (0.24 \times age\,(yr)) + 84.88$$

References

Chumlea W C, Roche A F, Mukherjee D (1984). Nutritional Assessment of the Elderly through Anthropometry. Ross Laboratories, Columbus, Ohio.

Chumlea W C, Roche A F, Steinbaugh M L (1985). Estimating stature from knee height for persons 60 to 90 years of age. Journal of the American Geriatrics Society 33: 116–120.

Lohman T G, Roche A F, Martorell R. (eds) (1988). Anthropometric Standardization Manual. Human Kinetics Books, Champagne, Illinois.

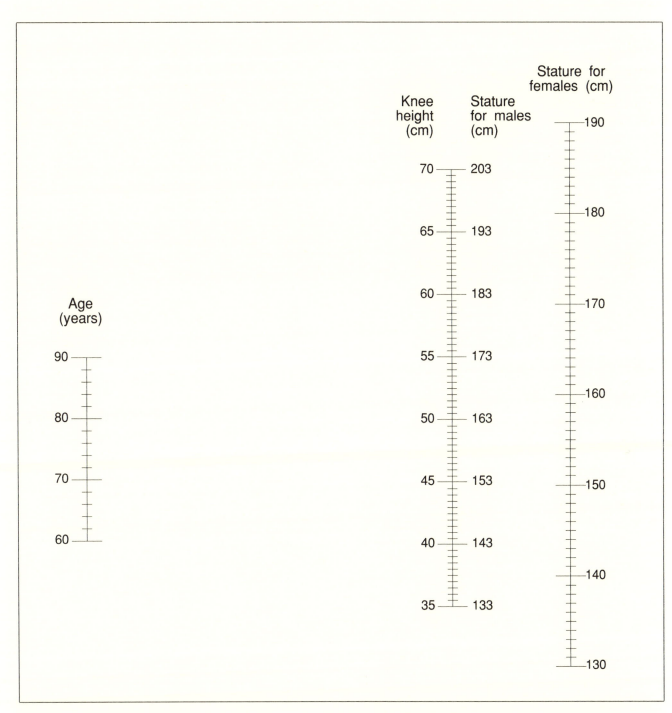

Fig. 4.8: Nomogram to estimate stature from knee height. To use the diagram, locate the person's age on the column furthest to the left, and the knee height on the next column. Then lay a rule or straightedge so that it touches these two points. The estimated stature is indicated at the intersection of the straightedge and the stature column for the appropriate sex. Reproduced with permission of Ross Laboratories, Columbus, OH 43216. From Nutritional Assessment of the Elderly through Anthropometry. Figure 9, page 11, © 1984 Ross Laboratories.

4.7 Elbow breadth

Principle

Elbow breadth measures skeletal breadth, and thus frame size independently of adiposity and age (Frisancho and Flegal, 1983). Elbow breadth is measured as the distance between the epicondyles of the humerus using a sliding caliper (Fig. 4.9) or Frameter (Lohman et al., 1988).

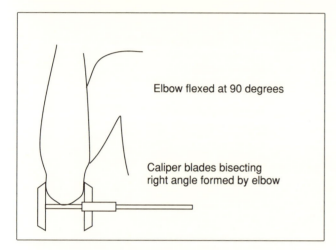

Fig. 4.9: Measurement of elbow breadth

Procedure

1. Stand in front of the subject and raise the subject's right arm forwards, to the horizontal. Then flex the subject's elbow to 90°, with the back of the hand facing the measurer.

2. Locate the lateral and medial epicondyles of the humerus.

3. Apply the blades of a flat-bladed sliding caliper to the epicondyles, with the blades pointing upwards to bisect the right angle formed at the elbow. Care must be taken to ensure that the caliper is held at a slight angle to the epicondyles and that firm pressure is exerted to minimize the influence of soft tissue on the measurement.

4. Record the measurement to the nearest millimeter.

5. Assess whether the subject has a small, medium or large frame size using the NHANES I data given in Table 4.14.

6. Determine, using the NHANES reference data (Table 4.15), in which percentile range the subject's elbow breadth falls.

Evaluation

Frame size by elbow breadth of U.S. black and Caucasian adults is given in Table 4.14. Data are from the NHANES I survey (1971–1974) and compiled by Frisancho and Flegel (1983). The frame size categories—small, medium and large—correspond to below the 15th, between the 15th

| Age (yr) | Frame Size | | |
	Small	Medium	Large
Caucasian males			
18–24	≤6.7	>6.7, <7.5	≥7.5
25–34	≤6.7	>6.7, <7.5	≥7.5
35–44	≤6.9	>6.9, <7.6	≥7.6
45–54	≤6.9	>6.9, <7.7	≥7.7
55–64	≤6.9	>6.9, <7.7	≥7.7
65–74	≤6.9	>6.9, <7.7	≥7.7
Caucasian females			
18–24	≤5.7	>5.7, <6.4	≥6.4
25–34	≤5.8	>5.8, <6.5	≥6.5
35–44	≤5.9	>5.9, <6.6	≥6.6
45–54	≤5.9	>5.9, <6.8	≥6.8
55–64	≤6.0	>6.0, <6.9	≥6.9
65–74	≤6.0	>6.0, <6.9	≥6.9
Black males			
18–24	≤6.7	>6.7, <7.6	≥7.6
25–34	≤6.8	>6.8, <7.6	≥7.6
35–44	≤6.7	>6.7, <7.7	≥7.7
45–54	≤6.9	>6.9, <7.9	≥7.9
55–64	≤6.9	>6.9, <7.9	≥7.9
65–74	≤6.9	>6.9, <7.8	≥7.8
Black females			
18–24	≤5.8	>5.8, <6.6	≥6.6
25–34	≤5.8	>5.8, <6.7	≥6.7
35–44	≤6.0	>6.0, <7.0	≥7.0
45–54	≤6.0	>6.0, <7.1	≥7.1
55–64	≤6.1	>6.1, <7.2	≥7.2
65–74	≤6.1	>6.1, <7.0	≥7.0

Table 4.14: Frame size as derived from elbow breadth measurements of United States black and Caucasian adults. Data from the NHANES I survey (1971–1974). Adapted from Frisancho and Flegel (1983). © Am. J. Clin. Nutr. American Society for Clinical Nutrition.

Age (yr)	Percentiles of elbow breadth (mm) by age							Percentiles of elbow breadth (mm) by age						
	5	10	25	50	75	90	95	5	10	25	50	75	90	95
	Male subjects							Female subjects						
1.0–1.9	36.0	37.0	39.0	40.0	42.0	44.0	45.0	34.0	35.0	37.0	39.0	41.0	42.0	43.0
2.0–2.9	38.0	39.0	41.0	42.0	44.0	46.0	47.0	36.0	37.0	39.0	41.0	42.0	44.0	45.0
3.0–3.9	40.0	41.0	43.0	44.0	46.0	48.0	50.0	38.0	39.0	41.0	42.0	44.0	46.0	47.0
4.0–4.9	42.0	43.0	44.0	46.0	48.0	50.0	52.0	40.0	41.0	42.0	44.0	46.0	48.0	49.0
5.0–5.9	43.0	44.0	46.0	48.0	50.0	52.0	53.0	42.0	43.0	44.0	46.0	48.0	50.0	52.0
6.0–6.9	45.0	46.0	48.0	51.0	52.0	55.0	56.0	43.0	44.0	46.0	48.0	50.0	52.0	53.0
7.0–7.9	47.0	48.0	49.0	52.0	54.0	56.0	57.0	45.0	46.0	48.0	50.0	52.0	54.0	55.0
8.0–8.9	48.0	49.0	51.0	54.0	56.0	59.0	60.0	46.0	47.0	49.0	51.0	54.0	56.0	58.0
9.0–9.9	50.0	51.0	53.0	56.0	58.0	61.0	62.0	48.0	50.0	51.0	54.0	56.0	59.0	60.0
10.0–10.9	52.0	53.0	55.0	58.0	61.0	64.0	65.0	50.0	51.0	53.0	56.0	58.0	61.0	62.0
11.0–11.9	53.0	55.0	57.0	60.0	62.0	65.0	67.0	52.0	53.0	55.0	58.0	60.0	63.0	64.0
12.0–12.9	55.0	57.0	60.0	63.0	66.0	69.0	72.0	53.0	55.0	57.0	59.0	62.0	64.0	66.0
13.0–13.9	58.0	60.0	62.0	66.0	69.0	72.0	74.0	54.0	56.0	58.0	60.0	62.0	65.0	66.0
14.0–14.9	61.0	63.0	66.0	68.0	71.0	74.0	76.0	54.0	56.0	58.0	60.0	63.0	65.0	66.0
15.0–15.9	63.0	64.0	67.0	70.0	72.0	75.0	77.0	54.0	56.0	58.0	61.0	63.0	66.0	67.0
16.0–16.9	64.0	66.0	68.0	71.0	73.0	76.0	77.0	55.0	56.0	59.0	61.0	64.0	66.0	67.0
17.0–17.9	64.0	66.0	68.0	71.0	73.0	76.0	77.0	55.0	56.0	59.0	61.0	64.0	66.0	68.0
18.0–24.9	64.0	66.0	69.0	71.0	74.0	76.0	78.0	55.0	56.0	59.0	61.0	63.0	66.0	67.0
25.0–29.9	65.0	67.0	69.0	71.0	74.0	77.0	79.0	56.0	57.0	59.0	61.0	64.0	66.0	68.0
30.0–34.9	65.0	67.0	69.0	72.0	74.0	77.0	79.0	56.0	57.0	59.0	62.0	64.0	67.0	70.0
35.0–39.9	65.0	67.0	70.0	72.0	75.0	77.0	80.0	56.0	58.0	60.0	62.0	65.0	68.0	71.0
40.0–44.9	66.0	68.0	70.0	73.0	75.0	78.0	80.0	57.0	58.0	60.0	63.0	66.0	69.0	71.0
45.0–49.9	66.0	68.0	70.0	73.0	76.0	79.0	80.0	57.0	59.0	61.0	63.0	66.0	69.0	72.0
50.0–54.9	66.0	68.0	71.0	73.0	76.0	78.0	80.0	57.0	59.0	61.0	64.0	67.0	70.0	73.0
55.0–59.9	67.0	68.0	71.0	73.0	77.0	80.0	81.0	58.0	59.0	61.0	64.0	67.0	71.0	73.0
60.0–64.9	67.0	68.0	71.0	73.0	76.0	79.0	81.0	58.0	60.0	62.0	64.0	67.0	70.0	72.0
65.0–69.9	66.0	68.0	70.0	73.0	76.0	79.0	81.0	58.0	59.0	62.0	64.0	67.0	71.0	73.0
70.0–74.9	67.0	68.0	71.0	73.0	76.0	79.0	81.0	58.0	60.0	62.0	64.0	68.0	71.0	72.0

Table 4.15: Percentiles of elbow breadth (mm) by age for males and females of one to seventy-four years. Data are from the NHANES I and NHANES II surveys and were compiled by Frisancho (1990).

and the 85th, and above the 85th sex- and age-specific percentiles of elbow breadth.

Percentiles of elbow breadth (mm) by age for U.S. males and females aged one to seventy four years are given in Table 4.15. Data are from the NHANES I (1971–1974) and NHANES II (1974–1980) surveys and were compiled by Frisancho (1990).

References

Frisancho A R (1990). Anthropometric Standards for the Assessment of Growth and Nutritional Status. The University of Michigan Press, Ann Arbor.

Frisancho A R, Flegel P N (1983). Elbow breadth as a measure of frame size for United States males and females. American Journal of Clinical Nutrition 37: 311–314.

Lohman T G, Roche A F, Martorell R (eds) (1988). Anthropometric Standardization Manual. Human Kinetics Books, Champagne, Illinois.

4.8　Frame index 2

Principle

Frame index 2 is derived from measurements of elbow breadth, height, and age. It is used as an alternative indicator of frame size which takes into account age-related changes in weight and height (Frisancho, 1990).

Procedure

1. Calculate Frame Index 2

$$\text{Frame Index 2} = \frac{\text{elbow breadth (mm)}}{\text{stature (cm)} \times 100}$$

2. Assess whether the subject has a small, medium or large frame size using the NHANES data given in Table 4.16

Evaluation

Classification of small, medium, and large frame size based on the Frame Index 2 for males and females by age are given in Table 4.16. Data are from the NHANES I (1971–1974) and NHANES II (1976–1980) surveys and were compiled by Frisancho (1990). The small, medium, and large frame sizes correspond to below the 25th, between the 25th to the 75th, and above the 75th percentiles of age and sex-specific Frame Index 2 values.

Age (yr)	Small	Medium	Large
Males			
18.0–24.9	<38.4	38.4–41.6	>41.6
25.0–29.9	<38.6	38.6–41.8	>41.8
30.0–34.9	<38.6	38.6–42.1	>42.1
35.0–39.9	<39.1	39.1–42.4	>42.4
40.0–44.9	<39.3	39.3–42.5	>42.5
45.0–45.9	<39.6	39.6–43.8	>43.8
50.0–54.9	<39.9	39.9–43.3	>43.3
55.0–59.9	<40.2	40.2–43.8	>43.8
60.0–64.9	<40.2	40.2–43.6	>43.6
65.0–69.9	<40.2	40.2–43.6	>43.6
70.0–74.9	<40.2	40.2–43.6	>43.6
Females			
18.0–24.9	<35.2	35.2–38.6	>38.6
25.0–29.9	<35.7	35.7–38.7	>38.7
30.0–34.9	<35.7	35.7–39.0	>39.0
35.0–39.9	<36.2	36.2–39.8	>39.8
40.0–44.9	<36.7	36.7–40.2	>40.2
45.0–45.9	<36.7	37.2–40.7	>40.7
50.0–54.9	<37.2	37.2–41.6	>41.6
55.0–59.9	<37.8	37.8–41.9	>41.9
60.0–64.9	<38.2	38.2–41.8	>41.8
65.0–69.9	<38.2	38.2–41.8	>41.8
70.0–74.9	<38.2	38.2–41.8	>41.8

Table 4.16: Classification of small, medium, and large frame size for males and females derived from Frame Index 2 by age. Data are from the NHANES I (1971–1974) and NHANES II (1976–1980) surveys and were compiled by Frisancho (1990).

References

Frisancho A R (1990). Anthropometric Standards for the Assessment of Growth and Nutritional Status. The University of Michigan Press, Ann Arbor.

Chapter 5
Assessment of fat-free mass

Contents

Introduction

Most anthropometric methods used to assess body composition are based on a model in which the body consists of two chemically distinct compartments: fat and fat-free mass. Anthropometric techniques can indirectly assess these two body compartments, and variations in their amount and proportion can be used as indices of nutritional status (Lohman, 1991).

The fat-free mass consists of the skeletal muscle, nonskeletal muscle and soft lean tissues, and the skeleton. The fat-free mass is estimated to have a density of $1.100 \, \text{g/cm}^3$ and a water content of 73.8% in reference man (Brŏzek et al., 1963). Body muscle is composed largely of protein. Hence, the assessment of body muscle can provide an index of the protein reserves of the body; these reserves become depleted during chronic under-nutrition, resulting in muscle wasting.

Mid-upper-arm muscle circumference and mid-upper-arm muscle area are both correlated with measures of total muscle mass and are therefore used to predict changes in total body muscle mass

and hence protein nutritional status. Unfortunately, the ratios of mid-upper-arm muscle circumference/area to fat-free mass are not constant, but change with age and certain disease states (Heymsfield and McManus, 1985). As a result, these anthropometric indices do not provide accurate measures of changes in body protein and cannot be used to detect small changes.

Arm muscle circumference and arm muscle area are both derived from the mid-upper-arm circumference and triceps skinfold measurements taken on the left arm. These indices can be used in clinical settings to identify hospital patients with chronic under- or over-nutrition, and to monitor long-term changes in body composition during nutritional support. They can also be used in public health to identify individuals who are vulnerable to under-nutrition, and also to evaluate the effectiveness of nutrition intervention programs designed to improve the proportion or amount of the fat-free mass.

References

Heymsfield S B, McManus C B (1985). Tissue components of weight loss in cancer patients. Cancer 55: 238–249.

Brŏzek J, Grande F, Anderson J T, Keys A (1963). Densitometric analysis of body compositions: Revisions of some quantitative assumptions. Annals of the New York Academy of Sciences 110: 113–140.

Lohman T G (1991). Anthropometric assessment of fat-free body mass. In: Himes J H (ed.) Anthropometric Assessment of Nutritional Status, Wiley-Liss Inc., New York, 173–183.

5.1 Mid-upper-arm circumference

Principle

The arm contains subcutaneous fat and muscle; a decrease in mid-upper-arm circumference may therefore reflect either a reduction in muscle mass, a reduction in subcutaneous tissue, or both. In less industrialized countries, where the amount of subcutaneous fat is frequently small, changes in mid-upper-arm circumference tend to parallel changes in muscle mass and hence are particularly useful in the diagnosis of protein-energy malnutrition or starvation. Changes in mid-upper-arm circumference measurements can also be used to monitor progress during nutritional therapy (Hofvander and Eksmyr, 1969), correlating positively with changes in weight. Arm circumference changes are easy to detect and require a minimal amount of time and equipment (Gurney and Jelliffe, 1973). Some investigators claim that mid-upper-arm circumference can differentiate normal children from those with protein-energy malnutrition as reliably as weight for age (Shakir and Morley, 1974).

Mid-upper-arm circumference measurements should be made taken a flexible, nonstretch tape made of fiberglass or steel; alternatively, a fiberglass insertion tape can be used (Fig. 5.1) (Lohman et al., 1988).

Procedure

1. Ask the subject to stand erect and sideways to the measurer, with the head in the Frankfurt plane, arms relaxed and legs apart. If the subject is wearing a sleeved garment, it should be removed or the sleeves rolled up.

2. Locate and mark the measurement point at the midpoint of the upper left arm, i.e. midway between the acromion process and the tip of the olecranon (Fig. 6.1).

3. Extend the left arm of the subject so that it is hanging loosely by the side, with the palm facing inwards.

4. Wrap the tape gently but firmly around the arm at the midpoint, care being taken to ensure that the arm is not squeezed (Fig. 5.1)

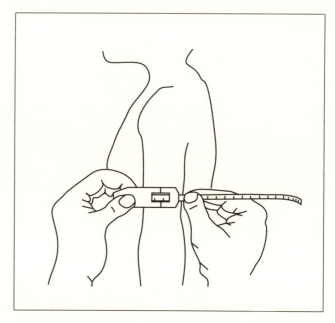

Fig. 5.1: Measurement of mid-upper-arm circumference

5. Take the measurement to the nearest millimeter.

6. Calculate the percentage of the median with the reference data cited below, using the appropriate age, sex, and median mid-upper-arm circumference.

$$\% \text{ Median} = \frac{100 \times \text{observed arm circ.}}{\text{median arm circ. for age and sex}}$$

7. Determine in which percentile range the subject's mid-upper-arm circumference falls using the same reference data.

If necessary, mid-upper-arm circumference can be measured with subjects in the recumbent position. In this case, a sandbag is placed under the elbow to raise the arm slightly off the surface of the bed (Chumlea et al., 1984). Precision of mid-upper-arm circumference measurements, both within and between trained examiners, can be high, even if the subjects are obese.

Evaluation

The percentiles for mid-upper-arm circumference (mm) for U.S. persons aged one to seventy-four years old are given in Table 5.1 Data are from the

Age (yrs)	Male subjects							Female subjects						
	5	10	25	50	75	90	95	5	10	25	50	75	90	95
1.0–1.9	142	147	152	160	169	177	182	136	141	148	157	164	172	178
2.0–2.9	143	148	155	163	171	179	186	142	146	154	161	170	180	185
3.0–3.9	150	153	160	168	176	184	190	144	150	157	166	174	184	190
4.0–4.9	151	155	162	171	180	187	193	148	153	161	170	180	190	195
5.0–5.9	155	160	166	175	185	195	205	152	157	165	175	185	200	210
6.0–6.9	158	161	170	180	191	207	228	157	162	170	178	190	205	220
7.0–7.9	161	168	176	187	200	218	229	164	167	175	186	201	216	233
8.0–8.9	165	172	181	192	205	226	240	167	172	182	195	212	232	251
9.0–9.9	175	180	190	201	218	245	260	176	181	191	206	222	250	267
10.0–10.9	181	186	197	211	231	260	279	178	184	195	212	234	261	273
11.0–11.9	185	193	206	221	245	276	294	188	196	206	222	251	279	300
12.0–12.9	193	201	215	231	254	285	303	192	200	215	237	258	283	302
13.0–13.9	200	208	225	245	266	290	308	201	210	225	243	267	301	327
14.0–14.9	216	225	238	257	281	300	323	212	218	235	251	274	309	329
15.0–15.9	225	234	251	272	290	312	327	216	222	235	252	277	300	322
16.0–16.9	241	250	267	283	306	327	347	223	232	244	261	285	316	335
17.0–17.9	243	251	268	286	308	333	347	220	231	245	266	290	328	354
18.0–24.9	260	271	287	307	330	354	372	224	233	248	268	292	324	352
25.0–29.9	270	280	298	318	342	366	383	231	240	255	276	306	343	371
30.0–34.9	277	287	305	325	349	367	382	238	247	264	286	320	360	385
35.0–39.9	274	286	307	329	351	369	382	241	252	268	294	326	368	390
40.0–44.9	278	289	310	328	349	369	381	243	254	272	297	332	372	388
45.0–49.9	272	286	306	326	349	369	382	242	255	274	301	335	372	400
50.0–54.9	271	283	302	323	345	368	383	248	260	280	306	338	375	393
55.0–59.9	268	281	304	323	343	366	378	248	261	282	309	343	380	400
60.0–64.9	266	278	297	320	340	360	375	250	261	284	308	340	373	396
65.0–69.9	254	267	290	311	332	353	366	243	257	280	305	334	365	385
70.0–74.9	251	262	285	307	326	348	360	238	253	276	303	331	358	375

Table 5.1: Percentiles for mid-upper-arm circumference (mm) for U.S. persons aged one to seventy-four years. Data are from the NHANES I (1971–1974) and NHANES II (1976–1980) surveys and were compiled by Frisancho (1990).

Age (yrs)	Male subjects							Female subjects						
	5	10	25	50	75	90	95	5	10	25	50	75	90	95
20–29	255	260	273	302	325	353	358	222	229	243	274	296	322	343
30–39	268	272	287	313	332	352	371	223	236	255	271	288	326	352
40–49	266	283	298	313	331	340	353	239	246	273	290	316	345	358
50–59	267	272	293	309	326	339	360	233	243	270	298	323	350	370
60–69	258	272	290	308	325	349	362	253	267	283	303	325	359	380
70+	234	248	270	287	306	327	342	231	248	273	297	323	344	384

Table 5.2: Percentiles for the mid-upper-arm circumference for Canadian adult males and females. Data are from the Nutrition Canada Survey and compiled by Jetté (1981) with permission.

NHANES I (1971–1974) and NHANES II (1976–1980) surveys and were compiled by Frisancho (1990).

Percentiles for the mid-upper-arm circumference for Canadian adult males and females are given in Table 5.2. Data are from Nutrition Canada and were compiled by Jetté (1981).

References

Chumlea W C, Roche A F, Mukherjee D (1984). Nutritional Assessment of the Elderly through Anthropometry. Ross Laboratories, Columbus, Ohio.

Frisancho A R (1990). Anthropometric Standards for the Assessment of growth and Nutritional Status. The University of Michigan Press, Ann Arbor.

Gurney J M, Jelliffe D B (1973). Arm anthropometry in nutritional assessment: nomogram for rapid calculation of muscle circumference and cross-sectional muscle and fat areas. American Journal of Clinical Nutrition 26: 912–915.

Hofvander Y, Eksmyr R (1969). Changes in upper arm circumference and body weight in a 2-year follow-up of children in an applied nutrition programme in a representative Ethiopian highland village. Journal of Tropical Pediatrics 15: 251–252.

Jetté M (1981). Guide for Anthropometric Classification of Canadian Adults for use in Nutritional Assessment. Health and Welfare, Ottawa.

Lohman T G, Roche A F, Martorell R (eds) (1988). Anthropometric Standardization Reference Manual. Human Kinetics Books, Champagne, Illinois.

Shakir A, Morley D (1974). Measuring malnutrition. Lancet 1: 758–759.

5.2 Mid-upper-arm muscle circumference

Principle

Mid-upper-arm muscle circumference is derived from measurements of both the mid-upper-arm circumference and triceps skinfold thickness. It represents the circumference of the inner circle of muscle mass surrounding a small central core of bone (Gurney and Jelliffe, 1973). Mid-upper-arm muscle circumference can be used to assess total muscle mass, and is frequently used for this purpose in field surveys. It can also be used to assess large changes in total body muscle mass, but is insensitive to small changes of muscle mass that might occur, for example, during a short illness. As muscle serves as the major protein store, assessment of muscle protein provides an index of the protein reserves of the body.

Procedure

1. Calculate the mid-upper-arm muscle circumference (C_2) using the following equation:

$$C_2 = mid-upper-arm\ circ\ (C_1) - \pi \times TSK)$$

   where TSK = triceps skinfold thickness (Fig. 5.2). Note that for this equation to be valid all measurements must be made in the same units (preferably millimeters). Alternatively a nomogram can be used to calculate mid-upper-arm muscle circumference (Fig. 5.3) (Gurney and Jelliffe, 1973).

2. Calculate the percentage of the median with the NHANES or Canadian reference data cited below, using the appropriate age, sex and median mid-upper-arm muscle circumference.

$$\%\ Median = \frac{100 \times observed\ muscle\ circ.}{median\ muscle\ circ.\ for\ age\ and\ sex}$$

3. Determine in which percentile range the subject's mid-upper-arm muscle circumference falls using the same reference data.

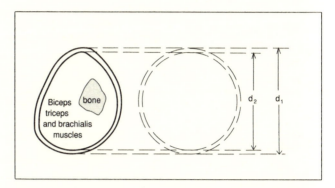

Fig. 5.2: Calculation of mid-upper-arm muscle circumference. Let C_1 = midupperarm circumference, TSK = triceps skinfold, d_1 = arm diameter and d_2 = muscle diameter. Then TSK = $2 \times$ subcutaneous fat = $d_1 - d_2$ and $C_1 = \pi d_1$. But muscle circumference (C_2) = πd_2 = $\pi(d_1 - (d_1 - d_2))$ = $\pi d_1 - \pi(d_1 - d_2)$. Hence $C_2 = C_1 - \pi \times TSK$. From Jelliffe DB. The Assessment of the Nutritional Status of the Community. Geneva, World Health Organization (1966). WHO Monograph Series, No. 53, page 77, Figure 44, with permission.

Both the equation and the nomogram for calculating mid-upper-arm muscle circumference are based on the same assumptions as those described for mid-upper-arm fat area Section 6.5. As variations in skinfold compressibility are ignored, and as the triceps skinfold of females is generally more compressible than that of males, female mid-upper-arm muscle circumferences may be underestimated (Clegg and Kent, 1967). As a further complication, the mid-upper-arm muscle circumference equation does not take into account inter-subject variation in the diameter of the humerus relative to mid-upper-arm circumference (Frisancho, 1981).

Evaluation

Percentiles for the mid-upper-arm muscle circumference for U.S. persons aged one to seventy-four years old are given in Table 5.3. Data are from the NHANES I (1971–1974) and NHANES II (1976–1980) surveys and were compiled by Frisancho (1990).

The percentiles for the mid-upper-arm muscle circumference (cm) for Canadian adult males and females are given in Table 5.4. Data are from the Nutrition Canada Survey and were compiled by Jetté (1981).

Age (yrs)	Male subjects							Female subjects						
	5	10	25	50	75	90	95	5	10	25	50	75	90	95
1–1.9	110	113	119	127	135	144	147	105	111	117	124	132	139	143
2–2.9	111	114	122	130	140	146	150	111	114	119	126	133	142	147
3–3.9	117	123	131	137	143	148	153	113	119	124	132	140	146	152
4–4.9	123	126	133	141	148	156	159	115	121	128	136	144	152	157
5–5.9	128	133	140	147	154	162	169	125	128	134	142	151	159	165
6–6.9	131	135	142	151	161	170	177	130	133	138	145	154	166	171
7–7.9	137	139	151	160	168	177	190	129	135	142	151	160	171	176
8–8.9	140	145	154	162	170	182	187	138	140	151	160	171	183	194
9–9.9	151	154	161	170	183	196	202	147	150	158	167	180	194	198
10–10.9	156	160	166	180	191	209	221	148	150	159	170	180	190	197
11–11.9	159	165	173	183	195	205	230	150	158	171	181	196	217	223
12–12.9	167	171	182	195	210	223	241	162	166	180	191	201	214	220
13–13.9	172	179	196	211	226	238	245	169	175	183	198	211	226	240
14–14.9	189	199	212	223	240	260	264	174	179	190	201	216	232	247
15–15.9	199	204	218	237	254	266	272	175	178	189	202	215	228	244
16–16.9	213	225	234	249	269	287	296	170	180	190	202	216	234	249
17–17.9	224	231	245	258	273	294	312	175	183	194	205	221	239	257
18–18.9	226	237	252	264	283	298	324	174	179	191	202	215	237	245
19–24.9	238	245	257	273	289	309	321	179	185	195	207	221	236	249
25–34.9	243	250	264	279	298	314	326	183	188	199	212	228	246	264
35–44.9	247	255	269	286	302	318	327	186	192	205	218	236	257	272
45–54.9	239	249	265	281	300	315	326	187	193	206	220	238	260	274
55–64.9	236	245	260	278	295	310	320	187	196	209	225	244	266	280
65–74.9	223	235	251	268	284	298	306	185	195	208	225	244	264	279

Table 5.3: Percentiles for mid-upper-arm muscle circumference (mm) for U.S. persons aged one to seventy-four years old. Data are from the NHANES I (1971–1974) survey. Data are from Frisancho (1981). © Am. J. Clin. Nutr. American Society for Clinical Nutrition.

Age (yrs)	Male subjects							Female subjects						
	5	10	25	50	75	90	95	5	10	25	50	75	90	95
20–29	232.4	237.1	249.0	263.1	291.5	299.8	306.4	179.3	184.3	196.4	210.3	223.7	243.1	251.4
30–39	235.7	248.7	262.8	274.3	292.4	304.7	308.8	180.8	186.0	197.1	212.0	224.6	241.3	257.7
40–49	244.3	250.8	261.4	279.0	293.8	299.1	304.5	195.3	198.1	210.8	229.7	242.7	263.0	276.3
50–59	241.1	245.7	259.4	273.3	286.3	299.3	309.0	181.7	190.3	206.1	225.0	241.6	262.3	279.6
60–69	229.5	239.5	254.7	274.0	286.7	298.7	314.7	190.5	198.8	214.5	233.1	248.0	262.7	289.1
70+	210.5	221.5	235.8	248.2	268.3	282.0	290.2	186.8	192.8	213.5	231.0	247.3	268.6	286.6

Table 5.4: Percentiles for the mid-upper-arm muscle circumference (cm) for Canadian adult males and females. Data are from the Nutrition Canada Survey and were compiled from Jetté (1981) with permission.

References

Clegg E J, Kent C (1967). Skin-fold compressibility in young adults. Human Biology 39: 418–429.

Frisancho A R (1981). New norms of upper limb fat and muscle areas for assessment of nutritional status. American Journal of Clinical Nutrition 34: 2540–2545.

Frisancho A R (1990). Anthropometric Standards for the Assessment of growth and Nutritional Status. The University of Michigan Press, Ann Arbor.

Gurney J M, Jelliffe D B (1973). Arm anthropometry in nutritional assessment: nomogram for rapid calculation of muscle circumference and cross-sectional muscle and fat areas. American Journal of Clinical Nutrition 26: 912–915.

Jelliffe D B (1966). The Assessment of the Nutritional Status of the Community. WHO Monograph Series No. 53. World Health Organization, Geneva.

Jetté M (1981). Guide for Anthropometric Classification of Canadian Adults for use in Nutritional Assessment. Health and Welfare, Ottawa.

5.3 Mid-upper-arm muscle area

Principle

Mid-upper-arm muscle area is also derived from measurements of mid-upper-arm circumference and triceps skinfold thickness. It provides a more valid index of body muscle mass and hence protein nutritional status than mid-upper-arm muscle circumference because it reflects more adequately the true magnitude of muscle tissue changes (Frisancho, 1981). Nevertheless, mid-upper-arm muscle area tends to overestimate body muscle in obese persons or those with triceps skinfold thickness above the 85th percentile for age and sex (Frisancho, 1990).

Procedure

1. The following equation may be used to estimate mid-upper-arm muscle area (AMA):

$$AMA = \frac{(C - (\pi \times TSK)^2)}{4\pi}$$

where C = mid-upper-arm circumference and TSK = triceps skinfold thickness. Consistent units, preferably millimeters, should be used throughout.

The equation is based on the following assumptions:

- the mid-upper-arm cross-section is circular;
- the triceps skinfold is twice the average fat rim diameter;
- the mid-upper-arm muscle compartment is circular in cross-section;
- bone atrophies in proportion to muscle wastage during protein-energy malnutrition;
- the cross-sectional areas of neurovascular tissue and the humerus are relatively small and ignored.

A nomogram can also be used to calculate mid-upper-arm muscle area when high precision is not essential (Fig. 5.3 and 5.4) (Gurney and Jelliffe, 1973).

2. Calculate the percentage of the median with the NHANES reference data cited below, using the appropriate age, sex, and median mid-upper-arm muscle area.

$$\% \text{ Median} = \frac{100 \times \text{observed arm muscle area}}{\text{median arm muscle area for age and sex}}$$

3. Determine in which percentile range the subject's mid-upper-arm muscle area falls using the same reference data.

Evaluation

Percentiles for mid-upper-arm muscle area (mm^2) by age and sex for U.S. persons aged one to seventy-four years old are given in Table 5.5. Data are from the NHANES I (1971–1974) and NHANES II (1976–1980) surveys and were compiled by Frisancho (1990). Arm muscle area generally increases up to age sixty-five years in women and up to middle age in men and then steadily decreases.

Frisancho (1990) has also devised a classification scheme for evaluating muscle status in association with linear growth and weight status using five reference limits based on percentiles or Z-scores and selected indices of growth and muscle status calculated from the NHANES I and NHANES II sex- and age-specific reference data (Table 5.6). The indices used are: height-for-age for linear growth, weight-for-age and/or frame size for weight, and mid-upper-arm muscle area by age and/or frame size, for muscle status.

References

Frisancho A R (1981). New norms of upper limb fat and muscle areas for assessment of nutritional status. American Journal of Clinical Nutrition 34: 2540–2545.

Frisancho A R (1990). Anthropometric Standards for the Assessment of growth and Nutritional Status. The University of Michigan Press, Ann Arbor.

Gurney J M, Jelliffe D B (1973). Arm anthropometry in nutritional assessment: nomogram for rapid calculation of muscle circumference and cross-sectional muscle and fat areas. American Journal of Clinical Nutrition 26: 912–915.

Age (yrs)	Male subjects							Female subjects						
	5	10	25	50	75	90	95	5	10	25	50	75	90	95
1.0–1.9	9.7	10.4	11.6	13.0	14.6	16.3	17.2	8.9	9.7	10.8	12.3	13.8	15.3	16.2
2.0–2.9	10.1	10.9	12.4	13.9	15.6	16.9	18.4	10.1	10.6	11.8	13.2	14.7	16.4	17.3
3.0–3.9	11.2	12.0	13.5	15.0	16.4	18.3	19.5	10.8	11.4	12.6	14.3	15.8	17.4	18.8
4.0–4.9	12.0	12.9	14.5	16.2	17.9	19.8	20.9	11.2	12.2	13.6	15.3	17.0	18.6	19.8
5.0–5.9	13.2	14.2	15.7	17.6	19.5	21.7	23.2	12.4	13.2	14.8	16.4	18.3	20.6	22.1
6.0–6.9	14.4	15.3	16.8	18.7	21.3	23.8	25.7	13.5	14.1	15.6	17.4	19.5	22.0	24.2
7.0–7.9	15.1	16.2	18.5	20.6	22.6	25.2	28.6	14.4	15.2	16.7	18.9	21.2	23.9	25.3
8.0–8.9	16.3	17.8	19.5	21.6	24.0	26.6	29.0	15.2	16.0	18.2	20.8	23.2	26.5	28.0
9.0–9.9	18.2	19.3	21.7	23.5	26.7	30.4	32.9	17.0	17.9	19.8	21.9	25.4	28.3	31.1
10.0–10.9	19.6	20.7	23.0	25.7	29.0	34.0	37.1	17.6	18.5	20.9	23.8	27.0	31.0	33.1
11.0–11.9	21.0	22.0	24.8	27.7	31.6	36.1	40.3	19.5	21.0	23.2	26.4	30.7	35.7	39.2
12.0–12.9	22.6	24.1	26.9	30.4	35.9	40.9	44.9	20.4	21.8	25.5	29.0	33.2	37.8	40.5
13.0–13.9	24.5	26.7	30.4	35.7	41.3	48.1	52.5	22.8	24.5	27.1	30.8	35.3	39.6	43.7
14.0–14.9	28.3	31.3	36.1	41.9	47.4	54.0	57.5	24.0	26.2	29.0	32.8	36.9	42.3	47.5
15.0–15.9	31.9	34.9	40.3	46.3	53.1	57.7	63.0	24.4	25.8	29.2	33.0	37.3	41.7	45.9
16.0–16.9	37.0	40.9	45.9	51.9	57.8	67.9	73.1	25.2	26.8	30.0	33.6	38.0	43.7	48.3
18.0–24.9	34.2	37.3	42.7	49.4	57.1	65.0	72.0	25.9	27.5	30.7	34.3	39.6	46.2	50.8
25.0–29.9	36.6	39.9	46.0	53.0	61.4	68.9	74.5	19.5	21.5	24.5	28.3	33.1	39.0	44.2
30.0–34.9	37.9	40.9	47.3	54.4	63.2	70.8	76.1	20.5	21.9	25.2	29.4	34.9	41.9	47.8
35.0–39.9	38.5	42.6	47.9	55.3	64.0	72.7	77.6	21.1	23.0	26.3	30.9	36.8	44.7	51.3
40.0–44.9	38.4	42.1	48.7	56.0	64.0	71.6	77.0	21.1	23.4	27.3	31.8	38.7	46.1	54.2
45.0–49.9	37.7	41.3	47.9	55.2	63.3	72.2	76.2	21.3	23.4	27.5	32.3	39.8	49.5	55.8
50.0–54.9	36.0	40.0	46.6	54.0	62.7	70.4	77.4	21.6	23.1	27.4	32.5	39.5	48.4	56.1
55.0–59.9	36.5	40.8	46.7	54.3	61.9	69.6	75.1	22.2	24.6	28.3	33.4	40.4	49.6	55.6
60.0–64.9	34.5	38.7	44.9	52.1	60.0	67.5	71.6	22.8	24.8	28.7	34.7	42.3	52.1	58.8
65.0–69.9	31.4	35.8	42.3	49.1	57.3	64.3	69.4	22.4	24.5	29.2	34.5	41.1	49.6	56.5
70.0–74.9	29.7	33.8	40.2	47.0	54.6	62.1	67.3	22.2	24.4	28.8	34.3	41.8	49.2	54.6

Table 5.5: Percentiles for mid-upper-arm muscle area (cm^2) by age and sex for U.S. persons aged one to seventy-four years old. Data are from the NHANES I (1971–1974) and NHANES II (1976–1980) surveys and were compiled by Frisancho (1990). Note that values for males and females aged 18 years and older have been adjusted for bone area by subtracting 10.0 cm^2 and 6.5 cm^2 respectively from the calculated mid-upper-arm muscle area.

Category	Percentile	Z-score [1]	Growth Status [2]	Weight Status [3]	Muscle Status [4]
I	0.0–5.0	Z < −1.645	Short	Low	Low, muscle wasted
II	5.0–15.0	−1.645 < Z < −1.036	Below average	Below average	Below average
III	15.0–85.0	−1.036 < Z < +1.036	Average	Average	Average
IV	85.0–95.0	+1.036 < Z < +1.645	Above average	Above average	Above average
V	90.0–100.0	Z > +1.645	Tall	Heavy	High; good nutrition

Table 5.6: Anthropometric classification and evaluation of height, weight and muscle status. Modified from Frisancho (1990), Table III.2. [1] Z-score = (standard's mean value - value of subject / standard deviation of standard). [2] Growth status defined with reference to sex specific standards of height. [3] Weight status defined with reference to sex specific standards of weight by age and/or frame size. [4] Muscle status defined with reference to sex specific standards of mid-upper-arm muscle area by age and/or frame size.

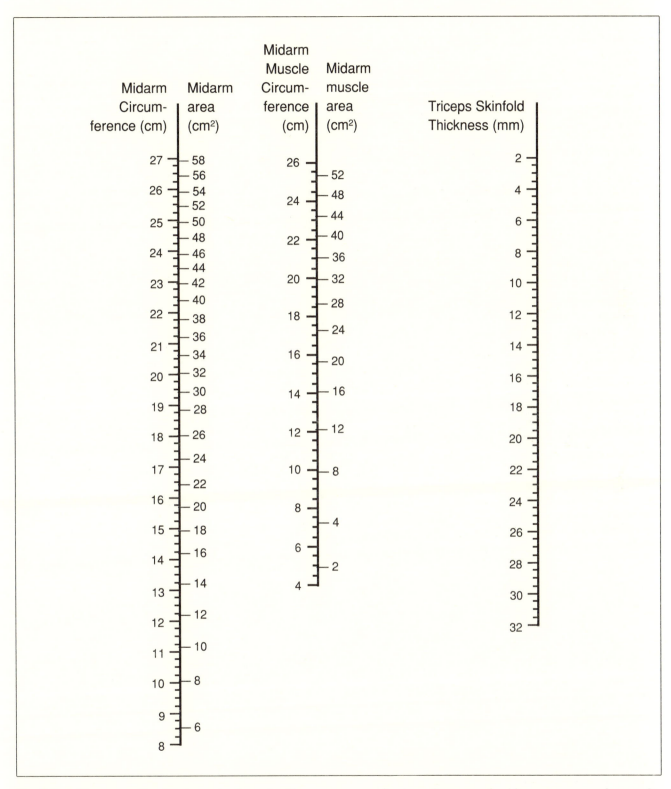

Fig. 5.3: Nomogram for the determination of mid-upper-arm muscle circumference and mid-upper-arm muscle area for children. To use the diagram, locate the child's mid-upper-arm circumference on the column furthest to the left, and the triceps skinfold on the right-hand column. Then lay a ruler so that it touches these two points. The estimated mid-upper-arm area, mid-upper-arm muscle circumference, and mid-upper-arm muscle area, are indicated at the intersection of the ruler and the appropriate column. From Gurney and Jelliffe (1973). © Am. J. Clin. Nutr. American Society for Clinical Nutrition.

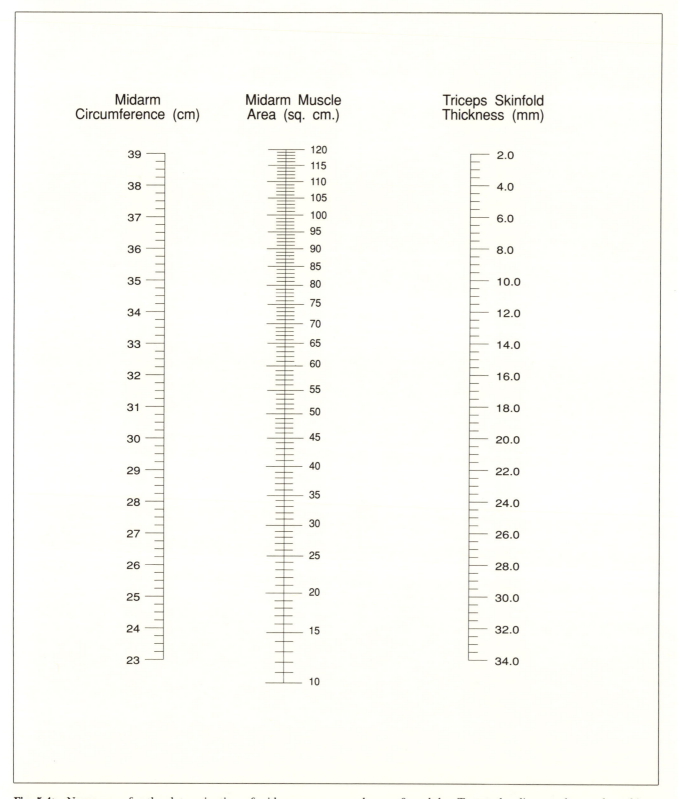

Fig. 5.4: Nomogram for the determination of mid-upper-arm muscle area for adults. To use the diagram, locate the subjects mid-upper-arm circumference on the column furthest to the left, and the triceps skinfold on the right-hand column. Then lay a ruler so that it touches these two points. The estimated mid-upper-arm muscle area is indicated at the intersection of the ruler and the appropriate column. Adapted from Gurney and Jelliffe (1973). © Am. J. Clin. Nutr. American Society for Clinical Nutrition.

5.4 Corrected mid-upper-arm muscle area

Principle

The equation shown in Section 5.3 overestimates mid-upper-arm muscle area by 20% to 25%, and, as a result, may underestimate the severity of muscle atrophy (Heymsfield et al., 1982). Instead, a revised equation which calculates absolute bone-free arm muscle area can be used. This revised equation takes into account errors resulting from the noncircular nature of the muscle compartment and the inclusion of nonskeletal muscle tissue (e.g. neurovascular tissue and bone). It reduces the average error for a given subject to 7% to 8% for mid-upper-arm muscle area. Nevertheless, Heymsfield et al. (1982) caution that even the corrected mid-upper-arm muscle area equation is only an approximation (e.g. $\pm 8\%$) of actual mid-upper-arm muscle area. Moreover, it is not appropriate for detecting small changes in mid-upper-arm muscle area such as those which may follow short-term nutritional support or deprivation because the estimated coefficient of variation for the measurement by trained examiners is 7%.

Procedure

1. Calculate corrected mid-upper-arm muscle area (cAMA) using the following equations:

$$cAMA = \frac{(C_1 - (\pi \times TSK))^2}{4\pi} - 10.0 \qquad \text{for men}$$

$$cAMA = \frac{(C_1 - (\pi \times TSK))^2}{4\pi} - 6.5 \qquad \text{for women}$$

where cAMA = the corrected mid-upper-arm muscle area, C_1 = mid-upper-arm circumference (cm), and TSK = triceps skinfold thickness (cm). These equations correct for bone area by subtracting $10.0 \, cm^2$ for males and $6.5 \, cm^2$ for females. They have not been validated for use with elderly persons and are not appropriate for obese patients. It should be noted that the equations assume that the measurements have been made in centimeters, and not millimeters, for conformity with the original reference.

2. Calculate the percentage of the median with the NHANES reference data cited below, using the median corrected mid-upper-arm muscle area for the appropriate age and sex:

$$\frac{100 \times \text{observed corrected muscle area}}{\text{median corrected muscle area for age and sex}}$$

3. Determine in which percentile range the subject's corrected mid-upper-arm muscle area falls using the NHANES reference data cited below.

Heymsfield et al. (1982) also developed an equation to predict total body muscle mass from height and corrected mid-upper-arm muscle area, using estimates of muscle mass derived from urinary creatinine excretion (Forbes and Bruining, 1976).

$$\text{Muscle mass (kg)} = \text{ht (cm)} \times (0.0264 + (0.0029 \times cAMA))$$

The error of this prediction ranges from 5% to 9%.

Evaluation

The percentiles for the bone-free mid-upper-arm muscle area, calculated using the corrected equation of Heymsfield et al. (1982), have been compiled for three categories of frame size for U.S. male and female adults eighteen to seventy-four years of age (Frisancho, 1990). Percentiles ranging from the 5th to the 95th are given in Table 5.7

References

Forbes G B, Bruining G J (1976). Urinary creatinine excretion and lean body mass. American Journal of Clinical Nutrition 29: 1359–1366.

Frisancho A R (1990). Anthropometric Standards for the Assessment of growth and Nutritional Status. The University of Michigan Press, Ann Arbor.

Heymsfield S B, McManus C B, Smith J, Stevens V, Nixon D W (1982). Anthropometric measurement of muscle mass: revised equations for calculating bone-free arm muscle area. American Journal of Clinical Nutrition 36: 680–690.

Age (yrs)	Male subjects with small frames							Female subjects with small frames						
	5	10	25	50	75	90	95	5	10	25	50	75	90	95
18.0–24.9	30.8	33.8	38.7	44.6	51.3	58.1	63.2	18.2	19.6	22.5	25.5	29.2	32.8	36.2
25.0–29.9	33.5	36.8	41.8	47.6	53.5	61.2	63.7	19.5	20.6	23.2	26.9	30.8	35.2	38.1
30.0–34.9	35.0	37.5	42.0	48.8	56.4	62.7	66.9	19.1	21.6	24.5	27.8	31.4	36.2	38.8
35.0–39.9	34.7	38.7	44.1	50.7	57.5	63.8	70.0	19.7	21.4	24.4	28.8	32.5	37.5	42.2
40.0–44.9	34.9	38.1	44.2	51.6	58.2	64.5	66.9	20.9	22.1	25.7	28.9	33.2	37.9	41.8
45.0–49.9	32.8	36.5	42.9	49.1	55.7	63.3	68.8	19.1	21.5	24.3	28.3	33.3	38.7	41.2
50.0–54.9	33.8	36.0	41.5	47.6	55.5	63.8	69.3	20.8	22.1	25.5	29.1	33.4	38.5	41.3
55.0–59.9	31.2	35.4	41.7	47.8	54.3	61.4	64.2	20.4	22.3	25.8	30.2	34.8	41.3	45.1
60.0–64.9	32.5	36.3	41.4	48.0	54.6	62.2	68.0	20.9	22.4	25.8	31.2	36.4	41.1	46.2
65.0–69.9	26.7	31.5	37.6	44.7	52.5	58.5	62.7	19.4	22.1	25.7	30.6	35.4	41.8	45.7
70.0–74.9	27.7	30.8	36.1	43.4	49.6	56.6	59.9	20.3	22.5	25.9	30.3	36.1	42.6	47.3

Age (yrs)	Male subjects with medium frames							Female subjects with medium frames						
	5	10	25	50	75	90	95	5	10	25	50	75	90	95
18.0–24.9	35.5	38.2	43.6	49.5	56.5	63.2	69.3	19.8	21.9	24.9	28.4	32.8	37.2	40.7
25.0–29.9	37.0	40.1	46.8	53.2	60.9	67.7	73.0	20.7	22.1	25.0	29.0	33.9	39.0	43.3
30.0–34.9	38.5	42.2	48.0	54.3	61.8	68.6	72.7	21.4	23.1	26.3	30.8	36.1	41.8	46.4
35.0–39.9	39.9	43.1	48.8	55.9	64.0	71.6	75.6	21.4	23.6	27.3	31.4	37.3	43.0	47.0
40.0–44.9	39.2	42.6	49.2	56.3	64.0	71.1	74.4	21.2	23.2	27.2	31.6	37.7	47.1	52.3
45.0–49.9	39.0	42.6	49.4	55.9	63.7	72.8	76.2	22.2	23.6	27.9	32.2	37.9	45.4	49.6
50.0–54.9	37.6	41.8	47.7	54.2	62.5	69.6	74.1	22.8	25.2	28.5	33.7	40.0	46.7	51.4
55.0–59.9	39.2	42.5	48.5	54.8	62.2	69.5	75.0	23.7	25.3	28.7	34.5	41.5	49.2	53.4
60.0–64.9	34.5	38.3	45.0	52.1	59.2	66.3	70.4	23.0	25.3	29.2	33.9	39.9	46.1	49.4
65.0–69.9	33.4	37.2	43.0	49.2	56.7	62.4	68.1	22.4	24.8	29.1	34.6	40.7	48.1	51.9
70.0–74.9	30.8	34.6	40.6	47.5	54.4	62.0	66.8	22.2	24.3	28.9	34.0	40.0	46.7	51.3

Age (yrs)	Male subjects with large frames							Female subjects with large frames						
	5	10	25	50	75	90	95	5	10	25	50	75	90	95
18.0–24.9	37.6	40.8	47.3	54.b	63.5	71.6	76.7	21.9	23.8	27.3	31.9	38.7	47.5	55.8
25.0–29.9	42.6	45.7	52.6	60.4	67.3	75.8	81.2	22.2	25.4	29.3	34.5	42.0	50.3	60.1
30.0–34.9	44.2	46.9	53.3	62.6	70.6	78.8	84.0	24.0	25.8	30.1	36.3	45.1	55.1	61.2
35.0–39.9	43.2	46.0	51.8	59.9	70.3	79.4	82.8	23.9	27.4	32.2	39.1	47.2	61.0	72.1
40.0–44.9	44.9	47.4	53.2	60.0	69.8	79.4	83.7	26.2	28.8	32.9	40.3	49.5	58.7	71.6
45.0–49.9	42.9	46.3	52.4	59.6	67.5	74.9	86.4	25.0	28.0	32.5	39.7	49.0	62.8	69.9
50.0–54.9	41.8	46.0	51.6	59.4	67.6	77.6	85.4	25.1	28.4	33.4	39.6	49.5	59.7	68.4
55.0–59.9	42.3	45.0	52.9	59.8	66.9	75.3	83.8	27.0	30.0	35.8	42.0	51.0	62.2	65.7
60.0–64.9	38.9	43.9	50.1	57.5	65.8	71.8	77.4	26.6	29.1	33.9	40.7	49.8	57.5	67.6
65.0–69.9	35.6	39.4	46.0	53.7	62.7	70.7	75.6	26.4	28.4	33.5	40.0	48.7	58.7	66.5
70.0–74.9	33.2	38.3	43.6	51.6	59.0	67.2	72.2	25.7	28.8	32.8	40.1	48.7	54.8	60.3

Table 5.7: Percentiles for muscle area (cm^2) by age for U.S. adult males and females with small, medium, and large frames. The values for males have been corrected for bone area by subtracting 10.0 cm^2 from the calculated mid-upper-arm muscle area. The corresponding adjustment for females is −6.5 cm^2. Data are from Frisancho (1990).

Chapter 6
Assessment of body fat

Contents

Introduction

The body fat content is the most variable component of the body, differing among individuals of the same sex, height, and weight. On average, the fat content of women is higher than that of men, representing 26.9% of their total body weight compared to 14.7% for men.

Body fat is deposited in two major types of storage sites: one for the essential lipids, and the other for general fat storage. Essential lipids are found in the bone marrow, central nervous system, mammary glands, and other organs, and are required for normal physiological functioning; fat from these sites makes up about 9% (4.9 kg) of body weight in reference woman and 3% (2.1 kg) in reference man. Storage fat consists of inter- and intramuscular fat, fat surrounding the organs and gastrointestinal tract, and subcutaneous fat (Lohman, 1981). The proportion of storage fat in males and females is relatively constant, and averages 12% of total body weight in males and 15% in females. One-third of the total body fat in reference man and woman is estimated to be subcutaneous fat (Allen et al., 1956).

Body fat can be measured either in absolute terms (the weight of total body fat, expressed in kilograms) or as a percentage of the total body weight (Roche et al., 1981). It can be assessed by using one or more skinfold thickness measurements. Empirical equations exist which relate skinfold measurements to body fat. Fat is the main storage form of energy in the body and is sensitive to acute malnutrition. Alterations in body fat content provide indirect estimates of changes in energy balance. A large and rapid loss of body fat is indicative of severe negative energy balance. Small changes in body fat (i.e. < 0.5 kg) cannot be measured accurately using anthropometry.

References

Allen T H, Peng M T, Chen K P, Huang T F, Chang C, Fang H S (1956). Prediction of total adiposity from skinfolds and the curvilinear relationship between external and internal adiposity. Metabolism 5: 346–352.

Lohman T G (1981). Skinfolds and body density and their relation to body fatness. A review. Human Biology 2: 181–225.

Roche A F, Siervogel R M, Chumlea W C, Webb P (1981). Grading body fatness from limited anthropometric data. American Journal of Clinical Nutrition 34: 2831–2838.

6.1 Triceps skinfold

Principle

The triceps skinfold is the single skinfold site most frequently selected to provide an indirect estimate of the size of the subcutaneous fat depot, which in turn is said to provide an estimate of the total body fat (Durnin and Rahaman, 1967).

The triceps skinfold site is chosen because it is assumed to be most representative of the whole of the subcutaneous fat layer. This assumption, however, is untrue; the distribution of subcutaneous fat is not uniform about the body and varies with sex, race, and age (Robson et al., 1971). Hence, the most representative skinfold site is not the same for both sexes, nor is it the same for all age and ethnic groups. Moreover, the thickness of the subcutaneous adipose tissue does not reflect a constant proportion of the total body fat. In fact, the relationship between subcutaneous and internal fat is nonlinear and varies with body weight, age, and disease states; very lean subjects have a smaller proportion of body fat deposited subcutaneously than obese subjects (Allen et al., 1956),

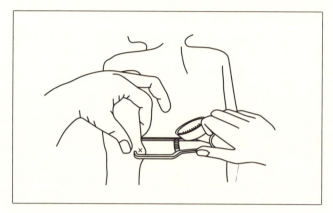

Fig. 6.2: Measurement of the triceps skinfold in the upright position using the Harpenden caliper. Modified from Robbins GE, Trowbridge FL. In: *Nutrition Assessment: A Comprehensive Guide for Planning Intervention* by M.D. Simko, C. Cowell, and J.A. Gilbride, p. 90, with permission of Aspen Publishers, Inc., © 1984.

and in malnourished persons there is probably a shift of fat storage from subcutaneous fat to deep visceral sites.

Procedure

1. Ask the subject to bend the left arm through 90° at the elbow, and then place the forearm across the body.

2. Locate and mark the tip of the acromion process of the shoulder blade at the outermost edge of the shoulder and the tip of the olecranon process of the ulna.

3. Measure the distance between these two points using a fiberglass insertion tape, and mark the midpoint with a soft pen or indelible pencil, directly in line with the point of the elbow and acromion process (Fig. 6.1).

4. Extend the subject's arm so that it is hanging loosely by the side.

5. Grasp a vertical fold of skin plus the underlying fat, 1 cm above the marked midpoint, in line with the tip of the olecranon process, using the thumb and forefinger.

6. Gently pull away the skinfold from the underlying muscle tissue, and apply the caliper jaws at right angles, exactly at the marked midpoint.

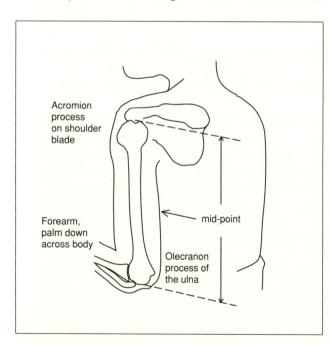

Fig. 6.1: Location of the midpoint of the upper arm. Reproduced from Robbins GE, Trowbridge FL. In: *Nutrition Assessment: A Comprehensive Guide for Planning Intervention* by M.D. Simko, C. Cowell, and J.A. Gilbride, p. 87, with permission of Aspen Publishers, Inc., © 1984.

7. Hold the skinfold between the fingers while the measurement is taken (Fig. 6.2).

8. Take two measurements; if differences are large, a third measurement should be taken and the mean of the closest pair recorded.

9. Calculate the percentage of the median with the NHANES or Canadian reference data, using the appropriate age, sex and median triceps skinfold.

$$\% \text{ Median} = \frac{100 \times \text{observed triceps skinfold}}{\text{median triceps skinfold for age \& sex}}$$

10. Determine in which percentile range the subject's triceps skinfold falls using the NHANES or Canadian reference data.

When the Lange, Harpenden, or Holtain calipers are used, pressure must be applied to open the jaws before the instrument is placed on the skinfold; the jaws will then close under spring pressure. As the jaws compress the tissue, the caliper reading generally diminishes for 2 to 3 seconds, and then the measurements are taken. When the McGaw skinfold calipers are used, they must be closed manually on the skinfold, using the thumb and forefinger, until the lines on the calipers are aligned. Skinfolds should be recorded to 0.2 mm on the Harpenden and Holtain skinfold calipers, 0.5 mm on the Lange, and to the nearest 1.0 mm on the McGaw caliper. Duplicate skinfold measurements made with precision calipers should normally agree to within 1 mm.

Evaluation

Percentiles for triceps skinfolds (mm) by age for U.S. persons aged one to seventy-four years are given in Table 6.1. Data are from the NHANES I (1971–1974) and NHANES II (1976–1980) surveys and were compiled by Frisancho (1990). Skinfold measurements for men are distributed over a narrower range than those for women. Moreover, the mean skinfold thickness measurements for women exceed those for men, irrespective of age. The triceps skinfold thickness percentiles derived from the NHANES I survey data are greater in adult women than corresponding percentiles derived from the earlier United States Health Examination Survey (HES) between 1960 and 1962. These trends may be associated with secular and/or age-related variations

(Frisancho, 1981) and emphasize the inadequacy of single sex-specific and/or outdated reference values to characterize the current triceps skinfold 'norm' for adult males and females.

Percentiles for triceps skinfolds (mm) by frame size and height for U.S. adults aged twenty-five to seventy-four years old are given in Tables 6.2 and 6.3. Data are from the NHANES I (1971–1974) and NHANES II (1976–1980) surveys and were compiled by Frisancho (1984). By using these reference data, investigators can distinguish a large-framed individual from a person who is truly obese, as indicated by excessive body weight and fat tissue. In the former, a large body weight is not associated with excessive fat tissue.

Percentiles for the triceps skinfold (mm) for Canadian adult males and females are given in Table 6.4. Data are from the Nutrition Canada Survey (1970–1972) and were compiled by Jetté (1981).

References

Allen T H, Peng M T, Chen K P, Huang T F, Chang C, Fang S (1956). Prediction of total adiposity from skinfolds and the curvilinear relationship between external and internal adiposity. Metabolism 5: 346–352.

Durnin J V G A, Rahaman M M (1967). The assessment of the amount of fat in the human body from measurements of skinfold thickness. British Journal of Nutrition 21: 681–689.

Frisancho A R (1981). New norms of upper limb fat and muscle areas for assessment of nutritional status. American Journal of Clinical Nutrition 34: 2540–2545.

Frisancho A R (1984). New standards of weight and body composition by frame size and height for assessment of nutritional status of adults and the elderly. American Journal of Clinical Nutrition 40: 808–819.

Frisancho A R (1990). Anthropometric Standards for the Assessment of Growth and Nutritional Status. The University of Michigan Press, Ann Arbor.

Jetté M (1981). Guide for Anthropometric Classification of Canadian Adults for use in Nutritional Assessment. Health and Welfare, Ottawa.

Robbins G E, Trowbridge F L (1984). Anthropometric techniques and their application. In: Simko M D, Cowell C, Gilbride J A (eds), Nutrition Assessment. Aspen Corporation, Rockville, Maryland, pp. 69–92.

Robson J R F, Bazin M, Soderstrom R (1971). Ethnic differences in skin-fold thickness. American Journal of Clinical Nutrition 24: 64–868.

Age (yr)	Triceps Skinfold Percentiles (mm)							Triceps Skinfold Percentiles (mm)						
	5	10	25	50	75	90	95	5	10	25	50	75	90	95
	Male subjects							Female subjects						
1.0–1.9	6.5	7.0	8.0	10.0	12.0	14.0	15.5	6.0	7.0	8.0	10.0	12.0	14.0	16.0
2.0–2.9	6.0	6.5	8.0	10.0	12.0	14.0	15.0	6.0	7.0	8.5	10.0	12.0	14.5	16.0
3.0–3.9	6.0	7.0	8.0	9.5	11.5	13.5	15.0	6.0	7.0	8.5	10.0	12.0	14.0	16.0
4.0–4.9	5.5	6.5	7.5	9.0	11.0	12.5	14.0	6.0	7.0	8.0	10.0	12.0	14.0	15.5
5.0–5.9	5.0	6.0	7.0	8.0	10.0	13.0	14.5	5.5	7.0	8.0	10.0	12.0	15.0	17.0
6.0–6.9	5.0	5.5	6.5	8.0	10.0	13.0	16.0	6.0	6.5	8.0	10.0	12.0	15.0	17.0
7.0–7.9	4.5	5.0	6.0	8.0	10.5	14.0	16.0	6.0	7.0	8.0	10.5	12.5	16.0	19.0
8.0–8.9	5.0	5.5	7.0	8.5	11.0	16.0	19.0	6.0	7.0	8.5	11.0	14.5	18.0	22.5
9.0–9.9	5.0	5.5	6.5	9.0	12.5	17.0	20.0	6.5	7.0	9.0	12.0	16.0	21.0	25.0
10.0–10.9	5.0	6.0	7.5	10.0	14.0	20.0	24.0	7.0	8.0	9.0	12.5	17.5	22.5	27.0
11.0–11.9	5.0	6.0	7.5	10.0	16.0	23.0	27.0	7.0	8.0	10.0	13.0	18.0	24.0	29.0
12.0–12.9	4.5	6.0	7.5	10.5	14.5	22.5	27.5	7.0	8.0	11.0	14.0	18.5	24.0	27.5
13.0–13.9	4.5	5.0	7.0	9.0	13.0	20.5	25.0	7.0	8.0	11.0	15.0	20.0	25.0	30.0
14.0–14.9	4.0	5.0	6.0	8.5	12.5	18.0	23.5	8.0	9.0	11.5	16.0	21.0	26.5	32.0
15.0–15.9	5.0	5.0	6.0	7.5	11.0	18.0	23.5	8.0	9.5	12.0	16.5	20.5	26.0	32.5
16.0–16.9	4.0	5.0	6.0	8.0	12.0	17.0	23.0	10.5	11.5	14.0	18.0	23.0	29.0	32.5
17.0–17.9	4.0	5.0	6.0	7.0	11.0	16.0	19.5	9.0	10.0	13.0	18.0	24.0	29.0	34.5
18.0–24.9	4.0	5.0	6.5	10.0	14.5	20.0	23.5	9.0	11.0	14.0	18.5	24.5	31.0	36.0
25.0–29.9	4.0	5.0	7.0	11.0	15.5	21.5	25.0	10.0	12.0	15.0	20.0	26.5	34.0	38.0
30.0–34.9	4.5	6.0	8.0	12.0	16.5	22.0	25.0	10.5	13.0	17.0	22.5	29.5	35.5	41.5
35.0–39.9	4.5	6.0	8.5	12.0	16.0	20.5	24.5	11.0	13.0	18.0	23.5	30.0	37.0	41.0
40.0–44.9	5.0	6.0	8.0	12.0	16.0	21.5	26.0	12.0	14.0	19.0	24.5	30.5	37.0	41.0
45.0–49.9	5.0	6.0	8.0	12.0	16.0	21.0	25.0	12.0	14.5	19.5	25.5	32.0	38.0	42.5
50.0–54.9	5.0	6.0	8.0	11.5	15.0	20.8	25.0	12.0	15.0	20.5	25.5	32.0	38.5	42.0
55.0–59.9	5.0	6.0	8.0	11.5	15.0	20.5	25.0	12.0	15.0	20.5	26.0	32.0	39.0	42.5
60.0–64.9	5.0	6.0	8.0	11.5	15.5	20.5	24.0	12.5	16.0	20.5	26.0	32.0	38.0	42.5
65.0–69.9	4.5	5.0	8.0	11.0	15.0	20.0	23.5	12.0	14.5	19.0	25.0	30.0	36.0	40.0
70.0–74.9	4.5	6.0	8.0	11.0	15.0	19.0	23.0	11.0	13.5	18.0	24.0	29.5	35.0	38.5

Table 6.1: Percentiles for triceps skinfolds (mm) by age for U.S. persons aged one to seventy-four years. Data are from the NHANES I (1971–1974) and NHANES II (1976–1980) surveys and were compiled by Frisancho (1990).

Male subjects 25–54 yr old (small frame)

Height in	cm	5	10	15	50	85	90	95
62	157				11			
63	160		6	10	17			
64	163		5	5	10	16	18	
65	165	4	5	6	11	17	19	21
66	168	5	6	6	11	18	18	20
67	170	5	6	6	11	18	20	22
68	173	5	6	6	10	15	16	20
69	175		6	6	11	17	20	
70	178			7	10	17		
71	180			7	10	16		
72	183				10			

Female subjects 25–54 yr old (small frame)

Height in	cm	5	10	15	50	85	90	95
58	147		12	13	24	30	33	
59	150	8	11	14	21	29	36	37
60	152	8	11	12	21	28	29	33
61	155	11	12	14	21	28	31	34
62	157	10	12	14	20	28	31	34
63	160	10	11	13	20	27	30	36
64	163	10	13	13	20	28	30	34
65	165	12	13	14	22	29	31	34
66	168		12		19	30		
67	170				18			
68	173				20			

Male subjects 25–54 yr old (medium frame)

Height in	cm	5	10	15	50	85	90	95
62	157				15			
63	160				11			
64	163		6	6	12	18	20	
65	165	5	7	8	12	20	22	25
66	168	5	6	7	11	16	18	22
67	170	5	7	7	13	21	23	28
68	173	4	5	7	11	18	20	24
69	175	5	6	7	12	18	20	24
70	178	5	6	7	12	18	20	23
71	180	4	5	7	12	19	21	25
72	183	5	7	7	12	20	22	26
73	185	6	7	8	12	20	24	27
74	188		6	9	13	21	23	

Female subjects 25–54 yr old (medium frame)

Height in	cm	5	10	15	50	85	90	95
58	147			20	25	40		
59	150	15	19	21	30	37	40	40
60	152	14	15	17	26	35	37	41
61	155	11	14	15	25	34	36	42
62	157	12	14	16	24	34	36	40
63	160	12	13	15	24	33	35	38
64	163	11	14	15	23	33	36	40
65	165	12	14	15	22	31	34	38
66	168	11	13	14	22	31	33	37
67	170	12	13	15	21	29	30	35
68	173	10	14	15	22	31	32	36
69	175		11	12	19	29	31	
70	178				19			

Male subjects 25–54 yr old (large frame)

Height in	cm	5	10	15	50	85	90	95
64	163							
65	165				14			
66	168			9	14	30		
67	170		7	7	11	23	27	
68	173		9	10	14	22	23	
69	175	6	7	8	15	25	29	31
70	178	7	7	7	14	23	25	30
71	180	6	8	10	15	25	27	31
72	183	5	6	7	12	20	22	25
73	185	5	6	7	13	19	22	31
74	188			8	12	19		

Female subjects 25–54 yr old (large frame)

Height in	cm	5	10	15	50	85	90	95
59	150				36			
60	152				38			
61	155		25	26	36	48	50	
62	157	16	19	22	34	48	48	50
63	160	18	20	22	34	46	48	51
64	163	16	20	21	32	43	45	49
65	165	17	20	21	31	43	46	48
66	168	13	17	18	27	40	43	45
67	170	13	16	17	30	41	43	49
68	173		16	20	29	37	40	
69	175			21	30	42		

Table 6.2: Percentiles for triceps skinfolds (mm) by frame size and height for U.S. adults aged twenty-five to fifty-four years old. Data are from the NHANES I (1971–1974) and NHANES II (1976–1980) surveys. From Frisancho (1984). © Am. J. Clin. Nutr. American Society for Clinical Nutrition.

Male subjects 55–74 yr old (small frame)

Height in	cm	5	10	15	50	85	90	95
62	157			6	9	12		
63	160		5	5	10	16	17	
64	163	4	4	4	9	20	21	22
65	165	5	6	7	11	18	19	24
66	168	5	6	7	11	16	20	20
67	170	5	6	6	10	15	17	25
68	173		5	5	10	15	17	
69	175			8	10	15		
70	178				11			

Female subjects 55–74 yr old (small frame)

Height in	cm	5	10	15	50	85	90	95
58	147		14	16	21	31	34	
59	150	11	13	15	21	30	31	33
60	152	10	11	13	20	29	31	35
61	155	10	12	14	22	29	29	32
62	157	11	11	12	21	29	30	32
63	160		12	13	20	29	30	
64	163		12	13	21	27	29	
65	165				18			
66	168				23			

Male subjects 55–74 yr old (medium frame)

Height in	cm	5	10	15	50	85	90	95
62	157			5	12	25		
63	160		7	7	11	20	23	
64	163	5	6	6	10	17	20	26
65	165	5	6	7	11	17	19	24
66	168	6	6	7	12	18	19	22
67	170	5	6	7	12	18	20	23
68	173	6	7	8	12	18	21	23
69	175	5	6	7	12	19	22	25
70	178	6	7	7	11	18	19	21
71	180	5	6	6	11	16	17	20
72	183		6	8	11	19	20	
73	185			8	13	16		

Female subjects 55–74 yr old (medium frame)

Height in	cm	5	10	15	50	85	90	95
58	147	5	13	17	28	40	40	41
59	150	12	15	18	26	34	38	41
60	152	13	17	18	25	33	34	38
61	155	13	16	18	25	35	37	42
62	157	13	15	17	24	33	36	39
63	160	12	14	16	24	32	35	38
64	163	12	14	16	25	33	34	37
65	165	14	16	17	24	33	35	39
66	168	12	13	16	24	33	33	36
67	170		17	17	27	35	35	
68	173				25			
69	175							

Male subjects 55–74 yr old (large frame)

Height in	cm	5	10	15	50	85	90	95
63	160				15			
64	163				21			
65	165			11	14	22		
66	168		7	8	13	21	25	
67	170	6	8	9	16	21	25	27
68	173	6	7	8	13	20	21	23
69	175	6	7	8	12	18	20	23
70	178	5	6	8	14	22	25	31
71	180		6	6	13	18	22	
72	183		8	8	13	23	26	
73	185				11			

Female subjects 55–74 yr old (large frame)

Height in	cm	5	10	15	50	85	90	95
58	147				45			
59	150				36			
60	152		25	26	35	44	45	
61	155	18	22	24	33	40	44	46
62	157	19	24	24	32	40	43	50
63	160	20	24	25	33	41	43	45
64	163	18	22	23	29	42	46	50
65	165	15	17	20	30	43	44	46
66	168		18	18	27	35	40	
67	170		22	32	44			
68	173							

Table 6.3: Percentiles for triceps skinfolds (mm) by frame size and height for U.S. adults aged fifty-five to seventy-four years old. Data are from the NHANES I (1971–1974) and NHANES II (1976–1980) surveys. From Frisancho (1984). © Am. J. Clin. Nutr. American Society for Clinical Nutrition.

Age (yr)	Triceps Skinfold Percentiles (mm)							Triceps Skinfold Percentiles (mm)						
	5	10	25	50	75	90	95	5	10	25	50	75	90	95
	Male subjects							Female subjects						
20–29	3	4	7	10	16	21	28	8	11	16	20	25	29	32
30–39	4	6	7	10	16	19	23	10	11	15	19	24	29	33
40–49	5	6	8	11	14	17	19	11	13	16	20	26	29	32
50–59	4	5	8	11	14	16	20	12	14	18	23	16	31	33
60–69	5	6	7	10	14	20	21	14	17	20	23	27	30	34
70+	5	6	8	11	14	19	21	11	13	17	21	25	30	31

Table 6.4: Percentiles for the triceps skinfold for Canadian adult males and females. Data are from the Nutrition Canada Survey and were compiled by Jetté (1981) with permission.

6.2 Subscapular skinfold

Principle

Subcutaneous fat is not uniformly distributed about the body. Hence, only a crude estimate of total body fat can be obtained from a single skinfold site. To account for the differing distribution of subcutaneous fat, a body skinfold site such as the subscapular skinfold, as well as a limb skinfold, are often used to improve the estimate of total body fat and provide information on the distribution of body fat. The latter has been associated with risk of certain diseases.

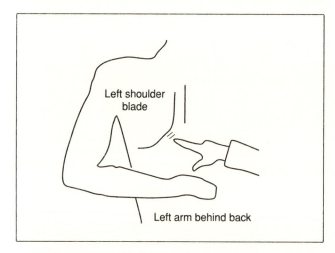

Fig. 6.3: Location of the subscapular skinfold site.

Procedure

1. Place the subject's left arm behind the back to assist in the identification of the measurement site for the subscapular skinfold.

2. Mark the measurement site which is just below and laterally to the angle of the left shoulder blade, with the shoulder and left arm relaxed at the side of the body Fig. 6.3.

3. Grasp the skinfold at the marked site with the fingers on top, thumb below, and forefinger on the site at the lower tip of the scapular. The skinfold should angle 45° from horizontal, in the same direction as the inner border of the scapula (i.e. medially upward, and laterally downward).

4. Take two readings; if the differences are large, take a third measurement and record the mean of the closest pair.

5. Calculate the percentage of the median with the NHANES reference data, using the appropriate age, sex, and median subscapular skinfold.

$$\% \text{ Median} = \frac{100 \times \text{observed subscapular skinfold}}{\text{median subscapular skinfold}}$$

6. Determine in which percentile range the subject's subscapular skinfold falls using the same reference data.

Evaluation

Percentiles for subscapular skinfolds (mm) for U.S. males and females of all races are shown in Table 6.5. The data are from the NHANES I (1971–1974) and the NHANES II (1976–1980) surveys conducted by NCHS and were compiled by Frisancho (1990).

Frisancho (1984) has also compiled age- and sex-specific percentile distributions for the subscapular skinfolds of U.S. adults twenty-five to seventy-four years. These are also based on the merged data from NHANES I and NHANES II and presented in relation to frame size and height (Tables 6.6 and 6.7). Subscapular reference percentiles for children and adults derived from the Nutrition Canada survey are not available.

Percentiles for sum of triceps and subscapular skinfold thicknesses (mm) by age for U.S. white and black males and females are shown in Tables 6.8, 6.9, and 6.10. Data are from the NHANES I (1971–1974) and NHANES II (1976–1980) surveys and were compiled by Frisancho (1990).

References

Frisancho A R (1984). New standards of weight and body composition by frame size and height for assessment of nutritional status of adults and the elderly. American Journal of Clinical Nutrition 40: 808–819.

Frisancho A R (1990). Anthropometric Standards for the Assessment of Growth and Nutritional Status. The University of Michigan Press, Ann Arbor.

Age (yr)	Percentiles of Subscapular Skinfolds (mm)							Percentiles of Subscapular Skinfolds (mm)						
	5	10	25	50	75	90	95	5	10	25	50	75	90	95
	Male subjects							Female subjects						
1.0–1.9	4.0	4.0	5.0	6.0	7.0	8.5	10.0	4.0	4.0	5.0	6.0	7.5	9.0	10.0
2.0–2.9	3.5	4.0	4.5	5.5	7.0	8.5	10.0	4.0	4.0	5.0	6.0	7.0	9.0	10.5
3.0–3.9	3.5	4.0	4.5	5.0	6.0	7.0	9.0	3.5	4.0	5.0	5.5	7.0	8.5	10.0
4.0–4.9	3.0	3.5	4.0	5.0	6.0	7.0	8.0	3.5	4.0	4.5	5.5	7.0	9.0	10.5
5.0–5.9	3.0	3.5	4.0	5.0	5.5	7.0	8.0	3.5	4.0	4.5	5.0	7.0	9.0	12.0
6.0–6.9	3.0	3.5	4.0	4.5	5.5	8.0	13.0	3.5	4.0	4.5	5.5	7.0	10.0	11.5
7.0–7.9	3.0	3.5	4.0	5.0	6.0	8.0	12.0	3.5	4.0	4.5	6.0	7.5	11.0	13.0
8.0–8.9	3.0	3.5	4.0	5.0	6.0	9.0	12.5	3.5	4.0	5.0	6.0	8.0	14.5	21.0
9.0–9.9	3.0	3.5	4.0	5.0	7.0	12.0	14.5	4.0	4.5	5.0	6.5	9.5	18.0	24.0
10.0–10.9	3.5	4.0	4.5	6.0	8.0	14.0	19.5	4.0	4.5	5.5	7.0	11.5	19.5	24.0
11.0–11.9	4.0	4.0	5.0	6.0	9.0	18.5	26.0	4.5	5.0	6.0	8.0	12.0	20.0	28.5
12.0–12.9	4.0	4.0	5.0	6.0	9.5	19.0	24.0	5.0	5.5	6.5	9.0	13.0	22.0	30.0
13.0–13.9	4.0	4.0	5.0	6.5	9.0	17.0	25.0	5.0	6.0	7.0	10.0	15.5	23.0	26.5
14.0–14.9	4.0	5.0	5.5	7.0	9.0	15.5	22.5	6.0	6.0	7.5	10.0	16.0	25.0	30.0
15.0–15.9	5.0	5.0	6.0	7.0	10.0	16.0	22.0	6.0	7.0	8.0	10.0	15.0	23.0	28.0
16.0–16.9	5.0	6.0	7.0	8.0	11.0	16.0	22.0	7.0	7.5	9.0	11.5	16.5	26.0	34.0
17.0–17.9	5.0	6.0	7.0	8.0	11.0	17.0	21.5	6.0	7.0	9.0	12.5	19.0	28.0	34.0
18.0–24.9	6.0	7.0	8.0	11.0	16.0	24.0	30.0	6.5	7.0	9.5	13.0	20.0	29.0	36.0
25.0–29.9	7.0	7.0	9.0	13.0	20.0	26.5	31.0	6.5	7.0	10.0	14.0	23.0	33.0	38.5
30.0–34.9	7.0	8.0	11.0	15.5	22.0	29.0	33.0	6.5	7.5	10.5	16.0	26.5	37.0	43.0
35.0–39.9	7.0	8.0	11.0	16.0	22.5	28.0	33.0	7.0	8.0	11.0	18.0	28.5	36.5	43.0
40.0–44.9	7.0	8.0	11.5	16.0	22.0	29.5	33.0	6.5	8.0	11.5	19.0	28.5	37.0	42.0
45.0–49.9	7.0	8.0	11.5	17.0	23.5	30.0	34.5	7.0	8.5	12.5	20.0	29.5	37.5	43.5
50.0–54.9	7.0	8.0	11.5	16.0	22.5	29.5	34.0	7.0	9.0	14.0	21.9	30.0	39.0	43.5
55.0–59.9	6.5	8.0	11.5	16.5	23.0	28.5	32.0	7.0	9.0	13.5	22.0	31.0	38.0	45.0
60.0–64.9	7.0	8.0	12.0	17.0	23.0	29.0	34.0	7.5	9.0	14.0	21.5	30.5	38.0	43.0
65.0–69.9	6.0	7.5	10.5	15.0	21.5	28.0	32.5	7.0	8.0	13.0	20.0	28.0	36.0	41.0
70.0–74.9	6.5	7.0	10.3	15.0	21.0	27.5	31.0	6.5	8.5	12.0	19.5	27.0	35.0	38.5

Table 6.5: Percentiles of subscapular skinfold thickness (mm) by age for males and females of one to seventy-four years. Data are from the NHANES I (1971–1974) and NHANES II (1976–1980) surveys and were compiled by Frisancho (1990).

Male & Female subjects 25–54 yr old (small frame)

Height (in cm)	5	10	15	50	85	90	95	Height (in cm)	5	10	15	50	85	90	95
			Male subjects 25–54 yr old (small frame)								Female subjects 25–54 yr old (small frame)				
62 157				16				58 147		10	12	23	34	38	
63 160		8	12	20				59 150	6	9	10	17	29	32	34
64 163		7	7	15	25	29		60 152	6	7	8	18	27	32	39
65 165	7	8	9	14	25	28	35	61 155	7	8	9	16	28	32	36
66 168	7	8	8	14	26	26	32	62 157	6	7	8	14	22	27	32
67 170	6	7	9	15	23	25	30	63 160	6	7	7	14	27	29	31
68 173	7	8	9	13	24	30	40	64 163	6	7	8	13	24	27	34
69 175		7	7	13	24	26		65 165	7	8	8	15	26	30	33
70 178			9	14	23			66 168			9	12	25		
71 180		8		13	22			67 170				13			
72 183				14				68 173				15			

Male & Female subjects 25–54 yr old (medium frame)

Height (in cm)	5	10	15	50	85	90	95	Height (in cm)	5	10	15	50	85	90	95
			Male subjects 25–54 yr old (medium frame)								Female subjects 25–54 yr old (medium frame)				
62 157				13				58 147			15	23	38		
63 160				18				59 150	10	12	13	29	38	39	43
64 163		7	9	17	30	32		60 152	8	10	11	22	35	37	41
65 165	8	9	10	16	26	29	32	61 155	7	9	10	19	32	36	42
66 168	7	7	9	16	25	27	33	62 157	7	9	10	18	33	37	40
67 170	8	9	10	18	26	30	33	63 160	7	8	10	18	31	34	38
68 173	7	8	9	16	25	28	31	64 163	7	7	8	16	31	35	38
69 175	7	8	9	16	25	27	31	65 165	7	8	8	15	29	33	38
70 178	7	8	9	15	24	27	30	66 168	7	8	9	14	28	30	35
71 180	7	8	9	14	24	27	30	67 170	7	8	8	15	28	32	37
72 183	7	8	9	15	26	30	32	68 173	8	8	9	15	29	33	35
73 185	8	9	9	15	25	29	32	69 175		8	8	12	25	29	
74 188		7	9	14	25	30		70 178				20			

Male & Female subjects 25–54 yr old (large frame)

Height (in cm)	5	10	15	50	85	90	95	Height (in cm)	5	10	15	50	85	90	95
			Male subjects 25–54 yr old (large frame)								Female subjects 25–54 yr old (large frame)				
65 165				21				60 152				42			
66 168		13		22	36			61 155		17	17	35	48	53	
67 170		8	11	20	36	40		62 157	13	16	18	32	48	51	55
68 173		12	14	20	31	35		63 160	11	14	16	32	44	48	50
69 175	9	10	11	18	31	32	38	64 163	10	12	15	28	42	46	50
70 178	7	10	11	17	31	35	38	65 165	10	12	14	29	42	48	52
71 180	9	11	11	20	35	40	46	66 168	8	9	11	25	36	40	45
72 183	8	9	9	19	28	30	36	67 170	7	10	11	25	41	46	55
73 185	7	9	9	18	27	28	30	68 173		10	12	21	45	48	
74 188			9	18	32			69 175		11	20	43			

Table 6.6: Percentiles for subscapular skinfolds (mm) by frame size and height for U.S. adults aged twenty-five to fifty-four years old. Data are from the NHANES I (1971–1974) and NHANES II (1976–1980) surveys. From Frisancho (1984). © Am. J. Clin. Nutr. American Society for Clinical Nutrition.

Height		Subscapular Skinfold Percentiles(mm)						Height		Subscapular Skinfold Percentiles (mm)					
		5	10	15	50	85	90	95			5	10	15	50	85	90	95
in	cm	Male subjects 55–74 yr old (small frame)							in	cm	Female subjects 55–74 yr old (small frame)						
62	157			11	16	23			58	147		8	9	18	32	33	
63	160		6	6	12	21	22		59	150	6	7	9	19	29	30	33
64	163	6	7	7	14	24	25	29	60	152	5	7	8	15	27	32	36
65	165	6	8	8	16	28	28	29	61	155	6	7	8	17	29	31	34
66	168	7	7	8	15	25	26	30	62	157	7	8	9	17	25	26	30
67	170	7	8	9	13	22	25	31	63	160		6	7	14	25	27	
68	173		7	7	13	21	22		64	163		6	7	18	24	25	
69	175			10	16	27			65	165				13			
70	178				13				66	168				13			
71	180				10				67	170							
in	cm	Male subjects 55–74 yr old (medium frame)							in	cm	Female subjects 55–74 yr old (medium frame)						
62	157			11	19	27			58	147	3	7	10	25	37	43	48
63	160		8	10	15	26	28		59	150	8	9	11	23	32	36	43
64	163	6	7	9	15	25	27	35	60	152	8	10	12	22	34	36	40
65	165	7	8	9	17	25	29	31	61	155	8	10	10	20	33	36	42
66	168	7	9	10	16	25	28	31	62	157	7	8	10	20	33	36	38
67	170	7	9	10	17	26	29	34	63	160	8	8	10	18	32	37	41
68	173	7	9	10	17	26	29	32	64	163	7	9	10	17	30	33	38
69	175	6	8	9	16	25	28	30	65	165	7	8	9	17	30	35	37
70	178	7	9	10	16	25	27	30	66	168	6	7	8	16	30	31	34
71	180	7	9	10	15	25	26	31	67	170		9	10	19	35	35	
72	183		8	10	16	28	30		68	173				16			
73	185			10	15	26			69	175							
in	cm	Male subjects 55–74 yr old (large frame)							in	cm	Female subjects 55–74 yr old (large frame)						
63	160				20				58	147				44			
64	163				31				59	150				31			
65	165			14	19	27			60	152		19	21	31	42	45	
66	168		9	11	20	31	35		61	155	13	16	19	29	40	43	48
67	170	8	11	12	20	35	35	38	62	157	13	19	22	30	39	48	53
68	173	8	10	11	18	27	30	32	63	160	13	15	16	29	40	45	51
69	175	7	11	11	19	27	30	33	64	163	10	12	16	24	41	46	55
70	178	9	11	13	20	30	33	37	65	165	8	9	12	26	42	46	48
71	180		8	9	15	30	30		66	168		9	12	26	34	36	
72	183		8	9	20	28	31		67	170			14	25	46		
73	185				19				68	173				21			
74	188				15				69	175							

Table 6.7: Percentiles for subscapular skinfolds (mm) by frame size and height for U.S. adults aged fifty-five to seventy-four years old. Data are from the NHANES I (1971–1974) and NHANES II (1976–1980) surveys. From Frisancho (1984). © Am. J. Clin. Nutr. American Society for Clinical Nutrition.

Age (yr)	Percentiles of Triceps + Subscapular (mm) by Age							Percentiles of Triceps + Subscapular (mm) by Age						
	5	10	25	50	75	90	95	5	10	25	50	75	90	95
	White male subjects							White female subjects						
1.0–1.9	11.0	12.0	14.0	16.5	19.0	22.5	24.0	10.5	12.0	14.0	16.5	19.5	23.0	25.0
2.0–2.9	10.0	11.5	13.0	15.5	18.0	21.5	24.0	11.0	12.0	14.0	16.5	19.0	23.5	25.5
3.0–3.9	11.0	11.5	13.0	15.0	17.5	20.5	23.0	10.5	12.0	14.0	16.5	19.0	22.0	25.0
4.0–4.9	10.0	10.5	12.0	14.0	17.0	19.0	22.5	10.5	11.5	13.5	16.0	18.5	22.0	24.0
5.0–5.9	9.5	10.0	11.5	13.5	16.5	19.2	22.0	10.5	11.5	13.5	16.0	18.5	23.5	28.5
6.0–6.9	8.6	9.5	11.0	13.0	16.0	21.0	28.0	10.0	11.0	13.5	16.5	19.5	24.0	28.0
7.0–7.9	8.5	9.5	11.0	14.0	17.5	23.0	28.5	10.0	11.5	14.0	16.5	20.5	26.0	32.5
8.0–8.9	9.0	9.5	11.0	14.0	17.0	25.0	29.5	10.5	11.5	14.0	17.5	23.0	32.0	41.5
9.0–9.9	9.0	10.0	12.0	15.0	21.0	31.0	35.5	11.5	12.5	16.0	20.0	26.5	40.0	49.0
10.0–10.9	9.5	10.0	13.0	16.5	23.5	33.5	42.5	12.0	13.0	15.5	20.5	28.5	41.0	50.5
11.0–11.9	9.5	10.5	13.0	17.5	26.0	41.5	55.0	13.0	14.0	17.0	22.0	31.0	42.5	55.0
12.0–12.9	9.5	10.5	13.0	17.5	24.0	41.0	53.0	13.0	14.5	18.0	23.0	31.0	41.0	52.0
13.0–13.9	10.0	11.0	13.0	16.0	23.5	41.0	49.0	12.5	14.0	18.5	24.5	36.0	46.0	56.5
14.0–14.9	9.5	11.0	13.0	16.0	23.0	35.0	47.0	15.0	16.5	20.5	27.0	38.0	48.5	61.5
15.0–15.9	10.0	11.0	12.0	15.0	21.5	32.5	42.0	15.5	18.0	21.5	27.0	34.5	48.0	60.5
16.0–16.9	10.0	11.5	13.0	16.5	23.5	35.5	46.5	17.5	20.0	24.0	29.5	39.5	53.5	64.5
17.0–17.9	10.5	11.5	13.0	16.0	23.5	32.0	39.0	17.0	19.0	23.0	31.5	42.0	56.5	69.0
18.0–24.9	11.0	12.5	16.0	21.5	30.5	42.0	50.5	17.0	19.4	24.5	32.0	43.5	57.0	69.0
25.0–29.9	12.0	13.5	17.5	25.5	35.5	46.0	53.0	17.5	20.0	25.0	34.0	47.0	63.5	73.0
30.0–34.9	12.5	15.0	20.5	28.5	38.5	48.5	56.5	18.5	22.0	28.0	38.0	52.0	68.5	80.5
35.0–39.9	12.5	15.0	21.0	29.0	37.0	47.0	52.0	19.0	22.5	29.5	39.5	54.0	69.0	81.0
40.0–44.9	13.0	15.5	21.5	28.5	37.0	47.5	55.0	20.0	23.5	30.5	41.0	54.5	70.0	77.5
45.0–49.9	14.0	16.5	21.5	29.5	39.0	47.5	55.0	21.0	24.0	33.0	44.5	58.0	71.5	80.0
50.0–54.9	13.5	16.0	21.5	28.5	37.5	48.0	55.5	21.0	25.5	35.0	46.0	59.0	73.0	79.5
55.0–59.9	12.5	16.0	21.0	29.0	37.0	46.0	52.5	21.0	26.0	34.5	46.5	60.0	72.0	80.0
60.0–64.9	13.0	16.0	21.5	29.0	37.5	47.0	55.0	22.5	27.0	35.0	46.5	60.0	73.0	82.5
65.0–69.9	11.5	14.0	20.0	27.5	36.0	46.5	53.0	21.0	25.0	33.5	43.0	56.0	69.0	76.5
70.0–74.9	12.0	15.0	20.0	27.0	35.0	44.5	51.0	18.5	23.5	32.5	42.5	55.0	66.5	74.5

Table 6.8: Percentiles of sum of triceps and subscapular skinfold thicknesses (mm) by age for white males and females of one to seventy-four years. Data are from the NHANES I (1971–1974) and NHANES II (1976–1980) surveys and were compiled by Frisancho (1990).

Age (yr)	Percentiles of Triceps + Subscapular (mm) by Age							Percentiles of Triceps + Subscapular (mm) by Age						
	5	10	25	50	75	90	95	5	10	25	50	75	90	95
	Black male subjects							Black female subjects						
1.0–1.9	10.0	12.0	14.0	16.5	19.0	22.0	24.0	10.0	12.0	13.5	17.0	19.0	22.0	24.5
2.0–2.9	9.0	10.5	12.5	15.5	18.0	21.0	24.5	10.5	11.0	13.0	15.5	18.5	24.0	25.0
3.0–3.9	9.5	10.5	11.5	14.0	17.0	19.0	21.5	9.0	10.5	12.0	14.0	17.0	20.5	22.0
4.0–4.9	8.5	9.5	11.0	12.5	15.0	17.5	19.5	9.0	10.0	12.0	14.0	18.0	22.5	26.0
5.0–5.9	7.5	8.5	10.0	11.5	14.0	16.5	21.0	9.0	10.0	11.0	13.5	18.0	25.0	29.0
6.0–6.9	7.0	7.0	9.0	11.0	13.0	16.0	24.0	8.0	10.0	11.0	14.0	17.0	19.0	33.5
7.0–7.9	8.0	8.0	9.0	10.5	13.0	17.0	24.0	9.0	11.0	12.5	14.5	18.0	23.0	29.0
8.0–8.9	7.5	8.0	10.0	12.0	14.0	20.0	26.0	9.5	10.5	12.0	14.0	16.5	31.0	33.0
9.0–9.9	7.0	8.0	10.0	11.0	15.0	19.0	27.5	10.0	10.5	12.0	15.5	23.0	32.0	42.0
10.0–10.9	9.0	10.0	11.0	13.0	17.0	27.0	40.0	10.5	12.0	13.5	18.0	28.0	39.0	54.0
11.0–11.9	8.0	9.5	11.0	14.0	17.0	38.0	46.0	9.5	12.5	14.5	19.0	28.5	43.0	55.0
12.0–12.9	7.5	8.5	11.0	13.0	18.0	38.0	43.0	11.5	13.0	16.0	21.5	34.0	55.0	67.0
13.0–13.9	7.0	9.0	10.5	13.0	17.0	22.5	34.5	13.0	14.0	19.0	25.5	35.5	50.0	60.5
14.0–14.9	8.5	9.0	11.0	13.0	15.0	23.0	27.0	12.5	14.0	19.0	24.0	35.0	53.5	65.5
15.0–15.9	10.0	10.0	12.0	14.5	19.0	35.0	45.0	13.0	15.0	18.0	24.0	33.0	52.0	66.2
16.0–16.9	10.0	11.0	13.0	15.5	18.0	27.5	28.5	18.0	20.0	23.0	32.5	41.0	62.0	72.5
17.0–17.9	9.5	10.5	11.5	14.0	19.5	24.5	31.0	14.0	17.0	21.0	25.0	36.5	49.0	58.0
18.0–24.9	10.0	11.0	13.0	17.0	27.0	39.0	51.0	15.5	18.0	22.5	32.5	47.5	63.0	74.0
25.0–29.9	10.5	11.0	14.0	19.0	29.5	49.0	61.0	17.5	20.0	28.0	42.0	57.0	68.0	77.5
30.0–34.9	10.0	12.5	17.5	26.0	37.0	49.0	59.5	15.0	22.0	30.5	50.0	66.0	84.0	91.0
35.0–39.9	11.0	13.0	19.0	26.5	38.0	47.0	57.0	18.0	22.0	36.5	53.2	67.0	79.0	86.0
40.0–44.9	12.0	13.0	16.5	27.0	35.0	47.0	50.5	19.0	26.0	39.0	54.0	68.0	82.0	89.0
45.0–49.9	10.0	11.0	16.0	26.0	39.5	48.0	59.0	18.5	24.0	36.5	55.0	70.5	81.5	91.0
50.0–54.9	10.0	11.5	15.0	26.0	41.0	49.0	56.0	21.0	30.0	45.5	60.2	76.5	86.5	93.8
55.0–59.9	9.0	10.0	15.5	25.5	38.0	52.0	57.0	17.0	23.0	41.0	57.0	71.5	87.0	98.5
60.0–64.9	10.0	13.0	18.0	25.5	37.0	53.0	61.0	21.5	27.5	40.0	55.5	67.5	81.5	92.0
65.0–69.9	10.0	11.0	15.0	23.5	33.5	48.0	57.0	18.0	24.5	36.5	49.5	62.0	77.5	85.5
70.0–74.9	10.0	11.5	15.0	23.0	32.5	46.0	49.5	19.0	24.0	33.0	46.5	61.0	69.5	78.5

Table 6.9: Percentiles of sum of triceps and subscapular skinfold thicknesses (mm) by age for black males and females of one to seventy-four years. Data are from the NHANES I (1971–1974) and NHANES II (1976–1980) surveys and were compiled by Frisancho (1990).

Age (yr)	Percentiles of Sum of Skinfolds (mm) by age							Percentiles of Sum of Skinfolds (mm) by age						
	5	10	25	50	75	90	95	5	10	25	50	75	90	95
	Male subjects							Female subjects						
1.0–1.9	11.0	12.0	14.0	16.5	19.0	22.0	24.0	10.5	12.0	13.5	16.5	19.5	23.0	25.0
2.0–2.9	10.0	11.0	13.0	15.5	18.0	21.5	24.0	11.0	12.0	14.0	16.0	19.0	23.5	25.5
3.0–3.9	10.5	11.0	13.0	14.5	17.5	20.5	23.0	10.5	11.5	13.5	16.0	18.5	21.5	25.0
4.0–4.9	9.5	10.5	12.0	14.0	16.5	19.0	21.5	10.0	11.0	13.0	15.5	18.5	22.5	24.5
5.0–5.9	9.0	10.0	11.0	13.0	16.0	19.0	22.0	10.0	11.0	12.5	15.0	18.5	24.0	28.5
6.0–6.9	8.0	9.0	10.5	13.0	15.2	20.0	28.0	10.0	10.5	12.5	15.5	18.5	23.5	28.0
7.0–7.9	8.5	9.0	10.5	13.0	16.0	23.0	26.6	10.0	11.0	13.5	16.0	20.0	26.0	32.5
8.0–8.9	8.5	9.0	11.0	13.5	17.0	24.5	30.5	10.5	11.0	13.0	17.0	22.5	31.0	41.5
9.0–9.9	8.5	9.5	11.0	14.0	19.0	29.0	34.0	11.0	12.0	14.5	19.0	25.5	39.0	48.9
10.0–10.9	9.0	10.0	12.0	15.5	22.0	33.5	42.0	12.0	12.5	15.0	20.0	28.5	40.5	51.0
11.0–11.9	9.0	10.0	12.5	16.5	25.0	40.0	53.5	12.0	13.5	16.0	22.0	30.0	42.0	55.0
12.0–12.9	9.0	10.0	12.5	17.0	24.0	40.5	53.0	13.0	14.0	18.0	23.0	31.0	44.0	57.0
13.0–13.9	8.5	10.5	12.5	15.0	21.0	37.0	48.0	12.5	14.0	18.5	24.5	35.5	47.5	56.5
14.0–14.9	9.0	10.0	12.0	15.0	22.0	33.0	45.0	14.5	16.0	20.0	26.0	37.0	48.5	62.0
15.0–15.9	10.0	10.5	12.0	15.0	21.0	32.5	43.0	15.0	17.0	20.5	26.5	34.5	48.5	62.5
16.0–16.9	10.0	11.5	13.0	16.0	22.5	33.5	44.0	17.5	20.0	24.0	30.0	39.5	53.5	69.5
17.0–17.9	10.0	11.0	13.0	16.0	22.0	31.5	41.0	16.5	18.5	23.0	31.0	42.0	55.5	67.4
18.0–24.9	11.0	12.0	15.0	21.0	30.0	41.5	50.5	16.7	19.0	24.0	32.0	44.0	58.5	70.0
25.0–29.9	11.5	13.0	17.0	24.5	35.0	46.0	54.5	17.5	20.0	25.5	35.0	48.5	64.5	73.9
30.0–34.9	12.0	14.5	20.0	28.0	38.0	49.0	58.0	18.0	22.0	28.5	39.0	55.0	71.0	83.0
35.0–39.9	12.0	14.5	21.0	29.0	37.0	47.0	54.5	19.0	22.5	30.0	42.0	57.5	72.2	82.5
40.0–44.9	13.0	15.0	20.5	28.5	37.0	47.5	55.0	20.0	23.5	31.0	43.0	58.0	73.0	80.0
45.0–49.9	12.5	15.0	20.5	29.0	39.0	48.0	55.0	21.0	24.0	33.5	45.0	59.5	74.5	81.0
50.0–54.9	13.0	15.0	20.5	28.0	37.5	48.0	55.5	21.0	26.0	35.5	47.0	61.0	75.3	83.5
55.0–59.9	12.0	15.0	21.0	28.5	37.0	47.0	53.5	21.0	26.0	35.0	47.5	62.0	75.0	85.0
60.0–64.9	13.0	15.5	21.0	29.0	37.5	47.0	55.5	22.0	27.0	35.5	48.0	61.0	74.0	83.5
65.0–69.9	11.0	13.5	19.5	27.0	36.0	46.5	53.5	21.0	25.0	34.0	44.0	57.0	70.0	78.0
70.0–74.9	11.5	14.0	19.0	26.0	35.0	45.0	51.0	19.0	23.5	32.0	43.0	56.0	67.0	75.5

Table 6.10: Percentiles of the sum of triceps and subscapular skinfold thicknesses (mm) by age for males and females of one to seventy-four years. Data are from the NHANES I (1971–1974) and NHANES II (1976–1980) surveys and were compiled by Frisancho (1990).

6.3 Biceps skinfold

Principle

Biceps and suprailiac skinfolds provide additional information on the distribution of subcutaneous fat. In addition, they are used in certain regression equations for estimating body density. From body density, the percentage of body fat can be calculated using empirical equations (Durnin and Womersley, 1974).

Procedure

1. Stand the subject facing the measurer, with the subject's arm hanging loosely by the side and the palm of the hand facing forwards.

2. Mark the measurement site on the front of the upper left arm, directly above the center of the cubital fossa, one superior to the mark for the triceps skinfold (Lohman et al., 1988).

3. Grasp a vertical fold at the marked level and apply the caliper jaws. Record the skinfold thickness to the nearest millimeter.

4. Use the biceps skinfold to calculate body density (D) (see Section 6.6) using the equation of Durnin and Womersley (1974).

Evaluation

No reference data for biceps skinfolds are known to the author.

References

Durnin J V G A, Womersley J (1974). Body fat assessed from total body density and its estimation from skinfold thickness: measurements on 481 men and women aged from 16 to 72 years. British Journal of Nutrition 32: 77–97.

Lohman T G, Roche A F, Martorell R (eds) (1988). Anthropometric Standardization Reference Manual. Human Kinetics Books, Champagne, Illinois.

6.4 Suprailiac skinfold

Principle

Suprailiac skinfolds provide additional information on the distribution of subcutaneous fat. In addition, they are used in certain regression equations for estimating body density. From body density, the percentage of body fat can be calculated (Durnin and Womersley, 1974).

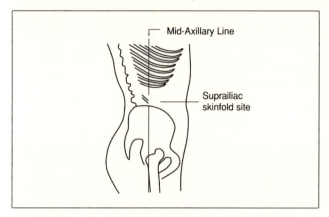

Fig. 6.4: Location of the suprailiac skinfold sites.

Procedure

1. Ask the subject to stand erect, feet together, with arms hanging loosely by the sides.

2. Mark the measurement site at the midaxillary line immediately superior to the iliac crest (Fig. 6.4).

3. Grasp the skinfold obliquely just posterior to the midaxillary line and parallel to the cleavage lines of the skin.

4. Apply the caliper jaws 1 cm from the fingers holding the skinfold, and record the thickness to the nearest millimeter (Lohman et al., 1988).

Evaluation

No reference data for suprailiac skinfolds are known to the author.

References

Lohman T G, Roche A F, Martorell R (eds) (1988). Anthropometric Standardization Reference Manual. Human Kinetics Books, Champagne, Illinois.

Durnin J V G A, Womersley J (1974). Body fat assessed from total body density and its estimation from skinfold thickness: measurements on 481 men and women aged from 16 to 72 years. British Journal of Nutrition 32: 77–97.

6.5 Mid-upper-arm fat area

Principle

Mid-upper-arm fat area, the cross-sectional area of the fat of the upper-arm, is calculated from the mid-upper-arm circumference and triceps skinfold thickness. It provides a better estimate of total body fat (i.e. fat weight) than a single skinfold thickness at the same site, because it is more highly correlated with total body fatness. In contrast, the estimation of percentage body fat from limb fat area is no better than the corresponding estimation by skinfold measurement, particularly in males (Himes et al., 1980).

Procedure

1. Calculate the mid-upper-arm fat area using the following equation:

$$A = \frac{SKF \times C_1}{2} - \frac{\pi \times (SKF)^2}{4}$$

where A = mid-upper-arm fat area (mm^2), C_1 = mid-upper-arm circumference (mm), and SKF = triceps skinfold thickness (mm). A nomogram can also be used to calculate mid-upper-arm fat area in the field (Gurney and Jelliffe, 1973).

2. Calculate the percentage of the median with the NHANES reference data, using the appropriate age, sex, and median mid-upper-arm fat area.

$$\% \text{ Median} = \frac{100 \times \text{observed arm fat area}}{\text{median arm fat area}}$$

3. Determine in which percentile range the subject's mid-upper-arm fat area falls using the same reference data.

4. Derive the arm fat index (AFI) (% of fat in the upper arm) from the mid-upper-arm fat area and the total arm area using the following equation:

$$AFI = \frac{\text{arm fat area} \times 100\%}{\text{total arm area}}$$

In this equation, 'total mid-upper-arm area' = $C^2/(4 \times \pi)$, where C = upper-arm circumference (mm).

Evaluation

Percentiles for arm fat area by age for U.S. persons aged one to seventy-four years are shown in Table 6.11. Data are from the NHANES I (1971–1974) and NHANES II (1976–1980) surveys and were compiled by Frisancho (1990).

Percentiles for arm fat index by age for U.S. persons aged one to seventy-four years are shown in Table 6.12. Data are from the NHANES I (1971–1974) and NHANES II (1976–1980) surveys and were compiled by Frisancho (1990).

A classification scheme (Table 6.13) for evaluating fat status has also devised using five reference limits based on percentiles or Z-scores of selected indices of fat status calculated from the NHANES I and NHANES II sex- and age-specific reference data (Frisancho, 1990). Up to four indices of fat status may be used. These are: sum of triceps and subscapular skinfold thickness, mid-upper-arm fat area, mid-upper-arm fat index, and/or percentage body fat. The use of three of these indices increases the validity of the classification of the fat status of the subject.

References

Frisancho A R (1990). Anthropometric Standards for the Assessment of Growth and Nutritional Status. The University of Michigan Press, Ann Arbor.

Gurney J M, Jelliffe D B (1973). Arm anthropometry in nutritional assessment: nomogram for rapid calculation of muscle circumference and cross-sectional muscle and fat areas. American Journal of Clinical Nutrition 26: 912–915.

Himes J H, Roche A F, Webb P (1980). Fat areas as estimates of total body fat. American Journal of Clinical Nutrition 33: 2093–2100.

Age (yr)	Mid-Upper Arm Fat Area Percentiles (cm^2)							Mid-Upper Arm Fat Area Percentiles (cm^2)						
	5	10	25	50	75	90	95	5	10	25	50	75	90	95
	Male subjects							Female subjects						
1.0–1.9	4.5	4.9	5.9	7.4	8.9	10.3	11.7	4.1	4.6	5.6	7.1	8.6	10.4	11.7
2.0–2.9	4.2	4.8	5.8	7.3	8.6	10.6	11.6	4.4	5.0	6.1	7.5	9.0	10.8	12.0
3.0–3.9	4.5	5.0	5.9	7.2	8.8	10.6	11.8	4.3	5.0	6.1	7.6	9.2	10.8	12.2
4.0–4.9	4.1	4.7	5.7	6.9	8.5	10.0	11.4	4.3	4.9	6.2	7.7	9.3	11.3	12.8
5.0–5.9	4.0	4.5	5.5	6.7	8.3	10.9	12.7	4.4	5.0	6.3	7.8	9.8	12.5	14.5
6.0–6.9	3.7	4.3	5.2	6.7	8.6	11.2	15.2	4.5	5.0	6.2	8.1	10.0	13.3	16.5
7.0–7.9	3.8	4.3	5.4	7.1	9.6	12.8	15.5	4.8	5.5	7.0	8.8	11.0	14.7	19.0
8.0–8.9	4.1	4.8	5.8	7.6	10.4	15.6	18.6	5.2	5.7	7.2	9.8	13.3	18.0	23.7
9.0–9.9	4.2	4.8	6.1	8.3	11.8	18.2	21.7	5.4	6.2	8.1	11.5	15.6	22.0	27.5
10.0–10.9	4.7	5.3	6.9	9.8	14.7	21.5	27.0	6.1	6.9	8.4	11.9	18.0	25.3	29.9
11.0–11.9	4.9	5.5	7.3	10.4	16.9	26.0	32.5	6.6	7.5	9.8	13.1	19.9	28.2	36.8
12.0–12.9	4.7	5.6	7.6	11.3	15.8	27.3	35.0	6.7	8.0	10.8	14.8	20.8	29.4	34.0
13.0–13.9	4.7	5.7	7.6	10.1	14.9	25.4	32.1	6.7	7.7	11.6	16.5	23.7	32.7	40.8
14.0–14.9	4.6	5.6	7.4	10.1	15.9	25.5	31.8	8.3	9.6	12.4	17.7	25.1	34.6	41.2
15.0–15.9	5.6	6.1	7.3	9.6	14.6	24.5	31.3	8.6	10.0	12.8	18.2	24.4	32.9	44.3
16.0–16.9	5.6	6.1	8.3	10.5	16.6	24.8	33.5	1.3	12.8	15.9	20.5	28.0	37.0	46.0
17.0–17.9	5.4	6.1	7.4	9.9	15.6	23.7	28.9	9.5	11.7	14.6	21.0	29.5	38.0	51.6
18.0–24.9	5.5	6.9	9.2	13.9	21.5	30.7	37.2	0.0	12.0	16.1	21.9	30.6	42.0	51.6
25.0–29.9	6.0	7.3	10.2	16.3	23.9	33.3	40.4	1.0	13.3	17.7	24.5	34.8	47.1	57.5
30.0–34.9	6.2	8.4	11.9	18.4	25.6	34.8	41.9	2.2	14.8	20.4	28.2	39.0	52.3	64.5
35.0–39.9	6.5	8.1	12.8	18.8	25.2	33.4	39.4	3.0	15.8	21.8	29.7	41.7	55.5	64.9
40.0–44.9	7.1	8.7	12.4	18.0	25.3	35.3	42.1	3.8	16.7	23.0	31.3	42.6	56.3	64.5
45.0–49.9	7.4	9.0	12.3	18.1	24.9	33.7	40.4	3.6	17.1	24.3	33.0	44.4	58.4	68.8
50.0–54.9	7.0	8.6	12.3	17.3	23.9	32.4	40.0	4.3	18.3	25.7	34.1	45.6	57.7	65.7
55.0–59.9	6.4	8.2	12.3	17.4	23.8	33.3	39.1	3.7	18.2	26.0	34.5	46.4	59.1	69.7
60.0–64.9	6.9	8.7	12.1	17.0	23.5	31.8	38.7	5.3	19.1	26.0	34.8	45.7	58.3	68.3
65.0–69.9	5.8	7.4	10.9	16.5	22.8	30.7	36.3	3.9	17.6	24.1	32.7	42.7	53.6	62.4
70.0–74.9	6.0	7.5	11.0	15.9	22.0	29.1	34.9	3.0	16.2	22.7	31.2	41.0	51.4	57.7

Table 6.11: Percentiles for mid-upper-arm fat area (cm^2) by age for U.S. persons aged one to seventy-four years old. Data are from the NHANES I (1971–1974) and NHANES II (1976–1980) surveys and were compiled by Frisancho (1990).

Age (yr)	Percentiles of Arm Fat Index by Age							Percentiles of Arm Fat Index by Age						
	5	10	25	50	75	90	95	5	10	25	50	75	90	95
	Male subjects							Female subjects						
1.0–1.9	24.5	26.1	30.3	36.1	41.4	46.2	48.7	24.0	26.2	30.5	36.8	41.8	47.8	51.2
2.0–2.9	22.3	24.3	28.2	34.0	39.4	44.9	49.0	24.0	26.4	30.9	36.1	41.1	45.8	49.9
3.0–3.9	22.5	24.6	28.0	32.9	37.3	43.1	46.1	23.7	25.6	29.6	35.0	39.8	44.3	47.8
4.0–4.9	20.3	22.4	25.5	30.0	35.2	39.4	43.5	22.0	24.5	28.4	33.6	38.8	43.5	46.0
5.0–5.9	17.9	20.5	23.8	27.7	33.2	38.4	42.1	20.5	23.6	27.2	32.2	37.7	42.8	46.6
6.0–6.9	15.7	18.3	22.0	26.2	32.6	37.5	40.4	20.1	22.7	26.2	31.3	37.2	41.8	45.5
7.0–7.9	15.0	17.2	20.8	25.2	31.2	38.7	43.8	20.1	22.8	26.5	32.3	37.0	44.3	48.2
8.0–8.9	16.3	17.4	21.1	26.0	31.3	39.4	44.4	19.4	22.3	26.4	32.8	38.5	45.3	51.6
9.0–9.9	15.3	17.3	20.8	25.9	33.5	40.1	44.9	20.6	22.6	27.6	33.8	41.0	48.1	52.3
10.0–10.9	15.8	17.5	21.6	27.6	34.9	44.1	48.4	20.7	23.3	26.9	33.7	41.9	49.6	52.6
11.0–11.9	14.3	16.8	21.5	26.7	36.4	45.2	50.3	20.2	22.9	27.6	34.0	41.0	48.0	52.3
12.0–12.9	12.9	16.2	20.0	26.9	34.3	45.6	50.3	20.3	23.2	28.2	33.6	41.0	47.5	50.3
13.0–13.9	11.8	12.9	16.8	22.3	29.9	40.3	44.9	19.4	21.4	28.0	35.3	42.2	48.5	52.3
14.0–14.9	10.5	11.8	15.4	20.1	27.2	37.4	42.8	21.3	23.9	28.9	34.9	42.6	49.4	53.0
15.0–15.9	10.8	11.7	13.8	17.4	23.4	34.3	42.1	20.7	23.4	28.5	36.2	42.7	48.7	53.5
16.0–16.9	9.5	10.7	13.7	17.3	23.8	32.2	39.6	24.8	26.9	32.4	39.2	45.0	51.3	53.9
17.0–17.9	9.6	10.4	12.9	15.7	21.8	28.8	34.1	22.0	25.3	30.5	38.4	45.1	51.6	55.2
18.0–24.9	9.2	10.5	13.6	19.1	26.3	33.4	38.3	22.5	26.0	32.0	38.8	46.2	53.0	56.0
25.0–29.9	8.7	10.7	14.2	20.1	27.4	34.6	39.6	24.1	27.4	33.6	40.8	48.4	54.3	57.4
30.0–34.9	9.2	11.6	15.7	21.9	28.5	35.3	40.0	24.7	28.7	35.7	43.4	50.0	55.6	59.2
35.0–39.9	9.4	11.3	16.0	21.6	27.7	33.9	38.7	25.9	29.8	37.0	43.9	50.6	56.5	59.2
40.0–44.9	10.5	12.1	15.7	21.2	27.7	35.2	40.0	27.1	30.1	37.5	44.8	50.8	55.6	59.1
45.0–49.9	10.4	12.2	16.0	21.2	27.6	34.6	39.1	27.4	31.7	38.4	45.5	52.1	57.2	59.3
50.0–54.9	10.6	12.5	16.1	20.9	26.7	34.9	39.1	26.8	31.7	39.7	45.8	51.7	57.0	59.5
55.0–59.9	9.7	11.8	15.9	21.1	26.9	33.6	39.1	26.7	31.2	38.9	45.4	52.0	56.5	59.0
60.0–64.9	10.6	12.6	16.3	21.3	27.9	34.2	38.2	28.1	32.6	39.2	45.7	51.4	56.5	59.0
65.0–69.9	9.8	11.9	15.7	21.3	27.4	33.7	38.5	27.0	30.6	37.3	43.9	50.2	54.7	57.6
70.0–74.9	10.5	12.3	16.3	21.5	27.1	33.4	37.8	25.2	29.4	36.0	43.0	49.0	53.8	57.6

Table 6.12: Percentiles of arm fat index (arm fat area / total fat area × 100) by age for males and females of one to seventy-four years. Data are from the NHANES I (1971–1974) and NHANES II (1976–1980) surveys and were compiled by Frisancho (1990).

Category	Percentile	Z-score [1]	Fat Status [2]
I	0.0–5.0	$Z < -1.645$	Lean
II	5.0–15.0	$-1.645 < Z < -1.036$	Below average
III	15.0–85.0	$-1.036 < Z < +1.036$	Average
IV	85.0–95.0	$+1.036 < Z < +1.645$	Above average
V	90.0–100.0	$Z > +1.645$	Excess fat

Table 6.13: Anthropometric classification and evaluation of fat status. Modified from Frisancho (1990), Table III.3. [1] Z-score = (standard's mean value – value of subject / standard deviation of standard). [2] Fat status defined with reference to sex- and age-specific standards of sum of triceps and subscapular skinfold thickness, mid-upper-arm fat area, mid-upper-arm fat index, and/or percentage body fat.

6.6 Calculation of body fat from skinfold measurements

Principle

Skinfold thickness measurements, preferably from multiple anatomical sites, can also be used to predict body density using an appropriate regression equation. A variety of population-specific and generalized regression equations are available. The former have been derived from small samples of specific population groups, homogeneous in terms of age, sex, and body fatness, and should not be applied to other age groups and populations (Sinning, 1978). In contrast, generalized regression equations have been developed based on large, heterogenous samples varying in age and degree of body fatness (Durnin and Womersley, 1974; Jackson and Pollock, 1978; Jackson et al., 1980). These allow the calculation of body density for specified age/sex groups from selected skinfold thickness measurements, and sometimes circumference measurements also. In some equations, age is included as an independent variable. Logarithmic or quadratic transformations and/or curvilinear equations are used, because the relationship between skinfold fat and body density is curvilinear over a wide range of densities.

From body density, the percentage of body fat can be calculated using empirical equations from the literature which relate fat content to body density. Several equations have been derived which use different values for the density of fat and the fat-free mass. More research is needed to identify appropriate empirical equations for specific population groups. Studies have shown that the density of the fat-free mass is not constant for all normal persons, as has been assumed when using most of the empirical equations. Instead, it varies in relation to obesity and muscular development, age, and disease state (Werdein and Kyle, 1960; Womersley et al., 1976). Once percentage body fat has been calculated, total body fat (fat weight in kilograms) can be determined by multiplying body weight by percentage fat (Brodie, 1988).

Procedure

The method involves four steps:

1. Measure the four skinfolds—triceps, subscapular, biceps, suprailiac—using the standardized techniques outlined in Section 6.1 to 6.4.

2. Calculate body density (D) using an appropriate regression equation. An example is given in Table 6.14 (Durnin and Womersley 1974). Select the appropriate values for 'c' and 'm' according to age, sex, and skinfold.

3. Calculate percentage body fat from body density, using the three empirical equations given below. All equations are based on the following assumptions: (a) the density of the fat-free mass is relatively constant; (b) the density of fat for normal persons does not vary among individuals; (c) the water content of the fat-free mass is constant; (d) the proportion of bone mineral (i.e. skeleton) to muscle in the fat-free body is constant. Different authors use different values for the density of fat and the fat-free mass.

Siri (1961):

$$\%F = \left\{ \frac{4.95}{D} - 4.50 \right\} \times 100\%$$

Brŏzek et al. (1963):

$$\%F = \left\{ \frac{4.570}{D} - 4.142 \right\} \times 100\%$$

Rathburn and Pace (1945):

$$\%F = \left\{ \frac{5.548}{D} - 5.044 \right\} \times 100\%$$

The Siri equation assumes that the density of fat is 0.900 g/cc and that the density of fat-free body is 1.100 g/cc. The equations of Brŏzek et al. (1963) and Rathburn and Pace (1945) are based on the concept of a reference man of a specified density and composition and avoid the requirement of estimating the density of fat-free mass.

4. Calculate the total body fat and/or the fat-free mass.

$$\text{Total body fat (kg)} = \frac{\text{body wt. (kg)} \times \% \text{ body fat}}{100}$$

$$\text{Fat-free mass (kg)} = \text{body wt. (kg)} - \text{body fat (kg)}$$

5. Compare total body fat calculated using the equations of Siri (1961), Brŏzek et al. (1963), and Rathburn and Pace (1945).

References

Brodie D A (1988). Techniques of measuring body composition. Part I and Part II. Sports Medicine 5: 11-40: 74–98.

Brŏzek J F, Grande F, Anderson J T, Keys A (1963). Densitometric analysis of body composition: revision of some quantitative assumptions. Annals of the New York Academy of Sciences 110: 113–140.

Durnin J V G A, Womersley J (1974). Body fat assessed from total body density and its estimation from skinfold thickness: measurements on 481 men and women aged from 16 to 72 years. British Journal of Nutrition 32: 77–97.

Jackson A S, Pollock M L (1978). Generalized equations for predicting body density of men. British Journal of Nutrition 40: 497–504.

Jackson A S, Pollock M L, Ward A (1980). Generalized equations for predicting body density of women. Medicine and Science in Sports and Exercise 12: 175–182.

Rathburn E N, Pace N (1945). Studies on body composition: I. The determination of total body fat by means of the body specific gravity. Journal of Biological Chemistry 158: 667–676.

Sinning W E (1978). Anthropometric estimation of body density, fat and lean body mass in women gymnasts. Medicine and Science in Sports and Exercise 10: 243–249.

Siri W E (1961). Body composition from fluid spaces and density: Analysis of methods. In: Techniques for Measuring Body Composition. National Academy of Sciences, National Research Council, Washington, D.C., pp. 223–244.

Werdein E J, Kyle L H (1960). Estimation of the constancy of density of the fat-free body. Journal of Clinical Investigation 39: 626–629.

Womersley J, Durnin J V G A, Boddy K, Mahaffy M (1976). Influence of muscular development, obesity and age on the fat-free mass of adults. Journal of Applied Physiology 41: 223–229.

Skinfold		Age (yrs)					
		17–19	20–29	30–39	40–49	50+	17–72
		Males					
Biceps	c	1.1066	1.1015	1.0781	1.0829	1.0833	1.0997
	m	0.0686	0.0616	0.0396	0.0508	0.0617	0.0659
Triceps	c	1.1252	1.1131	1.0834	1.1041	1.1027	1.1143
	m	0.0625	0.0530	0.0361	0.0609	0.0662	0.0618
Subscapular	c	1.1312	1.1360	1.0978	1.1246	1.1334	1.1369
	m	0.0670	0.0700	0.0416	0.0686	0.0760	0.0741
Suprailiac	c	1.1092	1.1117	1.1047	1.1029	1.1193	1.1171
	m	0.0420	0.0431	0.0432	0.0483	0.0652	0.0530
Biceps+	c	1.1423	1.1307	1.0995	1.1174	1.1185	1.1356
Triceps	m	0.0687	0.0603	0.0431	0.0614	0.0683	0.0700
Biceps+	c	1.1457	1.1469	1.0753	1.1341	1.1427	1.1498
Subscapular	m	0.0707	0.0709	0.0445	0.0680	0.0762	0.0759
Biceps+	c	1.1247	1.1259	1.1174	1.1171	1.1307	1.1331
Suprailiac	m	0.0501	0.0502	0.0486	0.0539	0.0678	0.0601
Triceps+	c	1.1561	1.1525	1.1165	1.1519	1.1527	1.1625
Subscapular	m	0.0711	0.0687	0.0484	0.0771	0.0793	0.0797
All four	c	1.1620	1.1631	1.1422	1.1620	1.1715	1.1765
skinfolds	m	0.0630	0.0632	0.0544	0.0700	0.0779	0.0744

Skinfold		Age (yrs)					
		16–19	20–29	30–39	40–49	50+	16–68
		Females					
Biceps	c	1.0889	1.0903	1.0794	1.0736	1.0682	1.0871
	m	0.0553	0.0601	0.0511	0.0492	0.0510	0.0593
Triceps	c	1.1159	1.1319	1.1176	1.1121	1.1160	1.1278
	m	0.0648	0.0776	0.0686	0.0691	0.0762	0.0775
Subscapular	c	1.1081	1.1184	1.0979	1.0860	1.0899	1.1100
	m	0.0621	0.0716	0.0567	0.0505	0.0590	0.0669
Suprailiac	c	1.0931	1.0923	1.0860	1.0691	1.0656	1.0884
	m	0.0470	0.0509	0.0497	0.0407	0.0419	0.0514
Biceps+	c	1.1290	1.1398	1.1243	1.1230	1.1226	1.1362
Triceps	m	0.0657	0.0738	0.0646	0.0672	0.0710	0.0740
Biceps+	c	1.1241	1.1314	1.1120	1.1031	1.1029	1.1245
Subscapular	m	0.0643	0.0706	0.0581	0.0549	0.0592	0.0674
Biceps+	c	1.1113	1.1112	1.1020	1.0921	1.0857	1.1090
Suprailiac	m	0.0537	0.0568	0.0528	0.0494	0.0490	0.0577
Triceps+	c	1.1468	1.1582	1.1356	1.1230	1.1347	1.1507
Subscapular	m	0.0740	0.0813	0.0680	0.0635	0.0742	0.0785
Biceps+	c	1.1549	1.1599	1.1423	1.1333	1.1339	1.1567
Suprailiac	m	0.0678	0.0717	0.0632	0.0612	0.0645	0.0717

Table 6.14: Parameters for linear regression equations for the estimation of body density $\times\ 10^3\,\mathrm{kg/m^3}$ from the logarithm of the skinfold thickness: density = c – m × log skinfold. From Durnin JVGA, Womersley J (1974). Body fat assessed from total body density and its estimation from skinfold thickness: measurements on 481 men and women aged 16 to 72 years. British Journal of Nutrition 32: 77–97. Reproduced with permission of Cambridge University Press.

6.7 Waist-hip circumference ratio

Principle

The waist-hip circumference ratio reflects the distribution of both subcutaneous and intra-abdominal adipose tissue (Larsson et al., 1984; Jones et al., 1986). It can be measured more precisely than skinfolds. Changes of waist-hip circumference ratio with age and excessive weight are not yet established. Jones et al. (1986) noted that the ratio increased with age (curvilinearly) and excessive weight, both separately and in combination, in a sample of 4349 British Caucasian men aged twenty to sixty-four years. Björntorp (1985) suggested that waist-hip ratios greater than 1.0 for men and 0.8 for women were indicative of increased risk of cardiovascular complications and related deaths.

Procedure

1. Ask the subject to fast overnight prior to the measurement and to wear little clothing while being measured.
2. Ask the subject to stand erect with the abdomen relaxed, arms at the sides, feet together and with the weight equally divided over both legs.
3. To perform the waist measurement, locate and mark with a felt tip pen the margin of the lowest rib.
4. Palpate and then mark the iliac crest in the midaxillary line.
5. Apply horizontally an elastic tape midway between the lowest rib margin and the iliac crest. Tie the tape firmly so that it stays in position around the abdomen about the level of the umbilicus.
6. Measure the waist circumference to the nearest millimeter by positioning a fiberglass tape over the elastic tape. Ask the subject to breathe normally, and to breathe out gently at the time of the measurement. This prevents the subject from contracting muscles or from holding their breath
7. Measure the hip circumference at the point yielding the maximum circumference over the buttocks (Jones et al., 1986), with the tape held in a horizontal plane, touching the skin but not indenting the soft tissue (Lohman et al., 1988).

References

Björntorp P (1985). Regional patterns of fat distribution: health implications. In: Health Implication in Obesity. A report on the US National Institutes of Health Consensus Development Conference. Bethesda, Maryland, pp. 35.

Jones P R M, Hunt M J, Brown T P, Norgan N G (1986). Waist-hip circumference ratio and its relation to age and overweight in British men. Human Nutrition: Clinical Nutrition 40C: 239–247.

Larsson B, SVardsudd B, Welin L, Wilhelmsen L, Björntorp P, Tibblin G (1984). Abdominal adipose tissue distribution, obesity and risk of cardiovascular disease and death: 13-year follow-up of participants in the study of men born in 1913. British Medical Journal 288: 1401–1404.

Lohman T G, Roche A F, Martorell R (eds.) (1988). Anthropometric Standardization Reference Manual. Human Kinetics Books, Champagne, Illinois.

General Laboratory Safety Guidelines

- A laboratory coat should be worn at all times while working in the laboratory, to provide some protection against minor spills.

- Long hair (shoulder length) should be tied back.

- Do not eat or smoke in the laboratory.

- Learn the location of the fire exits, fire extinguishers, eyewash, safety showers and sinks with running water, for use in emergencies.

- Read the instructions carefully before commencing any analytical procedure. If you are unsure of any part of the procedure, seek advice from the laboratory supervisor, instructor, teaching assistant, or technologist.

- Extreme caution should be exercised when handling blood, saliva, and urine samples to prevent inadvertent transmission of disease. Gloves should be worn at all times when handling these materials.

- No liquid should be pipetted by mouth. Always use the rubber pipet bulbs provided.

- The absence of a specific warning attached to a particular chemical or procedure should not be interpreted as an indication of safety. Caution should be exercised at all times.

- Safety glasses should be worn if handling strong acids and other corrosive liquids.

- When heating or mixing the contents of test tubes, hold these away from yourself or anybody else in the vicinity.

- If you cut yourself or spill any chemicals on your skin, rinse immediately with running tap water. If any chemicals get into your eyes again rinse immediately with tap water. Quickly inform the laboratory supervisor, instructor, teaching assistant, or technologist of any personal accidents in the laboratory.

- Never place your fingers in your mouth during laboratory work. Always rinse your hands after the laboratory session.

- Clean up any spills on the bench before leaving the laboratory. If possible, discard any broken glassware in special containers provided for this purpose. Seek advice from the laboratory supervisor, instructor, teaching assistant, or technologist on the disposal of any unused chemicals.

- Turn off all equipment after use.

Safety Procedures for Handling Radioactive Materials

- Use gloves while handling radioactive materials and wash hands thoroughly after use.

- Radioactive spills should be wiped up quickly with some absorbent material. The contaminated absorbent material should then be disposed of in the radioactive waste bin. Then a wipe test should be performed.

Part III
Biochemical Assessment

Contents

Overview

Biochemical assessment is used primarily to detect subclinical deficiency states or to confirm a clinical diagnosis. It provides an objective means of assessing nutritional status, independent of emotional and other subjective factors. Both static and functional tests can be used in biochemical assessment. The static tests have been classified into two major categories: measurement of a nutrient in biological fluids or tissues (e.g. whole blood or some fraction, urine, hair, saliva, fingernails), and measurement of the urinary excretion rate of a nutrient or its metabolite. Ideally, these tests reflect either the total body content of the nutrient or the size of the tissue store most sensitive to depletion. In practice, for many nutrients the ideal biopsy material is not accessible for routine use (i.e. liver), and/or the storage site most sensitive to depletion has not been identified.

Functional biochemical tests measure the extent of the functional consequences of a specific nutrient deficiency, and hence have greater biological significance than the static biochemical tests. Functional biochemical tests may involve measuring changes in the production of an abnormal metabolite, or changes in the activities of certain enzymes and/or blood components dependent on a specific nutrient. Other functional tests measure physiological (e.g. taste acuity) or behavioral (e.g. cognitive) functions dependent on specific nutrients, but are not included in this book. A complete classification of the functional tests can be found in Solomons and Allen (1983).

Biochemical tests are often affected by biological and technical factors other than depleted body stores of the nutrient, which may confound the interpretation of the result. These factors are listed below:

- Homeostatic regulation

- Diurnal variation

- Sample contamination

- Physiological state

- Infections

- Hormonal status

- Physical exercise

- Age, sex, ethnic group

- Recent dietary intake

- Hemolysis—for serum/plasma

- Drugs

- Disease states

- Nutrient interactions

- Inflammatory stress

- Weight loss

- Sampling and collection procedures

- Accuracy and precision of
  the analytical method

- Sensitivity and specificity
  of the analytical method

Frequently, their effects can be minimized or eliminated by standardizing the sampling and collection procedures, and by an appropriate experimental design.

Generally, a combination of static biochemical and/or functional tests should be used, rather than a single test for each nutrient. Several concordant abnormal values are more reliable than a single aberrant value in diagnosing a deficiency state. The type and number of biochemical tests selected will depend on a variety of factors including precision, accuracy, analytical specificity, analytical sensitivity, predictive value, validity, and the study objectives. Some of these factors are defined in the glossary at the back of this book.

Biochemical tests can be evaluated by comparing the results with reference limit values, often defined by percentiles drawn from a reference sample of healthy persons participating in a national nutrition survey (Pilch and Senti, 1984). Alternatively, cutoff points based on data from subjects with clinical and/or functional manifestations of a nutrient deficiency, can be used. Sometimes, several cutoff points are used to define levels of 'risk' of deficiency such as 'high risk', 'medium risk', and 'low risk', as used in the Nutrition Canada survey (Health and Welfare Canada, 1973). The U.S. Interdepartmental Committee on Nutrition for National Defense (ICNND, 1963) chose four levels, designated as 'deficient', 'low', 'acceptable', and 'high'. Several examples of the use of both reference limits and cutoff points to evaluate biochemical tests are given in the following chapters.

References

Health and Welfare Canada (1973). Nutrition Canada National Survey. Health and Welfare, Ottawa.

ICNND (Interdepartmental Committee on Nutrition for National Defense) (1963). Manual for Nutrition Surveys, US Government Printing Office, Washington, D.C.

Pilch SM, Senti FR (eds) (1984). Assessment of the iron nutritional status of the U.S. population survey based on data collected in the second National Health and Nutrition Examination Survey, 1976–1980. Life Sciences Research Office, Federation of the American Societies for Experimental Biology, Bethesda, Maryland.

Solomons NW, Allen LH (1983). The functional assessment of nutritional status: principles, practice and potential. Nutrition Reviews 41: 33–50.

Chapter 7
Assessment of protein status

Contents

Introduction

The adult human body of a 70 kg reference man contains about 10 to 13 kg of protein, which is widely distributed throughout the different tissues of the body (Table 7.1). Proteins are essential for structural (e.g. collagen and elastin) and regulatory (e.g. hormone and enzyme) functions. They also act as specific carrier proteins and mediators of the immune response.

	%		%
Muscle	22	Extracellular	17
Skeleton	20	Fat	6
Viscera & skin	18		

Table 7.1: The protein content of body tissues, calculated from Forbes et al. (1953) with permission. © The American Society for Biological Chemists, Inc.

There are no dispensable protein stores in humans, and therefore loss of body protein results in loss of essential structural elements as well as impaired function. Most of the body protein is concentrated in the skeletal muscle (approximately 30% to 50% of total body protein) and in the smaller visceral protein pool (Table 7.1). Visceral protein is made up of serum proteins, erythrocytes, granulocytes, and lymphocytes as well as the solid tissue organs such as the liver, kidneys, pancreas, and heart.

Loss of muscle mass (and adipose tissue) characterizes the marasmic form of protein-energy malnutrition, the form most frequently encountered in developing countries. It is generally the result of a prolonged reduction in food intake. The latter may also occur in hospital patients with chronic illnesses, or result from the prolonged use of clear fluid diets and hypocaloric intravenous infusions of 5% dextrose.

Kwashiorkor, another form of protein-energy malnutrition, also occurs in children from certain regions of developing countries, as well as in hospital patients. In developing countries, kwashiorkor is often precipitated by a series of infections occurring successively or concurrently in the presence of a diet with a low protein content relative to energy. In hospital patients, kwashiorkor tends to arise from inadequate intakes of dietary protein concomitant with acute protein losses induced by stress associated with hypermetabolism such as trauma and/or sepsis (Jeejeebhoy, 1981). Unlike

Protein	Half-Life	Pool Size (g/kg)
Serum albumin	14–20 days	3–5
Serum transferrin	8–10 days	<0.1
Serum retinol-binding protein (RBP)	12 hours	0.0002
Serum transthyretin (TTR)	2–3 days	0.010

Table 7.2: Half-life and body pool size (g/kg body weight) of serum proteins of hepatic origin.

marasmus, kwashiorkor does not result in a depletion of skeletal muscle protein; instead, the visceral protein pool is depleted and edema occurs.

Laboratory indices of protein status measure (a) visceral protein status; (b) somatic protein status; (c) metabolic changes induced by protein-energy malnutrition; (d) muscle function; and (e) immune function. Assessment of muscle and immune function are not included in this laboratory manual. Visceral protein status is frequently assessed by measuring total serum protein (Section 7.1) or one or more of the individual serum proteins, albumin, transferrin, retinol-binding protein, and transthyretin (Table 7.2). The main site of synthesis for most of these is the liver, one of the first organs to be affected by protein malnutrition. In such circumstances, the limited supply of protein substrate impairs the synthesis of serum proteins, resulting in a decline in serum protein concentrations.

Of the four serum proteins—albumin, transferrin, retinol-binding protein, and transthyretin—albumin and transferrin are most frequently used in hospital assessment protocols. Unfortunately, they are not necessarily the most appropriate, particularly for monitoring short-term changes in protein status. They—like most serum proteins—show a relatively slow response, which may be complicated by the effects of such confounding factors as stress, sepsis, and hydration, severely limiting their use in critically ill patients. As a result, serum albumin (Section 7.2) and transferrin are better used to monitor long-term changes during convalescence.

Short-term changes in visceral protein status during convalescence, should be monitored by measuring retinol-binding protein and transthyritin in the serum (Section 7.3). These proteins

have a smaller total body pool, a shorter half-life (Table 7.2), and a relatively high specificity, when compared to serum albumin and transferrin (Fischer, 1981). Future studies may suggest the measurement of serum somatomedin-C, which is said to be more sensitive to acute changes in protein status than the other serum proteins.

Indices of somatic protein status include urinary excretion of 3-methyl-histidine and of creatinine; the latter is frequently expressed as a creatinine height index (Section 7.4). The creatinine height index is used to assess the degree of depletion of muscle mass in marasmic patients; it may also be used to assess the degree of repletion after long-term nutrition intervention, provided that accurately timed seventy-two-hour urine collections are made. Urinary excretion of 3-methyl-histidine appears promising as a marker of muscle protein except in conditions of severe sepsis or major physical trauma, although it has not been widely used.

Metabolic changes occurring in protein-energy malnutrition may also be used as indices of protein status. For example, in field settings where both kwashiorkor and marasmus may occur, tests which differentiate between subclinical cases of these two forms of protein-energy malnutrition are desirable. The hydroxyproline index (Section 7.7), in combination with the serum nonessential:essential amino-acid (NEAA:EAA) ratio (Section 7.5), has been used in such circumstances. For hospital patients, urinary urea nitrogen excretion on at least three twenty-four-hour urine samples, in association with nitrogen intake data, can provide an estimate of nitrogen balance (Section 7.6). In field surveys, twenty-four-hour urine collections are impractical; instead, the urinary urea nitrogen:creatinine ratio on casual urine samples can be used to assess the adequacy of protein intake.

References

Fischer J E (1981). Plasma proteins as indicators of nutritional status. In: Levenson S M (ed). Nutritional Assessment— Present Status, Future Directions and Prospects. Ross Laboratories, Columbus, Ohio, pp. 25–26.

Forbes R M, Cooper A R, Mitchell H H (1953). Composition of adult human body as determined by chemical analysis. Journal of Biological Chemistry 203: 359–366.

Jeejeebhoy K N (1981). Protein nutrition in clinical practice. British Medical Bulletin 37: 11–17.

7.1   Serum protein

Principle

Cupric (Cu^{2+}) ions in alkaline tartrate solution (Biuret reagent) react with peptide bonds (−CONH) and produce a violet-colored peptide complex. The color intensity is directly proportional to the number of peptide bonds over a wide range of measurements. The complex is formed only if at least two peptide linkages (−CONH) are present. Consequently proteins react with Biuret reagent, whereas amino acids, ammonia, urea, and other simple nitrogen-containing compounds do not (Peters and Biamente, 1982).

Reagents

- Biuret reagent. Add approximately 800 mL of distilled water to a 1 L volumetric flask. Dissolve in this water: 9 g potassium-sodium-tartrate, 5 g potassium chloride, 8 g sodium hydroxide. Add to this solution 3 g of copper sulfate dissolved in 100 mL distilled water. Mix all components well and make up to volume with distilled water. Allow reagent to stand overnight. Filter if cloudy and store in a stoppered plastic container. Discard after six months.

- Protein standard. Use a commercial standard, containing known concentrations of protein. Keep frozen in 0.5 mL portions and do not refreeze once thawed.

- Sample. Serum is preferred. Plasma obtained using heparin or EDTA as anticoagulants can also be used.

- Certified reference serum, (e.g. Accutron Chemical Control, Sigma Chemical Co., St Louis, MO)

- Pooled serum sample (used to assess method precision).

Equipment

- Spectrophotometer.
- 5 mL pipets, 50 μL micro-pipets.
- Test tubes.
- Cuvets.

Procedure

1. Label test tubes for the standard, reference, pool, and for each test subject.
2. Add 3.0 mL biuret reagent to each tube.
3. To the standard tube, add 50 μL of standard solution; to the reference, add 50 μL of the reference serum; to the pool, add 50 μL of pooled serum; for each test subject, add 50 μL of test serum.
4. Mix each tube well and allow to stand in a dark cupboard for a minimum of ten minutes.
5. Set the spectrophotometer wavelength at 555 nm. Zero the spectrophotometer using a cuvet of biuret reagent as a reference blank.
6. Transfer the contents of each tube to a cuvet.
7. Read and record the absorbance of the standard, reference, pool and test samples.

Calculation of results

Results can be calculated as protein (g/dL) from the following equation:

$$C_{test} = \frac{A_{test}}{A_{standard}} \times C_{standard} \ (g/dL)$$

where C_{test} = concentration of protein in a test sample,

A_{test} = absorbance of the test,

$A_{standard}$ = absorbance of standard, and

$C_{standard}$ = concentration of standard (g/dL).

Alternatively, the absorbance at 555 nm can be converted to g/dL protein by reading directly from a prepared calibration curve. The conversion to SI units (g/L) = ×10.0.

Evaluation

Interpretive guidelines for the evaluation of total serum protein concentrations (g/dL) are given in Table 7.3. The values for protein in plasma are about 0.2 to 0.4 g/dL higher than those for serum because of the presence of fibrinogen.

Reference	Subjects	Less than Acceptable		Acceptable (low risk)
		Deficient (high risk)	Low (medium risk)	
Sauberlich et al. (1974)				
	Infants 0 to 11 months	—	<5.0	≥ 5.0
	Children 1 to 5 years	—	<5.5	≥ 5.5
	Children 6 to 17 years	—	<6.0	≥ 6.0
	Adults	<6.0	6.0–6.4	≥ 6.5
	Pregnant, 2nd and 3rd trimester	<5.5	5.5–5.9	≥ 6.0
Health and Welfare Canada (1973)				
	Infants 0 to 5 months	—	—	—
	6 months to 71 months	<5.0	5.0–6.0	>6.0
	≥ 6 years	<6.0	6.0–6.4	>6.4
	Pregnant Women	<5.5	5.5–6.0	>6.0

Table 7.3: Guidelines for the interpretation of total serum protein concentrations (g/dL). Conversion factor to SI units (g/L) = ×10.0. Reproduced with permission from Sauberlich H E, Dowdy R P, Skala J H (1974). Laboratory Tests for the Assessment of Nutritional Status. CRC Press, Inc., Boca Raton, FL., and the Minister of Supply and Services Canada.

Total serum protein is a rather insensitive index of visceral protein status. It is maintained initially within the normal range despite a restricted protein intake, and is significantly depleted only when clinical signs of protein malnutrition are apparent. The observed decline results largely from a marked decrease in the serum albumin concentrations which represent 50% to 60% of the total serum protein.

In severely ill hospital patients, blood products such as albumin are sometimes administered; this may significantly affect the concentration of total serum protein. Furthermore, many other factors influence the concentration of total serum protein and hence compromise the specificity and sensitivity of this index.

References

Health and Welfare Canada (1973). Nutrition Canada National Survey. Health and Welfare, Ottawa.

Peters T Jr, Biamente G T (1982). Protein (total protein) in serum, urine, and cerebrospinal fluid; albumin in serum. In: Faulkner W R, Meites S (eds). Selected Methods of Clinical Chemistry. Volume 9. American Association for Clinical Chemistry, Washington, D.C. pp. 317.

Sauberlich H E, Dowdy R P, Skala J H (1974). Laboratory Tests for the Assessment of Nutritional Status. CRC Press Inc., Cleveland, Ohio.

7.2 Serum albumin

Principle

Albumin is the major component of total serum proteins in normal healthy individuals. Serum albumin is assayed in most clinical laboratories via a dye-binding method using bromocresol green (BCG) (McPherson and Everard, 1972). Serum albumin binds specifically and quantitatively to bromocresol green to form a blue albumin-BCG complex which absorbs maximally at 600 nm.

Reagents

The reagents listed below can be obtained from the Sigma Chemical Co., St Louis, MO, as a kit. Follow the procedure given by the manufacturer if this differs from that outlined below.

- Buffered dye containing 150 μmol/L bromocresol green in a succinate buffer, pH 4.2, with nonreactive antimicrobial agents and surfactant. Use as supplied. Store at 20–25°C in the original container.
- Albumin standard, approximately 4 g/dL, containing purified Fraction V bovine serum albumin. The standard is reconstituted with 5.0 mL of deionized, purified water. Allow the vial to stand undisturbed for 15 minutes or until the protein cake is dissolved. Mix gently. The reconstituted albumin standard may be stored for up to three days at 2–8°C or frozen at −20°C for up to three months. Discard if the standard becomes cloudy.
- Sample. Serum is the specimen of choice; plasma specimens obtained using heparin or EDTA as anticoagulants can also be used. Specimens are stable for up to three days at room temperature, up to a month when refrigerated, or may be frozen up to six months.
- Certified reference serum, (e.g. Accutron Chemical Control, Sigma Chemical Co.)
- Pooled serum sample (to assess precision).

Equipment

- Spectrophotometer or colorimeter capable of measuring absorbance at a wavelength of 600 nm, and cuvets

- 20 μL micro-pipets.

Procedure

1. Label test tubes: blank, standard, reference, pool, and for each test subject.
2. Add 5.0 mL buffered dye reagent to each tube.
3. To the blank add 20 μL of distilled-deionized water. To the standard add 20 μL of standard solution. To the reference add 20 μL of the reference serum. To the pool add 20 μL of pooled serum. For each test subject add 20 μL of test serum.
4. Mix each tube well and allow to stand for two minutes.
5. Transfer contents of each test tube to a cuvet.
6. Set the spectrophotometer wavelength to 600 nm.
7. Zero the spectrophotometer using the reagent blank.
8. Read and record the absorbance of the standard, reference, pool, and test samples.

The final color developed is stable for at least one hour. Samples which have more than 6 g/dL albumin should be diluted with isotonic saline and assayed again. The results should then be corrected for this dilution.

Calculation of results

Results can be calculated as albumin (g/dL) from the following equation:

$$C_{test} = \frac{A_{test}}{A_{standard}} \times C_{standard} \ (g/dL)$$

where C_{test} = concentration of albumin in a test sample,

A_{test} = absorbance of the test,

$A_{standard}$ = absorbance of standard, and

$C_{standard}$ = concentration of standard (g/dL).

Alternatively, the absorbance at 600 nm can be converted to g/dL albumin by reading directly from a prepared calibration curve. The conversion factor to SI units $(g/L) = \times 10.0$.

Age (yr)	Percentiles of serum albumin (g/dL) by age							Percentiles of serum albumin (g/dL) by age						
	5	10	25	50	75	90	95	5	10	25	50	75	90	95
	Male subjects							Female subjects						
3–5	4.2	4.4	4.5	4.7	4.9	5.0	5.1	4.2	4.3	4.5	4.7	4.9	5.0	5.1
6–8	4.4	4.4	4.6	4.8	5.0	5.1	5.2	4.3	4.4	4.6	4.8	4.9	5.1	5.2
9–11	4.4	4.5	4.6	4.8	5.0	5.1	5.2	4.2	4.4	4.6	4.8	4.9	5.1	5.2
12–14	4.4	4.5	4.7	4.8	5.0	5.2	5.3	4.3	4.4	4.6	4.8	5.0	5.1	5.2
15–17	4.5	4.6	4.8	5.0	5.2	5.3	5.4	4.3	4.4	4.6	4.8	5.0	5.2	5.3
18–24	4.5	4.7	4.8	5.0	5.2	5.4	5.5	4.1	4.2	4.5	4.7	4.9	5.1	5.2
25–34	4.5	4.6	4.8	4.9	5.1	5.3	5.4	4.1	4.2	4.5	4.7	4.9	5.0	5.2
35–44	4.3	4.4	4.6	4.8	5.0	5.2	5.3	4.1	4.2	4.4	4.6	4.8	5.0	5.1
45–54	4.2	4.4	4.5	4.7	4.9	5.1	5.2	4.2	4.3	4.4	4.6	4.8	5.0	5.1
55–64	4.2	4.3	4.5	4.6	4.8	5.0	5.1	4.1	4.2	4.4	4.6	4.8	4.9	5.0
65–74	4.1	4.2	4.4	4.6	4.7	4.9	5.0	4.0	4.2	4.3	4.5	4.7	4.9	5.0

Table 7.4: Percentiles of serum albumin (g/dL) by age for males and females of all races of three to seventy-four years. Data are from the U.S. NHANES II (1976–80) survey and were compiled by Fulwood et al. (1982).

Evaluation

Percentiles for serum albumin (g/dL) from the NHANES II survey, compiled by Fulwood et al. (1982) are given in Table 7.4. Interpretive guidelines for the assessment of deficient and low serum albumin concentrations are given in Table 7.5. Serum albumin is not very sensitive to any short-term changes in protein status; it has a long half-life of 14–20 days. In addition, any reduction in hepatic synthesis of serum albumin is largely compensated by reduced catabolism.

Low serum albumin levels (hypo-albuminemia) may be generated in certain gastrointestinal and renal diseases by loss of protein, in liver disease and hypothyroidism by reduced protein synthesis, in congestive heart failure by increases in the plasma volume, and in pregnancy by hemodilution. Infection and zinc depletion also reduce serum albumin levels (Wahlqvist et al., 1981). In the presence of traumatic injury or ongoing stress, a shift of albumin from the intravascular to the extravascular

space also results in a transient fall in serum albumin, whereas in semistarvation the opposite effect occurs. Hence, serum albumin concentrations are artificially elevated in semistarvation (James and Hay, 1968). In patients with dehydration, hyperalbuminemia may also occur as a result of diminished plasma volume.

References

Fulwood R, Johnson C L, Bryner J D et al. (1982). Hematological and nutritional reference data for persons 6 months – 74 years of age: United States, 1976–80. Vital and Health Statistics Series 11, No.232 DHHS Publication No. 83-1682, Washington, DC.

James W P, Hay A M (1968). Albumin metabolism: effect of the nutritional state and the dietary protein intake. Journal of Clinical Investigation 47: 1958–1972.

McPherson I G, Everard D W (1972). Serum albumin estimation: modification of the bromocresol green method. Clinica Chimica Acta 37: 117–121.

Peters T Jr, Biamente G T (1982). Protein (total protein) in serum, urine, and cerebrospinal fluid; albumin in serum. In: Faulkner W R, Meites S (eds). Selected Methods of Clinical Chemistry. Volume 9. American Association for Clinical Chemistry, Washington, D.C. pp. 317.

Sauberlich H E, Dowdy R P, Skala J H (1974). Laboratory Tests for the Assessment of Nutritional Status. CRC Press Inc., Cleveland, Ohio.

Wahlqvist M L, Flint D M, Prinsley D M, Dryden P A (1981). Effect of zinc supplementation on serum albumin and folic acid concentrations in a group of hypo-albuminaemia and hypozincaemia aged persons. In: Howard A N, Baird I M (eds). Recent Advances in Clinical Nutrition. Volume 1. John Libbey, London, pp. 83–84.

Subjects	Deficient	Low	Acceptable
Infants 0 to 11 months	—	< 2.5	≥ 2.5
Children 1 to 5 years	< 2.8	< 3.0	≥ 3.0
Children 6 to 17 years	< 2.8	< 3.5	≥ 3.5
Adults	< 2.8	2.8 to 3.4	≥ 3.5
Preg., 1st trimester	< 3.0	3.0 to 3.9	≥ 4.0
Preg., 2nd & 3rd trim.	< 3.0	3.0 to 3.4	≥ 3.5

Table 7.5: Interpretive guidelines for serum albumin concentrations (g/dL). Conversion factor to SI units (g/L) = × 10.0. Reproduced with permission from Sauberlich HE, Dowdy RP, Skala JH. (1974).

7.3 Serum transthyretin

Principle

Transthyretin (TTR), formally known as thyroxine-binding pre-albumin (TBPA), serves as a transport protein for thyroxine (T_4), and as a carrier protein for retinol binding protein (RBP). Levels of TTR in serum are four to five times higher than those of RBP, and are easier to assay; a single radial immunodiffusion technique is used. For this technique, specific antibodies for the protein under investigation, are incorporated into an agar-gel layer of uniform thickness 1–3 cm which contains a series of small wells at spaced intervals. Three of the wells are filled with three different known concentrations of a specific antigen (i.e. the standard purified serum protein); other wells contain reference, pooled and test serum samples. The plates are left to stand at room temperature, during which time the antigen diffuses radially through the agar, reacts with the antibody incorporated into the agar gel, and eventually forms a diffuse precipitin zone around each well. The zone grows until all the antigen has formed a complex with the antibody. After 48 hours, the diameter of the precipitin zone is measured using a calibrated eyepiece. The concentration of the antigen varies directly with the area of the precipitin zone, which is proportional to the square of the diameter.

Reagents

- Physiological saline: 0.9% NaCl.
- Standard stabilized human serum (available from Behring Diagnostics, Somerville, NJ, 08876, USA). The TTR concentration is shown on the information sheet enclosed with each batch.
- Reference serum (Behring Diagnostics).
- Pooled serum sample (used to assess method precision).
- Sample. Undiluted plasma or serum, either fresh or previously frozen at −20°C.

Equipment

- Immunodiffusion plates. These are available from several companies. LC-Partigen plates for transthyretin are available from Behring Diagnostics. The plates can be used up to the date of expiry on the label. Once opened, a package of plates should be used within a four week period.
- Micropipets 5 μL: Accurate micropipets which will deliver microliter volumes are required (e.g. Hamilton microliter syringes or Eppendorf pipets).
- Partigen measuring device or magnifying glass (×7) with 0.1 mm graduations.
- Narrow beam lamp to illuminate the precipitin rings against a dark background.
- Linear graph paper.

Procedure

Note that care must be taken to ensure that the wells do not overflow. The plates should be stored in a horizontal position on a level surface at room temperature throughout the assay procedure.

1. Prepare, as described below, three different concentrations of the standard human serum with a known TTR concentration (e.g. 25 mg/dL); these are used for the standard curve.

   - Dilute one part standard human serum with three parts 0.9% NaCl giving a concentration of 6.25 mg/dL. Mix with a vortex mixer.
   - Dilute one part standard human serum with one part 0.9% NaCl giving a concentration of 12.5 mg/dL. Mix with a vortex mixer.
   - Use undiluted standard human serum with a concentration of 25 mg/dL.

2. Fill wells 1 to 3 with 5 μL of each of the three standard serum concentrations using a Hamilton syringe or an Eppendorf micropipet.

3. Fill well 4 with 5 μL of undiluted reference serum.

4. Fill well 5 with 5 μL of undiluted pooled serum.

– 111 –

5. Fill additional wells with 5 µL of each of the test serum samples.

6. After loading, allow the plates to stand open for about 10 to 20 minutes, and then close the plates with the plastic lid to protect them from desiccation during incubation.

7. Leave the plates to stand in a horizontal position on a level surface at room temperature for 48 hours. This incubation period allows the diffusion to reach the end-point (i.e. all available antigen has combined with the antibody).

8. After 48 hours, measure the diameter of the precipitin rings (to the nearest 0.1 mm) illuminated by the narrow beam lamp against a dark background using a magnifying glass. Alternatively, the Partigen measuring device can be used. When using the latter, place the device so that the precipitin ring touches both sides of the cone at its greatest diameter; take the measurement at the point of contact between the diameter of the precipitin ring and the markings of the measuring device. Two orthogonal measurements of each precipitin ring should be taken to minimize errors resulting from non-circular rings.

Calculation of results

1. Using linear graph paper, plot the standard concentrations of the antigen (mg/dL) as the abscissa against the mean diffusion ring diameter squared (mm^2) as the ordinate. The calibration line should be straight and intersect the ordinate at $22 \, mm^2 \pm 4.5$.

2. Square the diameter (d^2) of the precipitin ring produced by the reference, pool, and test serum samples, and read off the corresponding concentration of TTR in the serum directly from the standard curve.

3. If the values of d^2 for the rings produced by the reference, pool, or test serum samples lie below the range of the standard curve, then the procedure must be repeated using a lower concentration of the standard human serum.

4. Multiply the concentration of TTR by the appropriate dilution factor, if any, to obtain the correct concentration in the undiluted test serum.

Evaluation

Transthyretin values appear to vary according to age and sex (Carpentier and Ingenbleek, 1983), and possibly with ethnic group and geographical area (Ingenbleek et al., 1975). For this reason, values for TTR should be compared with those of a matched control group. Reported mean concentrations for healthy adult males and females vary widely: the normal lower limit appears to range from 10 mg/dL (Buckell et al., 1979) to 24 mg/dL (Carpentier and Ingenbleek, 1983). Age- and sex-specific interpretive values are not yet available. Tentative interpretive guidelines are: no protein deficit 15–29.6 mg/dL; mild deficit 10–15 mg/dL; moderate deficit 5–10 mg/dL; severe deficit <5 mg/dL (Grant et al., 1981). Ogunshina and Hussain (1980) have provided some preliminary data in relation to stages of protein-energy malnutrition (Fig. 7.1).

Serum TTR is a more sensitive index of protein status and responds more rapidly to dietary treatment than serum albumin or transferrin (Shetty et al., 1979). The presence of other conditions such as gastrointestinal disease, renal or kidney disease, surgical trauma, stress, inflammation, and

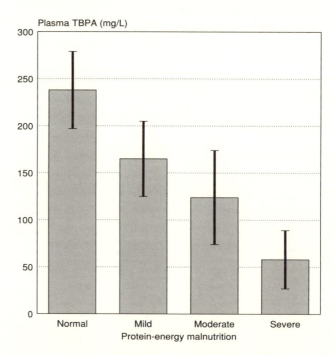

Fig. 7.1: Plasma TTR (mean ± SE) levels in children classified as normal, or with mild, moderate, and severe protein-energy malnutrition according to the Waterlow classification of protein-energy malnutrition. From Ogunshina and Hussain (1980). © Am. J. Clin. Nutr. American Society for Clinical Nutrition.

infection, leads to modifications in the metabolism of TTR and reduces its specificity as an index of protein status (Farthing, 1982). Furthermore, because TTR, like RBP, is extremely sensitive to even minor stress and inflammation, decreasing markedly in such conditions, it is not a very useful index for critically ill patients. Some patients with acute renal failure may have increased serum TTR values because of the role of the kidneys in transthyretin catabolism. Deficiencies of vitamin A, zinc, and iron do not affect the levels of transthyretin.

References

Buckell N A, Lennard-Jones J E, Hernandez M A, Kohn J, Riches P G, Wadsworth J (1979). Measurement of serum proteins during attacks of ulcerative colitis as a guide to patient management. Gut 20: 22–27.

Carpentier Y A, Ingenbleek Y (1983). Serum-thyroxine-binding pre-albumin: an unreliable index of nutritional status? Nutrition Research 3: 617–620.

Farthing M J G (1982). Serum thyroxine-binding pre-albumin: an unreliable index of nutritional status in chronic intestinal disease. Nutrition Research 2: 561–568.

Grant J P, Custer P B, Thurlow J (1981). Current techniques of nutritional assessment. Surgical Clinics of North America 61: 437–463.

Ingenbleek Y, Schrieck H G van den, De Nayer P L, De Visscher M (1975). Albumin, transferrin and the thyroxine-binding pre-albumin/retinol-binding protein (TBPA-RBP) complex in assessment of malnutrition. Clinica Chimica Acta 63: 61–67.

Ogunshina S O, Hussain M A (1980). Plasma thyroxine-binding prealbumin as an index of mild protein-energy malnutrition in Nigerian children. American Journal of Clinical Nutrition 33: 794–800.

Shetty P S, Jung R T, Watrasiewicz K E, James W P T (1979). Rapid-turnover transport proteins: an index of subclinical protein-energy malnutrition. Lancet 2: 230–232.

7.4 Urine creatinine

Principle

Creatinine is derived from the catabolism of creatine phosphate, a metabolite present principally in muscle. When kidney function is normal, creatinine excretion in the urine is used as an index of muscle mass.

Creatinine reacts with picric acid under alkaline conditions to form a characteristic yellow-orange complex (Cook, 1975). The color is derived from creatinine as well as certain non-specific substances likely to be present in the sample. However, when acid is added, the color contributed by creatinine is destroyed; only the color produced by non-specific substances remains. The difference in color intensity measured at 520 nm before and after acidification is proportional to the creatinine concentration. Urinary aceto-acetate interferes with this method, making the creatinine height index an unsuitable index for insulinopenic (type I) diabetic patients who excrete large amounts of the metabolite in their urine. Note that if proteinuria is present, the protein must be removed by precipitation prior to analysis.

Reagents

The reagents listed below can be obtained from the Sigma Chemical Co., St Louis, MO, as a kit. Follow the procedure given by the manufacturer if this differs from that outlined below.

- Sodium hydroxide solution (1.0 N). Store at room temperature.
- Creatinine color reagent. Contains picric acid 0.6%, sodium borate, and surfactant. Store at room temperature.
- Alkaline picrate solution. Prepare by mixing 5 volumes of creatinine color reagent with 1 volume of 1.0 N sodium hydroxide solution. Mixture is stable for at least 1 week if stored in the dark at room temperature. Solution darkens with time, but can still be used.
- Acid reagent. Contains sulfuric acid and acetic acid. Store at room temperature.
- Creatinine standard solution. Contains 3.0 mg/dL (0.26 mmol/L) creatinine in dilute acid solution. Store in refrigerator at 0–5°C.

- Pooled urine sample (used to assess method precision).
- Sample. Twenty-four-hour urine sample containing thymol-isopropanol or toluene. Stable for 24 hours at room temperature or several days at 0–5°C.

Equipment

- Spectrophotometer.
- 1.0 mL and 10 mL graduated pipets; 100 µL micro-pipets.
- Automatic dispensers for creatinine color reagent.

Procedure

1. Select a convenient day for the collection of a twenty-four-hour urine sample.

2. On the morning of the pre-selected day, ask the subject to empty his or her bladder, and discard this initial urine sample. Note the time (e.g. 7.00 a.m.)

3. Save all the urine voided by the subject subsequently, up to and including the urine voided at the same time (i.e. 7.00 a.m.) next day.

4. Measure and record the total volume of the twenty-four-hour urine collection using a 1 L measuring cylinder. Transfer some of the specimen to a storage bottle and label with the subject's name and date. Freeze immediately at −20°C. If the total volume of urine cannot be measured immediately after collection, add 5 mL thymol-isopropanol preservative.

5. Discard the remainder of the urine in the sink while flushing with cold water. Rinse out both the measuring cylinder and the urine collection bottle three times with cold tap water.

6. Dilute both pool and all test urine samples twenty times prior to use by using a pipet to transfer 0.5 mL of each urine into a bottle containing 9.5 mL distilled water. This provides a 1:20 dilution.

Height (cm)	Males Age (yr)							Females Age (yr)						
	20–29	30–39	40–49	50–59	60–69	70–79	80–89	20–29	30–39	40–49	50–59	60–69	70–79	80–89
140								858	804	754	700	651	597	548
142								877	822	771	716	666	610	560
144								898	841	790	733	682	625	573
146	1258	1169	1079	985	896	807	718	917	859	806	749	696	638	586
148	1284	1193	1102	1006	915	824	733	940	881	827	768	713	654	600
150	1308	1215	1123	1025	932	839	747	964	903	848	787	732	671	615
152	1334	1240	1145	1045	951	856	762	984	922	865	803	747	685	628
154	1358	1262	1166	1064	968	872	775	1003	940	882	819	761	698	640
156	1390	1291	1193	1089	990	892	793	1026	961	902	838	779	714	655
158	1423	1322	1222	1115	1014	913	812	1049	983	922	856	796	730	670
160	1452	1349	1246	1137	1035	932	829	1073	1006	944	877	815	747	686
162	1481	1376	1271	1160	1055	950	845	1100	1031	968	899	835	766	703
164	1510	1403	1296	1183	1076	969	862	1125	1054	990	919	854	783	719
166	1536	1427	1318	1203	1094	986	877	1148	1076	1010	938	871	799	733
168	1565	1454	1343	1226	1115	1004	893	1173	1099	1032	958	890	817	749
170	1598	1485	1372	1252	1139	1026	912	1199	1124	1055	980	911	835	766
172	1632	1516	1401	1278	1163	1047	932	1224	1147	1077	1000	929	853	782
174	1666	1548	1430	1305	1187	1069	951	1253	1174	1102	1023	951	872	800
176	1699	1579	1458	1331	1211	1090	970	1280	1199	1126	1045	972	891	817
178	1738	1615	1491	1361	1238	1115	992	1304	1223	1147	1065	990	908	833
180	1781	1655	1529	1395	1269	1143	1017	1331	1248	1171	1087	1011	927	850
182	1819	1690	1561	1425	1296	1167	1038							
184	1855	1724	1592	1453	1322	1190	1059							
186	1894	1579	1625	1483	1349	1215	1081							
188	1932	1795	1658	1513	1377	1240	1103							
190	1968	1829	1689	1542	1402	1263	1123							

Table 7.6: The expected creatinine excretion (mg/day) in males and females of ideal weight. Data from Imbembo A L, Walser M (1984). Nutritional assessment. In: Walser M, Imbembo A L, Margolis S, Elfert G A (eds). Nutritional Management. The Johns Hopkins Handbook. WB Saunders Co., Philadelphia, with permission.

7. Label test tubes: blank, standard, pool, and one for each test sample.

8. To blank add 0.3 mL of distilled-deionized water. To standard add 0.3 mL of the creatinine standard. To pool add 0.3 mL of the pooled urine sample (diluted as above). Add 0.3 mL of each diluted test urine sample to separate tubes.

9. Add 3.0 mL creatinine color reagent to each tube using an automatic dispenser. Mix and allow to stand for 10 to 15 minutes.

10. Set wavelength at 520 nm. Zero the spectrophotometer using the blank.

11. Read and record initial absorbance of standard, pool, and test urine sample. Return samples to tubes.

12. To all tubes add 0.1 mL of the acid reagent. Mix and allow to stand at room temperature for five minutes.

13. Read and record final absorbance of standard, pool, and test samples at 520 nm, again using the blank to zero the spectrophotometer.

Calculation of results

1. Calculate the concentration of creatinine (mg/dL) after dilution, using the formula:

$$\frac{AT_I - AT_F}{AS_I - AS_F} \times C$$

where AT_I = initial absorbance of test,
AT_F = final absorbance of test,
AS_I = initial absorbance of standard,
AS_F = final absorbance of standard,
C = concentration of creatinine standard (3.0 mg/dL).

The conversion to SI units (μmol/L) = ×88.40.

2. Multiply the above result by 20 (the original dilution of urine sample).

3. Divide result by 100 and multiply by the total volume of the twenty-four-hour urine collection (in mL). This gives the creatinine concentration in milligrams per 24 hours. The conversion to SI units (μmol per 24 hours) = ×88.40.

Evaluation

A variety of factors are known to affect daily creatinine excretion and thus limit the validity of urinary creatinine as an index of muscle mass. These include strenuous exercise, emotional stress, menstruation, age, infection, fever, trauma, chronic renal failure, and dietary intakes of creatine and creatinine from meat (Heymsfield et al., 1983).

Two methods for expressing urinary creatinine excretion, the creatinine height index and the creatinine height index as a percentage deficit, are discussed below.

The Creatinine height index (CHI) , expressed as a percentage, can be calculated using the following formula:

$$\frac{\text{Measured 24-hr urinary creat. (mg/day)} \times 100\%}{\text{Expected 24-hr urinary creat. for height, age, and sex}}$$

A creatinine height index of 60% to 80% is said to represent a moderate deficit in body muscle mass, whereas a value of less than 60% may indicate a severe deficit of muscle mass (Blackburn et al., 1977).

Creatinine excretion is generally expressed in relation to height in preference to body weight because height is not affected by adipose tissue and fluid imbalances (e.g. edema). The expected creatinine excretion (mg/day) in males and females of ideal weight, used to determine an age-corrected CHI, is given in Table 7.6.

The CHI is most frequently used to assess the degree of depletion of muscle mass in children with the marasmic form of protein-energy malnutrition. In such subjects, CHI will be lower as a result of loss of lean body mass to maintain serum protein levels. The CHI can also be used to monitor the effects of long-term nutritional intervention on repletion of lean body mass in hospital patients. It is not sensitive to weekly changes in lean body mass and should be used over longer periods. The CHI is also useful for patients for whom measurements of weight and/or skinfolds are unobtainable or inaccurate (e.g. in patients with severe edema, marked obesity, and/or pendulous skinfolds).

The creatinine height index as a percentage deficit is calculated from the CHI using the formula below. A CHI deficit of between 5 and 15% is considered 'mild', 15–30% 'moderate', >30% 'severe'.

$$\text{Percentage deficit} = 100 - \text{CHI}\,(\%)$$

References

Blackburn G L, Bistrian B R, Maini B S, Schlamm H T, Smith M F (1977). Nutritional and metabolic assessment of the hospitalized patient. Journal of Parenteral and Enteral Nutrition 1: 11–22.

Cook J G H (1975). Factors influencing the assay of creatinine. Annals of Clinical Biochemistry 12: 219–232.

Heymsfield S B, Arteaga C, McManus C B, Smith J, Moffitt S (1983). Measurement of muscle mass in humans: validity of the twenty-four-hour urinary creatinine method. American Journal of Clinical Nutrition 37: 478–494.

Imbembo A L, Walser M (1984). Nutritional assessment. In: Walser M, Imbembo A L, Margolis S, Elfert G A (eds). Nutritional Management. The Johns Hopkins Handbook. W.B. Saunders Co., Philadelphia pp. 9–30.

7.5 Amino acid screening test

Principle

A simplified technique to determine serum amino-acid ratios using a finger-prick blood sample and one-dimensional paper chromatography was developed for field survey use by Whitehead and Dean (1964a). For this technique, a small volume of deproteinized serum is streaked onto a piece of chromatography paper and allowed to dry, and then a suitable solvent is allowed to flow (by capillary attraction) over the mixture. As the solvent flows, the amino acids in the serum dissolve and are carried along by the solvent *at different rates*. The separated amino acids are then detected by spraying the dried chromatogram with a solution of ninhydrin in acetone. The amino acids combine with the ninhydrin to give a blue-violet colored compound and so appear as blue-violet spots on the paper. Only the spots corresponding to the NEAA glycine, and the EAA's leucine + valine are cut out, eluted, and the absorption of the eluate measured spectrophotometrically. The following ratio is then calculated:

$$\text{Simplified amino-acid ratio} = \frac{\text{Glycine}}{\text{Leucine} + \text{valine}}$$

Reagents

- Solvent. Mix together thoroughly: 30 mL acetic acid, 120 mL iso-butanol, and 50 mL distilled water. Use the upper layer for developing the chromatogram. The same solution may be used for three runs.

- Ninhydrin 0.2%. Dissolve 0.2 g of ninhydrin in 100 mL of acetone. Use this solution once only.

- Copper nitrate solution: Mix 100 mL of 96% ethyl alcohol with 1 mL of a saturated solution of copper nitrate and add 0.2 mL of 10% nitric acid.

- Methanol.

- 10% Isopropanol.

- Standard amino acids: leucine, valine, glycine.

- Sample. Serum or plasma from a fasting blood sample is preferred. Alternatively, blood samples should be taken four hours after the most recent meal. N.B. Do not use serum that has been refrozen after thawing.

Equipment

- Centrifuge tubes (15 mL); boiling tubes.
- 5 mL pipets; Eppendorf pipets.
- Flat-bottomed tubes (20 × 50 mm).
- Whatman No. 1 chromatography paper.
- Chromatography tank.
- Boiling water bath; electric fan; oven; hair dryer.
- Spectrophotometer.

Procedure

1. Pipet into separate 15 mL centrifuge tubes 100 μL of each test serum. Add rapidly to each tube 4 mL 90% ethyl alcohol. Mix the tubes vigorously, allow to stand for 10 minutes, and then centrifuge for about 10 minutes to precipitate the protein.

2. Transfer the supernatant liquid from each centrifuge tube to a flat-bottomed tube (20 × 50 mm) and evaporate to dryness on a boiling water bath. Remove the tube from the water bath *immediately* after the alcohol has evaporated because prolonged heating causes considerable loss of the amino acids. An electric fan may be used in place of a water bath.

3. Completely dissolve the residue in each flat-bottomed tube in 100 μL of 10% isopropanol. As the residue is fatty, the last remnants must often be dislodged with a glass rod.

4. Transfer 25 μL of the 100 μL extract from each flat-bottomed tube to a Whatman No. 1 chromatography paper on a line 5 cm from the bottom and apply it as a streak 2 cm long (Fig. 7.2). Dry the streak with a hair dryer between applications. An exact quantitative transfer is not necessary, as it is the ratio that is estimated, not the absolute amounts.

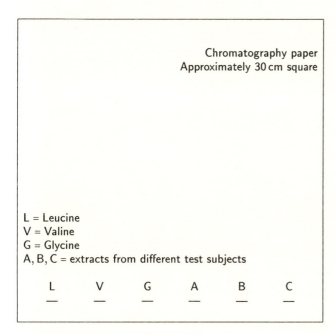

Fig. 7.2: Diagram showing the positioning of the sample and standards on a typical one dimensional ascending chromatography sheet when used in the amino-acid screening test.

5. Streak on 25 µL of the three standard amino acids—leucine, valine, and glycine—2 cm apart at the left hand side of the paper.

6. Run the paper in a tank overnight in the solvent. A satisfactory separation has been achieved when the solvent front has risen about 20 cm.

7. Remove the paper from the tank and dry it with an electric fan. The acetic acid must be completely evaporated before staining and the paper should not smell of acetic acid when dry.

8. Rapidly soak or spray the paper in the solution of ninhydrin-acetone and dry for five minutes.

9. When the acetone has evaporated, after a few minutes drying time at room temperature, develop the amino-acid spots in an oven at $105 \pm 5°C$ for five minutes. The temperature should not fall below 90°C during this development process.

10. Stabilize the color by dipping the paper through a copper nitrate solution. Dry the paper at room temperature; the blue ninhydrin spots will become red-brown.

11. Ring the compounds selected for analysis with a pencil. The non-essential amino-acid spot is not well separated from its neighbours, but it

is easily identified as the largest spot on the chromatogram.

12. Cut out each of the spots containing leucine + iso-leucine (Rf 0.67), valine + methionine (Rf 0.51), and glycine + glutamine + serine (Rf 0.13) (Fig. 7.3).

13. Place the paper containing each spot in a separate boiling tube.

14. Extract the color, using 4 mL of methanol for twenty minutes, occasionally gently agitating the boiling tubes to complete the extraction.

15. Read the absorbance at 507 nm. Use methanol as the blank to zero the spectrophotometer. The color is stable for at least four hours in daylight.

Calculation of results

The ratio of the non-essential: essential amino-acids ratio (NEAA : EAA) is calculated as the absorbance of the eluate for:

$$\frac{\text{Glycine} + \text{Glutamine} + \text{Serine}}{\text{Leucine} + \text{Iso-leucine} + \text{Valine} + \text{Methionine}}$$

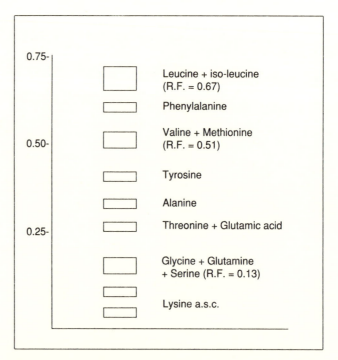

Fig. 7.3: The separation of the more important amino-acids on a chromatogram.

Evaluation

Serum NEAA:EAA ratios >3.0 for all ages are considered high risk for kwashiorkor, ratios 2.0–3.0 medium risk, and those <2.0 low risk for kwashiorkor (Sauberlich et al., 1974). The ratio of NEAA to EAA rises in the serum of children with kwashiorkor because the the branched-chain amino acids leucine, iso-leucine, and valine, as well as methionine, fall to low concentrations whereas the NEAA, especially glycine, tend to remain normal or even rise. Such changes in serum amino-acid levels are not found in normal children, or those with marasmus (Whitehead and Dean, 1964b). Nevertheless, the ratios are not always consistent with the type or severity of protein-energy malnutrition because of the confounding effects of infections, diarrhea, energy deficits, etc. The resulting rather low sensitivity and specificity of the NEAA:EAA ratio has limited its use (Simmons, 1970).

The absence of elevated serum NEAA:EAA ratios in children with marasmus may result from a metabolic adaptation to an inadequate energy intake. Children with marasmus have low serum insulin concentrations in response to their reduced food intake (Coward and Lunn, 1981). Low serum insulin concentrations may induce the release of energy metabolites from endogenous sources; as a result, EAA are released from skeletal muscle for gluconeogenesis and probably for serum protein synthesis in the liver, maintaining the serum amino-acid ratio within normal levels.

References

Coward W A, Lunn P G (1981). The biochemistry and physiology of kwashiorkor. British Medical Bulletin 37: 19–24.

Sauberlich H E, Dowdy R P, Skala J H (1974). Laboratory Tests for the Assessment of Nutritional Status. CRC Press Inc., Cleveland, Ohio.

Simmons W K (1970). The plasma amino acid ratio as an indicator of the protein nutrition status: A review of recent work. Bulletin of the World Health Organization 42: 480–484.

Whitehead R G, Dean R F A (1964a). Serum amino acids in kwashiorkor. An abbreviated method of estimation and its application. American Journal of Clinical Nutrition 14: 320–330.

Whitehead R G, Dean R F A (1964b). Serum amino acids in kwashiorkor. I. Relationship to clinical conditions. American Journal of Clinical Nutrition 14: 313–319.

7.6 Urinary urea nitrogen

Principle

The enzyme urease splits urea into carbon dioxide and ammonia.

$$H_2N\text{-}CO\text{-}NH_2 + H_2O \rightarrow 2NH_3 + CO_2$$

The ammonia liberated is determined using the reaction of Berthelot. The ammonia reacts with phenol-hypochlorite reagent to give a blue colored complex which is measured at 624 nm. Sodium nitroprusside is added as a catalyst (Searcy et al., 1965). The room used for the determination must be free of other sources of ammonia vapour, as these interfere with the determination.

Reagents

The reagents listed below can be obtained from the Sigma Chemical Co., St Louis, MO, as a kit. Follow the procedure given by the manufacturer if this differs from that outlined below.

- Phosphate buffer, pH 6.8. Dissolve 3.6 g of KH_2PO_4 and 6.4 g of $Na_2HPO_4.12H_2O$ in 500 mL deionized water.

- Urease solution. Dissolve 75 mg urease (Sigma Type III from jack beans) in 50 mL of phosphate buffer. Alternatively, completely dissolve a 50 mg urease tablet in 35 mL of buffer. Refrigerate for up to one month.

- Urea nitrogen standard, 20 mg/dL. Dry about 1 g of reagent grade urea in a desiccator overnight. Dissolve exactly 0.2145 g of the urea in distilled water and make up to 500 mL. Add a few drops of chloroform as preservative and store in a brown bottle in a refrigerator.

- Phenol reagent. Dissolve 10 g of phenol and 50 mg of sodium nitroprusside in distilled water and make up to 200 mL. Store in a brown bottle in a refrigerator. Stable for about two months. The reagent must not come into contact with the skin.

- Hypochlorite reagent. In a 200 mL volumetric flask, dissolve 5.0 g of sodium hydroxide in about 50 mL distilled water. Add 4 mL of 'Chlorox' or 'Purex' or a similar commercial bleach containing about 5.25% sodium hypochlorite, and make up to the 200 mL mark with distilled water. Store in a brown bottle in the refrigerator. Stable for about one month.

- Pooled urine sample (to assess precision).

- Sample. Twenty-four-hour urine sample containing thymol-isopropanol or toluene. Stable for 24 hours at room temperature or several days at 0–5°C.

Equipment

- Spectrophotometer.
- Waterbath at 37°C.
- Micro-pipets: 20 μL; 200 μL.
- 10 mL pipets.
- Automatic dispensers.
- Stop watch; vortex mixer.
- Large test tubes.

Procedure

1. Select a convenient day for the collection of a twenty-four-hour urine sample.

2. On the morning of the pre-selected day, ask the subject to empty his or her bladder, and discard this initial urine sample. Note the time (e.g. 7.00 a.m.)

3. Save all the urine voided by the subject subsequently, up to and including the urine voided at the same time (i.e. 7.00 a.m.) next day.

4. Measure and record the total volume of the twenty-four-hour urine collection using a 1 L measuring cylinder. Transfer some of the specimen to a storage bottle and label with the subject's name and date. Freeze immediately at −20°C. Note that if the total volume of urine cannot be measured immediately after collection, add 5 mL thymol-isopropanol preservative.

5. Discard the remainder of the urine in the sink while flushing with water. Rinse the measuring cylinder and the urine collection bottle three times with cold tap water.

6. Dilute both pool and all test urine samples twenty times prior to use by using a pipet to transfer 0.5 mL of each urine into a bottle containing 9.5 mL distilled water. This provides a 1:20 dilution.

7. Prepare and label a series of large test tubes: blank, standard, pool and one for each test sample.

8. To the blank add 20 µL of distilled deionized water. To the standard add 20 µL of the urea-nitrogen standard. To pool add 20 µL of the pooled diluted urine sample. Add 20 µL of each of the diluted test urine samples to separate tubes.

9. Pre-incubate the large test tubes for about five minutes in a water bath at 37°C.

10. Add 200 µL urease solution to each tube at exactly one minute intervals.

11. Mix by rotating the tubes in a near horizontal position. Then incubate each tube for exactly 15 minutes in a water bath at 37°C.

12. At the end of the incubation period, add, at the timed interval, 1 mL of phenol reagent and 1 mL hypochlorite reagent to each tube with an automatic dispenser. Note that the phenol reagent should be added first.

13. Develop the color by incubating the tubes for exactly five minutes more in the water bath at 37°C.

14. Add 8.0 mL distilled water to each tube and mix with a Vortex mixer.

15. Set the wavelength at 625 nm. Zero the spectrophotometer using the reagent blank.

16. Read and record the absorbance of the standard, pool and test samples. If the absorbance exceeds 1.00, dilute quantitatively with distilled water.

Calculation of results

1. The concentration of urea nitrogen in the test sample is given by the following formula:

$$\text{Urea-nitrogen (mg/dL)} = \frac{A_{test} \times C_{standard}}{A_{standard}}$$

where A_{test} = absorbance of test sample,
$A_{standard}$ = absorbance of standard, and
$C_{standard}$ = urea-nitrogen concentration in standard (e.g. 20 mg/dL)

2. Multiply the above result by 20 (original dilution of urine sample).

3. Divide the result by 100 and multiply by the total volume of the twenty-four-hour urine collection (in mL). This gives urea-nitrogen in milligrams per 24 hours. Divide result by 1000 to give the urea-nitrogen in grams per 24 hours. The conversion to SI units (mmol/24 hours) = ×35.70.

Evaluation

The concentration of urea-nitrogen in the urine depends on the protein intake, kidney function, and urine volume. The normal range for urinary urea-nitrogen excretion is from 9.3–16.2 g/day.

The estimated nitrogen balance indicates the net change in the total body protein mass. It can be calculated from the urinary urea nitrogen by employing the equation shown below. At least three consecutive, complete twenty-four-hour urine collections are required.

Balance = Prot. intake (g)/6.25 − Urinary urea N_2 (g) + 4 g

In this equation, nitrogen intake is estimated from the protein intake, assuming that protein contains 16% nitrogen in a mixed diet. If parenteral solutions containing free amino acids are used, specific conversion factors should be used to calculate their nitrogen content exactly. The constant (4 g) in the equation above represents two correction factors: (a) 2 g for dermal and fecal losses of nitrogen which occur but are not measured; and (b) 2 g for the non-urea nitrogen components of the urine (e.g. ammonia, uric acid, and creatinine) (MacKenzie et al., 1985).

When the method is used in hospital patients, it is preferable to use at least three consecutive, complete twenty-four-hour urine collections because intra-subject variation for urinary nitrogen excretion can be large. Care must be taken to avoid spills, discards, or inadvertent omissions of urine during collection, because these lead to a positive error in the nitrogen balance.

Healthy adults with adequate energy and nutrient intakes should be in nitrogen balance (i.e. intakes are adequate to replace the endogenous nitrogen losses and for the growth of the hair and nails). When nitrogen intake exceeds nitrogen output, subjects are in positive balance.

This occurs during growth, late pregnancy, athletic training, and recovery from illness. In contrast, when nitrogen output exceeds nitrogen intake, subjects are in negative nitrogen balance. A negative nitrogen balance of 1 g/day is equivalent to a reduction in total body protein of 6.25 g/day. If the negative balance persists, the resultant protein depletion may have adverse effects on all organ systems. Factors which may precipitate a negative nitrogen balance include: inadequate protein and/or energy intakes; an imbalance in EAA:NEAA; conditions of accelerated protein catabolism (e.g. trauma, infection, sepsis, and burns) and excessive losses of nitrogen arising from fistulas or excessive diarrhea. The range of nitrogen balance values observed in hospital patients can vary from $+4$ to -20 grams of nitrogen per day. An estimate of the change in nitrogen balance, rather than a single measurement, is preferred to monitor the effectiveness of nutritional therapy.

The estimated nitrogen balance equation is not appropriate in certain circumstances. In patients with malabsorption, fecal nitrogen losses may be as high as 3.5 g/day, making the correction factor of two grams for dermal and fecal losses of nitrogen inappropriate. During severe energy restriction or starvation, the production of renal ammonia is increased to such an extent that the non-urea nitrogen correction factor of two grams is inadequate (Winterer et al., 1980). When protein intakes are low, urinary urea nitrogen excretion is no longer a valid index of total urinary nitrogen excretion because it accounts for a decreasing percentage of total urinary nitrogen excretion (e.g. 61% to 70% compared to more than 80% to 90% on a normal mixed diet) (Allison and Bird, 1977). In contrast, increased excretion of urea (ureagenesis) occurs when diets are based on proteins of low biological value, or when parenteral or enteral solutions containing certain amino acids (e.g. arginine and glutamine) are administered.

The adjusted nitrogen balance takes into account changes in body urea nitrogen (BUN) in nitrogen-retention diseases such as renal or hepatic failure. It can be calculated using the following equations:

$$\text{Measured N balance} - \text{change in BUN}$$

where the change in BUN equals:

$$((SUN_f - SUN_i) \times BW_i \times 0.6) + ((BW_f - BW_i) \times SUN_f)$$

$$\text{where BW} = \text{body weight (kg)}$$
$$SUN = \text{serum urea nitrogen (g/L)}$$

In this equation the suffixes i and f indicate the initial and final values of the measurement (Harvey et al., 1980). The fraction of the body weight that is water is assumed to be 0.6. Unfortunately, this fraction varies with the age and condition of the patient and no simple corrections are available. For example, in lean patients or those with edema, the fraction (i.e. 0.6) is too low whereas in obese or very young persons, the fraction is too high (Kopple, 1987).

The apparent net protein utilization can be calculated using the following formula:

$$\left(\frac{P}{6.25} - (UUN + 2) - N_L \right) \div \frac{P}{6.25}$$

$$\text{where P} = \text{protein intake (g)}$$
$$UUN = \text{urinary urea nitrogen (g)}$$
$$\text{and } N_L = \text{obligatory nitrogen loss}$$

N_L is approximately 0.1 g for each kilogram of ideal body weight (Blackburn et al., 1977).

The urinary urea nitrogen:creatinine ratio indicates the abundance of urea nitrogen relative to creatinine in the urine. It is calculated using the following formula:

$$\frac{\text{mg urea nitrogen/mL urine}}{\text{mg creatinine/mL urine}}$$

A ratio of >12.0 is defined as 'acceptable' (low risk), 6.0–12.0 as 'low' (medium risk), and <6.0 as 'deficient' (high risk) (Sauberlich et al., 1974). These values are, however, tentative because of the uncertain effects of age.

The urinary urea nitrogen:creatinine ratio is used in field surveys to assess the adequacy of recent dietary protein intake (Simmons, 1972). It does not provide an index of long-term protein status. The next urine sample after the first-voided morning fasting sample should be used to calculate this ratio. Creatinine excretion is measured to take into account variations in urine volume, on the assumption that excretion of creatinine is relatively constant over a twenty-four-hour period.

Several extraneous factors can affect urinary urea nitrogen:creatinine ratios. Those specific for creatinine are noted in Section 7.4. Conditions such as trauma, sepsis, infections, burns, fistulas, and diarrhea all increase the level of urinary nitrogen excretion and hence, in turn, excretion of urea. The latter is also influenced by the presence of urinary tract infections which reduce the glomerular filtration rate.

References

Allison J B, Bird J W C (1977). Elimination of nitrogen from the body. In: Munro H N, Allison J B (eds). Mammalian Protein Metabolism. Volume 1. American Medical Association, Chicago, pp. 141–146.

Blackburn G L, Bistrian B R, Maini B S, Schlamm H T, Smith M F (1977). Nutritional and metabolic assessment of the hospitalized patient. Journal of Parenteral and Enteral Nutrition 1: pp. 11–22.

Harvey K B, Blumenkrantz M J, Levine S E, Blackburn G L (1980). Nutritional assessment and treatment of chronic renal failure. American Journal of Clinical Nutrition 33: 1586–1597.

Kopple J D (1987). Uses and limitations of the balance technique. Journal of Parenteral and Enteral Nutrition 1: pp. 27–29.

MacKenzie T A, Clark N G, Bistrian B R, Flatt J P, Hallowell E M, Blackburn G L (1985). A simple method for estimating nitrogen balance in hospitalized patients: a review and supporting data for a previously proposed technique. Journal of the American College of Nutrition 4: pp. 575–581.

Sauberlich H E, Dowdy R P, Skala J H (1974). Laboratory Tests for the Assessment of Nutritional Status. CRC Press Inc., Cleveland, Ohio.

Searcy R L, Simms N M, Foreman J A, Bergquist L M (1965). A study of the specificity of the Berthelot color reaction. Clinica Chimica Acta 12: pp. 170–175.

Simmons W K (1972). Urinary urea nitrogen-creatinine ratio as an indicator of recent protein intake in field studies. American Journal of Clinical Nutrition 25: pp. 539–542.

Winterer J, Bistrian B R, Bilmazes C, Blackburn G L, Young V R (1980). Whole body protein turnover studied with 15N-glycine, and muscle protein breakdown in mildly obese subjects during a protein-sparing diet and a brief total fast. Metabolism 29: pp. 575–581.

7.7 Urinary hydroxyproline

Principle

Urinary 3-hydroxyproline, mainly in the peptide form, is an excretory product derived from the soluble and insoluble collagens of both the soft and calcified tissues. Urinary hydroxproline excretion levels are low in malnourished children with impaired growth, irrespective of the type of malnutrition. In adults, levels of 3-hydroxyproline in the urine are often used to diagnose certain bone and connective tissue or endocrine disorders. The colorimetric method used for rapid assay of 3-hydroxyproline in urine is based on the oxidation of hydroxyproline to pyrrole, which is then coupled with ρ-dimethylamino-benzaldehyde to form a red chromophore (Prockop and Udenfriend, 1960). In the method outlined below, chloramine-T is employed as the oxidant (Dabev and Struck, 1971).

Reagents

The three buffer solutions listed below are stable at 4°C for several months.

- Buffer-stock solution pH 6.0. In a 250 mL beaker containing 100 mL of double distilled deionized water, dissolve 12.5 g citric acid, 3 mL 96% acetic acid and 30.0 g sodium acetate (trihydrate), successively. Adjust the pH of this solution to pH 6.0 using 50% w/v solution of sodium hydroxide. Then transfer to a 250 mL volumetric flask and dilute to volume with double distilled deionized water.

- Buffer for chloramine-T solution. To 100 mL of the buffer-stock solution, add 20 mL distilled water and 30 mL 1-propanol.

- Buffer for color reaction. To 100 mL of the buffer stock solution add 80 mL of distilled water and 100 mL 1-propanol.

- Chloramine-T solution. 282 mg of chloramine-T (sodium N-chloro-p-toluenesulfonamide) should be dissolved in 2 mL distilled water in a 50 mL volumetric flask. Then add 2 mL 1-propanol, and make up to 50 mL with buffer. Store in a dark bottle. Stable for 2–3 weeks at 4°C. For best results make fresh weekly.

- Perchloric acid (60%). Add 85.7 mL of 70% perchloric acid to 10 mL disilled water and bring the volume to 100 mL with distilled water.

- Color reagent. In a 50 mL beaker suspend 3 g of ρ-dimethylamino-benzaldehyde in 12 mL 1-propanol. Add 5.2 mL 60% perchloric acid and then adjust the volume to 20 mL with 1-propanol. Make fresh daily.

- Charcoal and resin. Mix 20 g Zeolite with 10 g Norite. Wash the mixture four times with about 100 mL 6N hydrochloric acid in a coarse sintered glass funnel, four times with ethanol, and then four times with about 100 mL ether. Dry the mixture at 60°C overnight.

- 1-Propanol

- Sodium hydroxide solution 50% w/v. In a beaker dissolve 50 g sodium hydroxide in 100 mL distilled water. Store in a plastic bottle.

- Hydrochloric acid solution (0.001 N). Add 0.08 mL hydrochloric acid to 100 mL distilled water and make up the volume to 1 L with distilled water.

- Hydroxyproline stock solution. Dissolve 10.0 mg L-hydroxyproline in 100 mL 0.001 N hydrochloric acid. Stable at 4°C for one month.

- Hydroxyproline solutions for standard curve. Prepare three standard solutions containing 1, 2, and 5 µg/mL hydroxyproline by diluting 1, 2, and 5 mL of hydroxyproline solution respectively to 100 mL with 0.001 N hydrochloric acid. Must be prepared daily.

- Pooled urine sample (used to assess method precision).

- Sample. Twenty-four-hour urine sample containing thymol-isopropanol or toluene. Stable for 24 hours at room temperature or several days at 0–5°C.

Equipment

- Micro-pipets: 200–1000 µL.
- Glass screw cap culture tubes (12 × 75 mm).

- Adjustable water bath.

- Test-tube rack.

- Spectrophotometer and microcuvets.

Procedure

1. Select a convenient day for the collection of a twenty-four-hour urine sample.

2. On the morning of the pre-selected day, ask the subject to empty his or her bladder, and discard this initial urine sample. Note the time (e.g. 7.00 a.m.)

3. Save all the urine voided by the subject subsequently, up to and including the urine voided at the same time (i.e. 7.00 a.m.) next day.

4. Measure and record the total volume of the twenty-four-hour urine collection using a 1 L measuring cylinder. Transfer some of the specimen to a storage bottle and label with the subject's name and date. Freeze immediately at $-20°$C. Note that if the total volume of urine cannot be measured immediately at the end of collection, then 5 mL of thymol-isopropanol should be added as a preservative.

5. Discard the remainder of the urine in the sink while flushing with cold water. Rinse both the measuring cylinder and the urine collection bottle three times with cold tap water.

6. Prepare and label a series of culture tubes: blank 1, blank 2, standard 1 (1 µg/mL), standard 2 (2 µg/mL) and standard 5 (5 µg/mL), pool, and one for each test sample.

7. To the blanks add 500 µL of distilled water. To the standards add 500 µL of the standard solutions containing 1, 2, and 5 µg hydroxyproline per mL. sample. To pool add 1 mL of pooled urine sample. To each test add 1 mL of the appropriate test urine sample.

8. Add 1 mL concentrated hydrochloric acid to each tube and heat tubes for 24 hours in an 120°C oven.

9. Cool tubes and then add approximately 0.25 g charcoal and resin into each tube. Shake each tube and then allow to stand for ten minutes.

10. Centrifuge the tubes and then transfer 2 × 0.5 mL aliquots of the clear supernatant from each tube into a labeled 12 × 75 mm glass culture tube. Dry each aliquot at room temperature under a stream of air.

11. Dissolve each dried sample in 500 µL distilled water and then mix with 500 µL of the color reaction buffer and 200 µL chloramine-T-solution at room temperature.

12. After 20 minutes, add 200 µL of the color reagent to each tube, shake, and then incubate samples in a water bath for 15 minutes at 60°C.

13. Cool tubes under tap water. Set the wavelength of the spectrophotometer to 560 nm. Zero the spectrophotometer using the reagent blank.

14. Read and record absorbance of the standards, pool and test samples within 45 minutes.

15. Plot the standard concentrations (µg/mL) as the abscissa against their absorbance as the ordinate.

Calculation of results

1. Read the hydroxyproline concentrations of the test and pooled urine samples (µg/mL) directly from the calibration curve.

2. Divide the result by 1000 and multiply by the appropriate total twenty-four-hour volume of urine (in mL). This gives the hydroxyproline in milligrams per 24 hours. The conversion to SI units (µmol/24 hours) = ×76.26.

Evaluation

Marked changes in hydroxyproline excretion with age and sex occur. As a result, investigators have developed methods for evaluating urinary hydroxyproline excretion which are independent of age.

The hydroxyproline : creatinine ratio may be calculated using the formula

$$\frac{\text{Hydroxyproline (mg) per 24 hr}}{\text{Creatinine (mg) per 24 hr}}$$

This ratio corrects at least partially for differences in adult body size. As a result, ratios in adults are independent of age and are the same for males and females aged 20 to 70 years (F: 0.028 ± 0.002;

M: 0.025 ± 0.002) (Allison et al., 1966). For children, however, the ratio changes rapidly with age; hydroxyproline decreases with age while creatinine excretion increases. Such age-related changes in hydroxyproline excretion are associated with differences in growth velocity. Other factors influencing urinary hydroxyproline excretion include the ingestion of collagen or gelatin, the presence of certain disease states, and hookworm and/or malarial infestation (Le Roy, 1967).

The hydroxyproline index takes body weight into account, forms an age-independent interpretive standard for children, and is given by the formula:

$$\frac{\text{mg hydroxyproline per mL urine}}{\text{mg creatinine per mL urine}} \times \text{kg body weight}$$

Interpretive guidelines for the index, applicable to infants and children from three months to ten years of age are: deficient (high risk) <1.0; low (medium risk) 1.0–2.0; and acceptable (low risk) >2.0 (Sauberlich et al., 1974).

In normal children between one and six years of age, the hydroxyproline index is relatively constant and is approximately 3.0. In malnourished children, however, the hydroxyproline index is low, irrespective of the type of malnutrition, but is statistically related to the extent of the growth deficit (Whitehead, 1965).

References

Allison D J, Walker A, Smith Q T (1966). Urinary hydroxyproline: creatinine ratio of normal humans at various ages. Clinica Chimica Acta 14: 729–734.

Dabev D, Struck H (1971). Microliter determination of free hydroxyproline in blood serum. Biochemical Medicine 5: 17–21.

Le Roy E C (1967). The technique and significance of hydroxyproline measurement in man. Advances in Clinical Chemistry 10: 213–253.

Prockop D J, Udenfriend S (1960). Analysis of hydroxyproline in tissues and urine. Analytical Biochemistry 1: 228–239.

Sauberlich H E, Dowdy R P, Skala J H (1974). Laboratory Tests for the Assessment of Nutritional Status. CRC Press Inc., Cleveland, Ohio.

Whitehead R G (1965). Hydroxyproline creatinine ratio as an index of nutritional status and rate of growth. Lancet 2: 567–570.

Whitehead R G (1967). Biochemical tests in differential diagnosis of protein and calorie deficiencies. Archives of Disease in Childhood 42: 475–484.

Chapter 8
Hematology

Contents

Introduction

Hematology is the study of blood, a mixture of red cells (erythrocytes), white cells (leukocytes), and platelets (thrombocytes) suspended in the plasma, a straw-colored aqueous fluid containing minerals and proteins. The hematological parameters most frequently used in nutritional assessment are included in a complete blood count (CBC), but erythrocyte sedimentation rate, reticulocyte count, osmotic fragility, blood coagulation, and bone marrow characteristics are also used (Wintrobe et al., 1981; Brown, 1988; Chanarin, 1989). The CBC consists of a hemoglobin, hematocrit, red cell count, platelet count, the number and type of white blood cells (i.e. differential leukocyte count), and three red cell indices: mean cell volume (MCV), mean cell hemoglobin (MCH), and mean cell hemoglobin concentration (MCHC).

Measurement of the concentration of hemoglobin in whole blood is probably the most widely used screening test for iron-deficiency anemia (Chapter 9). A low hemoglobin concentration is associated with hypochromia, a characteristic feature of iron-deficiency anemia. The hematocrit is defined in SI units as the volume fraction of packed red cells. It also falls during iron deficiency, but only after hemoglobin formation has become impaired. The red blood cell count is the number of red blood cells in one liter. The count is low in severe anemia but high in polycythemia.

Red cell indices are used to characterize three types of anemias: (a) normocytic, normochromic; (b) microcytic, hypochromic; and (c) macrocytic, normochromic. Vitamin B-12 and/or folic acid deficiencies are associated with macrocytic normochromic anemias, and microcytic hypochromic anemias with deficiencies of iron and vitamin B-6.

Measurements may involve the collection of venous and/or capillary blood specimens, preparation and staining of peripheral blood smears, and the collection and staining of bone marrow specimens.

References

Brown B A (1988). Hematology: Principles and Procedures. Lea and Febiger, Philadelphia, pp. 87–92.

Chanarin I (ed) (1989). Laboratory Haematology An Account of Laboratory Techniques. Churchill Livingstone, Edinburgh, pp. 11–12.

Wintrobe M M, Lee G R, Boggs D R, Bithell T C, Foerster J, Athens J W, Lukens J N (eds) (1981). Clinical Hematology. Eighth edition, Lea and Febiger, Philadelphia.

8.1 Blood smear

Principle

A microscopic examination of a stained blood smear provides information on the red cell (erythrocyte), platelet, and white cell (leukocyte) status of the subject (Turgeon, 1988). It can also be used for a neutrophil lobe count.

The erythrocytes are produced in the bone marrow by a process termed erythropoiesis, during which hemoglobin is synthesized in the erythrocytes. The heme pigment of hemoglobin is responsible for transporting oxygen to the tissues and carbon dioxide from the tissues. Protein, iron, vitamin B-12, vitamin B-6, folic acid, and cobalt are required for normal erythrocyte and hemoglobin production. Hence, deficiencies of these nutrients may result in abnormalities in the size, shape, color, and distribution of erythrocytes, all apparent in a stained blood smear. The presence of certain inclusions in erythrocytes, such as malarial parasites, can also be seen.

Mature platelets (thrombocytes) are produced from megakaryocytes in the bone marrow. They respond to vascular damage by adhering to the subendothelial lining and exposed collagen of the intima of the blood vessel, when they undergo aggregation. The latter is accompanied by the release of active constituents which promote further platelet aggregation, vaso-constriction of blood vessels, and acceleration of blood coagulation. Megaloblastic anemias arising from deficiencies of vitamin B-12 and folic acid, and iron deficiency anemia, cause a decrease in the production of platelets (i.e. thrombocytopenia).

Differential leukocyte counts on stained blood smears determine the relative number of each type of the three major classes of leukocytes: granulocytes, monocytes, and lymphocytes. Granulocytes can be further subdivided into neutrophils, eosinophils, and basophils, all of which function in phagocytosis, a body defense mechanism. Monocytes also function in phagocytosis, and when mature, are the largest cells in the peripheral blood. Monocytes also synthesize various substances such as transferrin, complement, interferon, and certain growth factors. Normal healthy children and adults have a relatively consistent population of each of the granulocytic and monocytic types of leukocytes.

Lymphocytes are produced in the bone marrow and in the thymus. B-lymphocytes are derived from the bone marrow, and, in general, are responsible for humoral immunity, producing antibodies (IgM, -A, -D, -E, -G) in response to specific antigens. B-lymphocytes make up 20% to 30% of peripheral blood lymphocytes. Lymphocytes originating from the thymus are called T-cells; they are responsible for mediating cell-mediated immunity reactions. Subjects suffering from malnutrition may develop lymphocytopenia—a reduction in the blood lymphocyte count.

Reagents

- Alcohol (70%) and alcohol wipes.
- EDTA-anticoagulated whole blood or free-flowing capillary blood. Note: If EDTA is used, prepare smears within one hour of blood collection.
- Wright's stain.

Equipment

- Sterile disposable blood lancets.
- Disposable gloves; sterile gauze.
- Clean glass slides–plain with one frosted end.
- Staining rack.
- Manual cell counter designed for differential counts.
- Microscope, immersion oil, lens paper.
- Set of reference slides.

Procedure

Prepare duplicate blood smears for each subject, using the following procedure. The thinner, more uniform of the two smears should be used for measurements.

1. Massage the third or fourth finger of the subject several times to warm the finger and to ensure a free flow of blood. Alternatively, place a warm cloth around the finger for a few minutes to increase the circulation of blood.

2. Clean the finger tip with 70% alcohol and dry with a sterile gauze.

3. Hold the finger with the thumb and index finger of a gloved hand and puncture the finger tip across the creases of the finger-print with a sterile lancet. Discard lancet in a puncture-proof container.

4. Wipe away the first drop of blood because it is mixed with lymphatic fluid and possibly alcohol.

5. Apply *gentle* pressure just below the finger tip to obtain subsequent drops of blood free of lymphatic fluid.

6. Place a small drop of blood (approximately 2 mm diameter) near the frosted end of a clean glass slide.

7. Place the slide on a flat surface with the blood specimen to the right.

8. Place a second spreader glass slide at an angle of 45°, just in front of the drop of blood.

9. Gently draw the spreader slide back towards the drop of blood and allow the blood to spread three-fourths along the bevel edge of the spreader slide but not to the edges. Gently push the spreader slide evenly forward (away from the drop), continuing to the end of the slide (Fig. 8.1).

10. Allow the blood smear to air dry before stain-ing, and label the frosted end with a pencil with the subject identifier.

11. Place the dried slide on a level staining rack with the smear side facing upward.

12. Use a pasteur pipet to place freshly filtered Wright's stain slowly on the slide until the smear is completely covered.

13. After two to three minutes, slowly add two to three volumes of buffer solution to the stain with a pasteur pipet, taking care to avoid washing off the stain. The buffer should form a large 'blob' on the slide.

14. Mix the diluted stain by gently blowing on the slide. A metallic scum should appear on the surface of the diluted stain.

15. Let the slide stand for three to five minutes and then wash off the stain and buffer with a gentle flow of tap water.

16. Wipe the underside of the slide to remove any stain and air dry. The slide must not be blotted dry.

17. Focus the microscope on the slide using the ×10 (low power) objective. Scan the blood smear to check for a thin area where the red cells are barely overlapping.

18. Add a drop of immersion oil, and switch to the high power (×100) (oil immersion) objective.

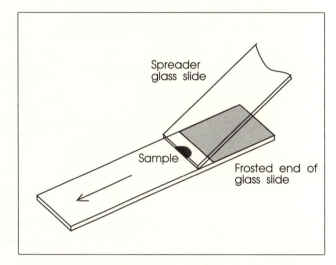

Fig. 8.1: The preparation of a blood smear using two glass slides, the upper smearing a drop of blood as a film over the surface of the lower slide.

Evaluation

Erythrocytes vary in size, shape, and color and should be examined for any abnormali-ties. In general, erythrocytes may be normocytic (i.e. normal in size), macrocytic (i.e. larger than normal), or microcytic (i.e. smaller than normal). In vitamin B-12 or folic acid deficiency anemias, the mature red cells are usually macrocytic whereas in iron deficiency anemia, microcytic red cells are present. The shape of the red cells on a stained blood smear may also differ from that of the normal, round, biconcave appearance. In such cases, poikilocytosis is said to occur. Poikilocytes can assume many shapes, each with distinctive features associated with specific disorders.

The normal color for an erythrocyte stained with a conventional blood stain is pinkish red with a lighter colored center, termed the 'central pallor' which does not normally exceed one-third of the cell's diameter. The color reflects the

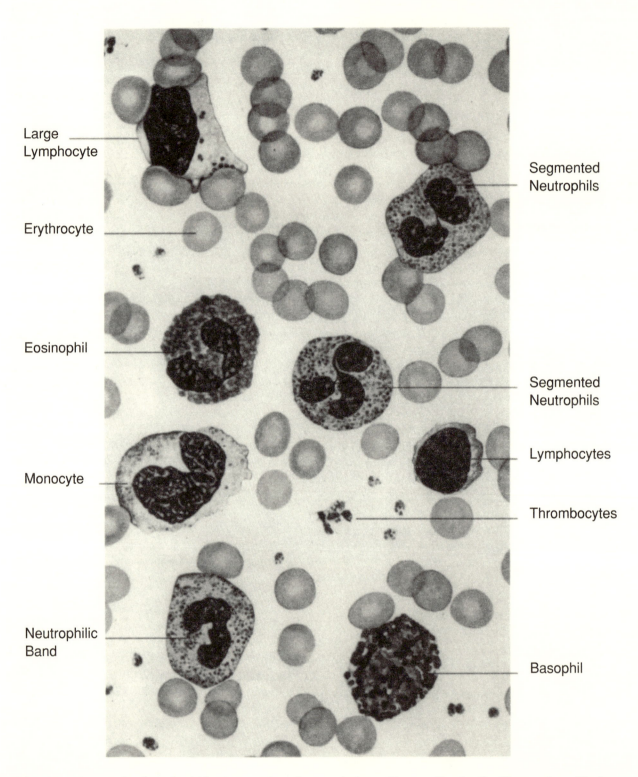

Fig. 8.2: Photomicrograph of a stained blood smear show the morphology of human blood cells. The number of leukocytes in relation to erythrocytes and thrombocytes is greater than would normally occur in a typical microscopic field of view. From Diggs LW, Sturm D, Bell A (1970). The Morphology of Human Blood Cells. Abbott Laboratories, North Chicago, IL. With permission.

amount of hemoglobin in the cell. When there is a decrease in hemoglobin synthesis, as occurs in iron deficiency anemia, the red cells are pale, and hypochromia is said to occur.

Platelets should be examined and their abundance estimated by counting a stained blood smear. Generally, 8 to 10 platelets per field can be expected when a ×100 oil-immersion objective is used. At least ten fields should be examined. The estimated platelet concentration = average platelet number × 20,000. Abnormalities in platelet size should also be noted.

Differential leukocyte counts determine the relative proportion of the types of leukocytes present. Count at least 100 leukocytes using a tracking pattern shown in Fig. 8.3.

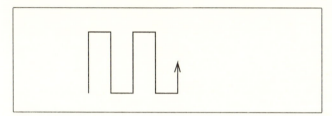

Fig. 8.3: The method of slide examination in the differential leukocyte count.

Each leukocyte should be identified as a: neutrophil (band), neutrophil (segmented) or polymorphonuclear neutrophil (PMN), lymphocyte, monocyte, eosinophil, or basophil using Fig. 8.2 or the colored version of the same figure

	Average (Cells/mm³)	Normal Range (Cells/mm³)	% Total White Cells
Total WBC	9000	4000-11,000	
Granulocytes			
Neutrophils	5400	3000–6000	50–70
Eosinophils	275	150–300	1–4
Basophils	35	0–100	0.4
Lymphocytes	2750	1500–4000	20–40
Monocytes	540	300–600	2–8

Table 8.1: Classes of leukocytes in the peripheral blood of the average adult. Conversion factor to SI units $(10^9/L)$= ×0.0001.

(Diggs et al., 1970, p.8). The results should be expressed as a percentage of the total leukocytes counted.

There are no significant age or sex differences in differential leukocyte counts after puberty. Normal adult values for mature leukocytes in peripheral blood are shown in Table 8.1. Several clinical disorders are associated with increases in normal leukocyte types; none are specifically related to nutritional deficiencies.

References

Diggs L W, Sturn D, Bell A (1970). The Morphology of Human Blood Cells. Abbott Laboratories, North Chicago, IL.

Turgeon M L (1988). Clinical Hematology Theory and Procedures. Little, Brown and Company, Boston.

8.2 Hematocrit

Principle

To assess hematocrit, whole blood is centrifuged and the ratio of the height of the red cell column to that of the whole blood sample in a hematocrit tube is measured. This ratio represents the packed red cell volume (PCV) and is expressed as a percent or decimal fraction of the total blood volume.

The PCV is used to detect anemia, polycythemia, hemodilution, or hemoconcentration. It is a relatively easy and rapid test, and is often used as a screening test for iron-deficiency anemia.

Equipment

- Heparinized capillary tubes.
- Clay-type tube sealer.
- Hematocrit centrifuge.
- Hematocrit reader.

Procedure

The determination should be completed in duplicate using capillary blood or venous blood anticoagulated with EDTA. When using the latter, blue-banded capillary tubes containing no anticoagulant are used.

1. Place one end of a capillary tube in a drop of the blood to be tested, so that the blood is drawn into the tube by capillary action. Fill the tube to within 10 mm of the opposite end. Wipe the outside of the tube with a wipe. (Note: Air bubbles in the tube will not affect the results).

2. Seal the empty end of the tube with a small plug of sealer by placing the dry end of the hematocrit tube into the sealant in the vertical position.

3. Place the sealed end of the capillary tube against the rim of the head of the centrifuge, and the tube in a radial groove. Note the position number of the specimen.

4. Repeat items 1 to 3 above for each test sample.

5. Fasten the lid of the centrifuge on top of the capillary tubes securely. Close the top and secure the latch. Centrifuge for five minutes at 10,000 to 15,000 rpm. Note that a balancing capillary tube should also be loaded into the head of the centrifuge if only one test is performed.

6. Remove the tubes from the centrifuge.

7. Measure the height of the red cells with the hematocrit reader at once. Do not include the buffy coat in reading the packed erythrocyte column. If it is not convenient, the capillary tube can be kept undisturbed in an upright position. Repeat the determination if the duplicates differ by more than 1% or if the sample has been spoilt during centrifugation.

Calculation of results

Express the result as a percentage of whole blood (packed red-cell length / total length). This is the packed red cell volume (PCV). The conversion factor to SI units = ×0.01.

Evaluation

Hematocrit values are dependent on age and sex, so that age- and sex-specific interpretive reference data must be used. Cutoff values for hematocrit, compiled by Dallman (1977), are given in Table 8.2. During iron deficiency, the hematocrit

Age (yr)		Mean	Lower limit
0.5–2		36	33
2–6		37	34
6–12		40	35
12–18			
	Female	41	36
	Male	43	38
18–49			
	Female	41	36
	Male	47	41

Table 8.2: Normal values for the mean and lower limit (mean − 2 SD) of normal for hematocrit (%). From Dallman PR (1977). New approaches to screening for iron deficiency. Journal of Pediatrics 90: 678–681 with permission. The conversion factor to SI units = ×0.01.

falls only after hemoglobin formation has become impaired. Consequently, in early cases of moderate iron deficiency, a marginally low hemoglobin value may be associated with a near-normal hematocrit (Graitcer et al., 1981). Only in more severe iron-deficiency anemia are both hemoglobin and hematocrit reduced.

The hematocrit is not a very sensitive index of iron status; it declines only during the final stage in the development of iron deficiency. It also lacks specificity. Low hematocrit values also occur in chronic infections and inflammations, hemorrhage, protein-energy malnutrition, thalassemia minor, vitamin B-12 or folate deficiency, hemoglobinopathies, pregnancy, and other states in which there is overhydration or acute plasma volume expansion. In contrast, elevated hematocrit values occur in polycythemia and hemoconcentration caused by dehydration.

The precision of the hematocrit method is poor, particularly when capillary blood samples are used. The low precision is often associated with improper mixing of blood caused by intermittent blood flow from the puncture site; poorly packed iron-deficient cells resulting in spuriously elevated values; excessive anticoagulant in the collection tube; and elevated white blood cell counts leading to a poorly defined boundary between the red blood cells and the plasma in the hematocrit tube (Graitcer et al., 1981).

References

Dallman P R (1977). New approaches to screening for iron deficiency. Journal of Pediatrics 90: 678–681.

Graitcer P L, Goldsby J B, Nichaman M Z (1981). Hemoglobins and hematocrits: are they equally sensitive in detecting anemias? American Journal of Clinical Nutrition 34: 61–64.

8.3 Hemoglobin

Principle

Iron is an essential component of hemoglobin, the oxygen-carrying pigment of the red blood cells. The hemoglobin molecule is a conjugate of a protein (globin) and four molecules of heme. Measurement of the concentration of hemoglobin in whole blood is probably the most widely used screening test for iron-deficiency anemia. The cyanmethemoglobin method is the most reliable assay for hemoglobin. All the usually encountered forms of hemoglobin in blood (oxyhemoglobin, methemoglobin, carboxyhemoglobin) are first oxidized to methemoglobin by potassium ferricyanide and then converted to stable cyanmethemoglobin by potassium cyanide (Drabkin and Austin, 1932). The absorbance of the pigment is measured spectrophotometrically at 540 nm.

Reagents

- Modified Drabkin's reagent: highly poisonous, contains cyanide. Handle with care.

- Aqueous certified standard solution of cyanmethemoglobin. This contains 80 mg/dL cyanmethemoglobin (equivalent to 20 g/dL hemoglobin). Stable for at least one year at 4°C.

- Sample. Capillary blood or venous blood of test subjects, anticoagulated with EDTA or heparin. Note that the hemoglobin concentration is lower when the blood is collected with the patient in the supine position compared to a sitting position. The variation may be as great as 15 g/dL.

- Pool blood sample for assessing the precision of the determination.

Equipment

- Test tubes; cuvets.
- Pipets:
  - 0.02 mL (Sahli);
  - 5 mL volumetric;
  - 10 mL graduated.

Procedure

1. Prepare the following standard dilutions in duplicate using Drabkin's reagent:

Tube No.	Volume of reagent (mL)	Volume of standard (mL)	g/dL
Blank	6.0	0	0
1	4.5	1.5	5
2	3.0	3.0	10
3	1.5	4.5	15
4	0	6.0	20

2. Label additional test tubes for each subject and one for the pool sample, then add exactly 5.0 mL of Drabkin's reagent to each.

3. For each subject and the pool sample, draw up with the Sahli pipet exactly 0.02 mL (20 μL) of blood. Wipe the outside of the Sahli pipet with a tissue and then quickly transfer the blood into the Drabkin's reagent in the appropriate test tube. Rinse the pipet three times with the reagent in the test tube to ensure transfer of all of the blood.

4. Allow all the tubes to stand for at least ten minutes to form the cyanmethemoglobin. The color is stable for 9–12 months.

5. Set the wavelength at 540 nm. Zero the spectrophotometer to zero absorbance using a cuvet containing only Drabkin's reagent as a reference blank.

6. Transfer the test, pool, and standard samples to a cuvet in turn and read the absorbance.

7. Construct a standard curve. Plot a graph with the standard concentrations (g/dL) as the abscissa against the absorbance as the ordinate.

Calculation of results

Read the hemoglobin value of the test and pool samples in g/dL directly from the standard curve. The conversion factor to SI units (g/L) = ×10.0

Evaluation

Hemoglobin values are dependent on age, sex, and race (Yip et al., 1984). Individuals of African descent have hemoglobin values which are 0.3 to 1.0 g/dL (3 to 10 g/L) lower than Caucasians, irrespective of age and income (Garn et al., 1981). Therefore, age, sex, and race-specific interpretive criteria must be used. Three different sets of interpretive criteria are given in Table 8.3.

The hemoglobin cutoff points derived from the U.S. NHANES II data are based on the distribution of hemoglobin values in venous blood obtained from a white, ostensibly healthy, nonpregnant population (Pilch and Senti, 1984). All subjects with evidence of iron deficiency and chronic disease were excluded. The hemoglobin cutoff points represent the lower limit of the 95% confidence interval for each age/sex group for white subjects (i.e. below the 2.5th percentile). As the sample size was small for young children, the value obtained for three- and four-year-old children was also used for subjects aged one to four

Age (yrs)	Hemoglobin Percentiles (g/dL)						
	5	10	25	50	75	90	95
Children							
1–2		11.3	11.6	12.2	12.6	13.0	
3–4	11.1	11.4	11.9	12.4	12.9	13.4	13.8
5–10	11.5	11.8	12.3	12.9	13.5	13.9	14.3
Males							
11–14	12.1	12.4	13.1	13.8	14.5	15.1	15.4
15–19	13.3	13.6	14.2	15.0	15.6	16.3	16.6
20–44	13.7	14.0	14.6	15.3	15.9	16.5	16.8
45–64	13.5	13.8	14.4	15.1	15.8	16.4	16.8
65–74	13.1	13.6	14.3	15.0	15.7	16.5	17.1
Females							
11–14	11.8	12.1	12.7	13.3	13.9	14.3	14.7
15–19	12.0	12.3	12.8	13.4	14.0	14.7	15.0
20–44	12.0	12.3	12.9	13.5	14.2	14.8	15.1
45–64	12.1	12.4	13.0	13.7	14.5	15.2	15.5
65–74	12.1	12.5	13.1	13.8	14.5	15.1	15.6

Table 8.4: Hemoglobin (g/dL) percentiles for persons one to seventy-four years (all races). Percentiles are for the NHANES II 'reference population'. Abstracted from the more comprehensive tabulations of Pilch and Senti (1984).

years. This approach was not used for American Negro subjects because too few were included in the survey for reliable determinations of the 95% confidence interval.

Selected percentiles for hemoglobin derived from the U.S. NHANES II reference population for persons aged one to seventy-four years, are given in Table 8.4. Persons with evidence of iron deficiency and chronic disease are excluded.

Normal mean and lower limit (mean − 2 SD) of normal for hemoglobin (g/dL) have also been compiled by Dallman (1977). These values are given in Table 8.5.

	Hemoglobin (g/dL)		
Age (yr)	Males and Females	Males	Females
NHANES II. (Pilch and Senti, 1984) [a]			
1–2	10.9	—	—
3–4	10.9	—	—
5–10	11.2	—	—
11–14	—	12.0	11.8
15–19	—	13.1	11.7
20–44	—	13.4	11.9
45–64	—	13.2	11.8
65–74	—	12.6	11.9
WHO. (World Health Organization, 1972) [b]			
0.5–6	11.0	—	—
6–14	12.0	—	—
>14	—	13.0	12.0
Nutrition Canada. (Health and Welfare Canada, 1973) [c]			
0–1	10.0	—	—
2–5	11.0	—	—
6–12	11.5	—	—
13–16	—	13.0	11.5
>17	—	14.0	12.0

Table 8.3: Three different sets of criteria used for analysis of hemoglobin data. [a] Hemoglobin cutoff points derived from the NHANES II population (white subjects only). [b] Concentrations of hemoglobin below which anemia is likely to be present. [c] Criteria given as the upper limit of 'moderate' risk of deficiency. Conversion factor to SI units (g/L) = ×10. Reproduced with permission of the World Health Organization and the Minister of Supply and Services Canada.

Age (yr)		Mean	Lower limit
0.5–2		12.0	11.0
2–6		12.5	11.0
6–12		13.5	11.5
12–18			
	Female	14.0	12.0
	Male	14.5	13.0
18–49			
	Female	14.0	12.0
	Male	15.5	13.5

Table 8.5: Normal values for the mean and lower limit (mean − 2 SD) of normal for hemoglobin (g/dL). From Dallman PR (1977). New approaches to screening for iron deficiency. Journal of Pediatrics 90: 678–681 with permission.

A low hemoglobin concentration is associated with hypochromia, a characteristic feature of iron-deficiency anemia. Hemoglobin, like the hematocrit, is also relatively insensitive; considerable overlap exists in the hemoglobin values of normal nonanemic and iron-deficient individuals (Garby et al., 1969). Specificity is also poor. It is affected by the same factors influencing the hematocrit.

Hemoglobin concentrations are also modified by a variety of other factors, including diurnal variation and cigarette smoking. Hemoglobin values tend to be lower in the evening than in the morning, by amounts of up to $1.0\,g/dL$ ($10\,g/L$). Cigarette smoking is associated with higher concentrations of hemoglobin (0.3 to $0.5\,g/dL$) (3 to $5\,g/L$) in adults (Pilch and Senti, 1984).

References

Dallman P R (1977). New approaches to screening for iron deficiency. Journal of Pediatrics 90: 678–681.

Drabkin D L, Austin J H (1932). Spectrophotometric studies: spectrophotometric constants for common hemoglobin derivatives in human, dog and rabbit blood. Journal of Biological Chemistry 98: 719–733.

Garby L, Irnell L, Werner I (1969). Iron deficiency in women of fertile age in a Swedish community. III. Estimation of prevalence based on response to iron supplementation. Acta Medica Scandinavica 185: 113–117.

Garn S M, Ryan A S, Owen G M, Abraham S (1981). Income matched black-white hemoglobin differences after correction for low transferrin saturations. American Journal of Clinical Nutrition 34: 1645–1647.

Health and Welfare Canada (1973). Nutrition Canada National Survey. Health and Welfare, Ottawa.

Pilch S M, Senti F R. (eds) (1984). Assessment of the iron nutritional status of the US population based on data collected in the second National Health and Nutrition Examination Survey, 1976–1980. Life Sciences Research Office, Federation of the American Societies for Experimental Biology, Bethesda, Maryland.

WHO (World Health Organization) (1972). Nutritional Anemia. WHO Technical Report Series No. 3. World Health Organization, Geneva.

Yip R, Johnson C, Dallman P R (1984). Age-related changes in laboratory values used in the diagnosis of anemia and iron deficiency. American Journal of Clinical Nutrition 39: 427–436.

8.4 Red blood cell count

Principle

The red blood cell count is the number of red blood cells in one liter of whole blood. The method depends on accurately counting the number of red blood cells in a precisely measured volume of blood, which has been accurately diluted with an isotonic diluent (Chanarin, 1989). The measured volume is obtained by placing the diluted sample of blood into a counting chamber of a Neubauer hemocytometer. Two methods are used for determining the red blood cell count; the manual method and the electronic cell counter method. The manual method is described below.

Reagents

- Hayems red blood cell count diluting fluid: sodium sulfate 2.50 g; sodium chloride 0.50 g; mercuric chloride 0.25 g; distilled water 100 mL.
- Sample. Whole blood, with EDTA as the anticoagulant. Alternatively, capillary blood may be used provided it is diluted immediately upon collection.

Equipment

- Neubauer hemocytometer and cover slip. The red cells are counted in squares 5A, B, C, D, E (Fig. 8.4).
- Microscope.
- Pipet shaker.
- Red cell pipet.
- Hand-held cell counter.

Procedure

1. Ensure that the coverslip for the hemocytometer is free of dust, grease and protein. Apply the coverslip firmly to the counting chamber so that Newton's rings are visible where it is in contact with the chamber.

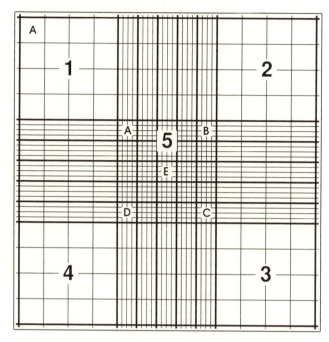

Fig. 8.4: Improved Neubauer counting chamber. Solid lines are triple lines. Red cells are counted in squares 5A, B, C, D, and E; white cells in squares 1, 2, 3 and 4.

2. Gently draw the blood up to exactly the 0.5 mark of the red cell pipet. If the blood goes beyond the mark, do not attempt to blow out the excess, but tap the tip of the pipet against the finger nail, until the blood is at the 0.5 mark. Wipe the pipet with a disposable wipe. (Do not touch the tip of the pipet).

3. Quickly[1] draw up Hayems diluting fluid to the 101 mark, and then mix the blood and the diluting fluid in the bulb by rotating the pipet horizontally between the hands for two minutes. This results in a dilution of 1 : 200.

4. Place the pipet on a pipet shaker for five to ten minutes.

5. Remove the pipet from the shaker. Expel the first four drops of the contents of the pipet onto a piece of gauze.

6. Gently place the tip of the pipet at the junction of the counting chamber and its cover slip, allowing a small quantity of diluted blood

---

[1]It is important to carry out stage 1 and 2 before the blood sample clots. If the blood clots, then the pipet must be discarded and steps 1 and 2 repeated.

to be drawn into the counting chamber by capillary attraction. This step must be undertaken smoothly, in an uninterrupted fashion and stopped at the right moment: fluid must not be allowed to overflow into the moat. Avoid introducing air bubbles.

7. Place the chamber inside a moistened petri dish for about three minutes to allow the red blood cells to settle before proceeding to the next step.

8. Set up the microscope by lowering the condenser a little, and partly closing the diaphragm, to reduce the amount of light. Using the low power ($\times 10$ objective), place the large center square in the middle of the field of vision. Examine the large square to confirm that the distribution of the red cells is even.

9. Change to the high power objective ($\times 40$). Move the counting chamber to ensure that the small upper left corner square (5A), subdivided into sixteen smaller squares, is completely in the field of vision.

10. Count the number of red cells in each of the sixteen squares making up the small upper left corner square (5A). To avoid counting the same cells twice, include in the total for each small square only cells lying on the upper and left dividing lines of each small square, but not those on the lower and right dividing lines.

11. Repeat the counting procedure for the squares 5B, 5C, 5D, and 5E.

Calculation of results

Calculate the average number of red blood cells (10^{12}/L) counted in the two sides of the counting chamber as follows:

$$\text{Red cell count} = \frac{\text{Cell count}}{\text{volume counted}} \times \text{dilution} \times 10^6 \text{ per liter}$$

For example, if the number of red blood cells counted in the five small squares = 400; the dilution = 1 : 200; volume counted = 5 small squares (0.02 µL); conversion to liters = $\times 10^6$

$$\begin{aligned} \text{RBC} &= (400/0.02) \times 200 \times 10^6 \text{ per liter} \\ &= 4.0 \times 10^{12} \text{ per liter} \end{aligned}$$

When the red blood cell count is very high, as in polycythemia, a 1 : 333 dilution should be used. Draw the blood to the 0.3 mark in the red cell pipet and dilute to the 101 mark. Alternatively, if the subject has severe anemia and the red blood cell count is low, a 1 : 100 dilution should be used. Draw the blood to the 1.0 mark and dilute to the 101 mark. In both cases, adjust the calculation accordingly.

Evaluation

Normal ranges for red blood cell counts for infants and adults are shown in Table 8.6.

Subject Group	Sex	Normal Range
Adults	Males Females	3.6–5.6 $\times 10^{12}$/L 4.2–5.8 $\times 10^{12}$/L
Infants at birth Infants 1 year	M + F M + F	5.0–6.5 $\times 10^{12}$/L 4.3 ± 0.8 $\times 10^{12}$/L

Table 8.6: Normal range for red blood cell counts. From: Brown BA (1988). Hematology: Principles and Procedures. Lea and Febiger, Philadelphia, pp. 87–92.

References

Brown BA (1988). Hematology: Principles and Procedures. Lea and Febiger, Philadelphia, pp. 87–92.

Chanarin I (ed) (1989). Laboratory Haematology An Account of Laboratory Techniques. Churchill Livingstone, Edinburgh, pp. 11–12.

8.5 Red cell indices

Principle

Three red cell indices—mean cell volume, mean cell hemoglobin concentration, and mean cell hemoglobin—are derived from measurements of hemoglobin, hematocrit, and/or red blood cell count. They are used to define cell size and the concentration of hemoglobin within the cell so that different types of anemia can be diagnosed. A comparison of the expected changes in red cell indices during iron-deficiency anemia, macrocytic anemia resulting from vitamin B-12 and/or folic acid deficiency, and the anemia of chronic disease is summarized in Table 8.7.

Red Cell Index	Iron Deficiency Anemia (microcytic hypochromic)	Macrocytic Anemia (normo-chromic)	Anemia of Chronic Disease (normocytic normochromic)
MCV	Low	High	Normal
MCHC	Low	Normal	Normal
MCH	Low	High	Normal

Table 8.7: Expected changes in red cell indices during iron-deficiency anemia, macrocytic anemia, and anemia of chronic disease. From Wintrobe MM, Lee GR, Boggs DR, Bithell TC, Foerster J, Athens JW, Lukens JN (eds) (1981). Clinical Hematology. Eight edition, Lea and Febiger, with permission.

Mean cell volume (MCV)

This is a measure of the average volume of the red blood cell expressed in femtoliters (fl).

$$\text{MCV(fL)} = \frac{\text{Hematocrit (volume fraction)}}{\text{Red blood cell count } (10^{12}/\text{L})} \times 1000$$

This index is useful to identify and classify anemias. Cells may be abnormally large (macrocytosis) as in vitamin B-12 and folic acid deficiency, or abnormally small (microcytosis) as in iron and vitamin B-6 deficiency. In the NHANES II survey, a MCV cutoff value of 80 fL was accepted as the lower limit of normal for adults; for children, cutoff values for four age groups were set (Pilch and Senti, 1984). Values greater than 98 fL indicate macrocytosis. The mean cell volume changes progressively during infancy, childhood, and early adult life (Yip et al., 1984). Mean cell volume (fL)

percentiles for persons one to seventy-four years (all races) are given in Table 8.8.

Mean cell hemoglobin concentration (MCHC)

This refers to the concentration of hemoglobin in the red blood cells.

$$\text{MCHC (g/L)} = \frac{\text{Hemoglobin (g/L)}}{\text{Hematocrit (volume fraction)}}$$

Values in normal adults range from 320–360 g/L. Values of less than 300 g/L indicate hypochromia and are associated with advanced iron deficiency. Values are normal in the macrocytic anemia of vitamin B-12 and folic acid deficiency and the anemia of chronic disease. After the first few months of life, mean cell hemoglobin concentration is less affected by age than any other red cell index. Nevertheless, it is the least useful of the red cell indices: it is the last to fall during iron deficiency.

Mean cell hemoglobin (MCH)

This refers to the absolute hemoglobin content of an average red blood cell. It is usually measured

Age (yrs)	Mean Cell Volume Percentiles (fL)						
	5	10	25	50	75	90	95
Children							
1–2	73.3	75.3	77.2	79.6	82.2	84.6	86.7
3–4	74.3	76.0	78.4	81.0	83.7	86.6	88.5
5–10	76.4	77.8	80.3	83.0	85.6	88.6	90.7
Males							
11–14	77.6	79.0	81.1	83.9	87.3	89.8	92.8
15–19	79.7	81.7	84.3	87.2	90.1	93.1	94.5
20–44	81.3	83.2	85.8	88.8	91.8	94.8	97.2
45–64	82.8	84.0	86.9	90.2	93.9	97.5	99.2
65–74	82.6	84.6	87.4	90.7	94.2	98.1	101.0
Females							
11–14	78.6	80.1	82.7	86.0	89.1	92.6	93.8
15–19	80.6	82.5	85.4	88.5	91.6	94.8	96.6
20–44	81.9	84.1	87.2	90.4	93.8	96.6	98.9
45–64	82.5	84.1	87.1	90.3	94.1	96.9	99.3
65–74	82.6	84.1	87.0	90.3	94.0	97.8	99.8

Table 8.8: Mean cell volume (fL) percentiles for persons one to seventy-four years (all races). Percentiles are for the NHANES II 'reference population'. Abstracted from the more comprehensive tabulations of Pilch and Senti (1984).

in picograms (pg) and is derived from the ratio of hemoglobin to the red blood cell count.

$$MCH\,(pg) = \frac{\text{Hemoglobin (g/L)}}{\text{Red blood cell count } (10^{12}/L)}$$

The MCH changes progressively from infancy to adulthood, when values range from 27–32 pg. It undergoes similar changes in iron-deficiency anemia to the MCV; it is low in iron-deficiency anemia but high in the macrocytic anemias of vitamin B-12 and folate deficiency (Table 8.7). In the latter, the red blood cells are laden with hemoglobin but are reduced in number. In severe iron deficiency, the relative fall in MCH is greater than the corresponding fall in MCV (Dallman, 1977).

References

Dallman P R (1977). New approaches to screening for iron deficiency. Journal of Pediatrics 90: 678–681.

Pilch S M, Senti F R (eds) (1984). Assessment of the iron nutritional status of the US population based on data collected in the second National Health and Nutrition Examination Survey, 1976–1980. Life Sciences Research Office, Federation of the American Societies for Experimental Biology, Bethesda, Maryland.

Wintrobe M M, Lee G R, Boggs D R, Bithell T C, Foerster J, Athens J W, Lukens J N (eds) (1981). Clinical Hematology. Eighth edition, Lea and Febiger, Philadelphia.

Yip R, Johnson C, Dallman P R (1984). Age-related changes in laboratory values used in the diagnosis of anemia and iron deficiency. American Journal of Clinical Nutrition 39: 427–436.

8.6   White cell count

Principle

The white blood cell count is the number of white blood cells in one liter of whole blood. The count is made by first diluting the blood with a weak acid solution to hemolyze the red blood cells. The number of white blood cells in a known volume of the diluted blood are then accurately counted using a Neubauer hemocytometer. Both manual and electronic cell counting methods can be used. The manual method (Chanarin, 1989) is described below.

Reagents

- White blood cell count diluting fluid. This lyses the red blood cells so that they will not obscure the white blood cells. Three commonly used diluting fluids are:
  - Acetic acid 2% v/v in distilled water
  - Hydrochloric acid, 1% v/v in distilled water
  - Turk's diluting fluid: Glacial acetic acid 3 mL; 1% wt/vol aqueous gentian violet 1 mL; distilled water 100 mL

- Sample. Whole blood preferably using EDTA as the anticoagulant. Alternatively, capillary blood may be used.

Equipment

- Neubauer hemocytometer and cover slip. The white cells are counted in the four large corner squares 1, 2, 3 and 4 (Fig. 8.4), each of which is subdivided into sixteen smaller squares.

- Microscope.

- Pipet shaker.

- White cell pipet.

- Hand-held counter.

Procedure

1. Gently mix the blood specimen by inversion.

2. Ensure that the coverslip for the hemocytometer is free of dust, grease, and protein. Apply the coverslip firmly to the counting chamber so that Newton's rings are visible where the cover slip is in contact with the chamber.

3. Gently draw the blood up to exactly the 0.5 mark of the white cell pipet. If the blood goes beyond the mark, do not attempt to blow out the excess, but tap the tip of the pipet against the finger nail, until the blood is at the 0.5 mark. Wipe the blood from the outside of the pipet with a tissue, making sure that no blood is withdrawn from the stem of the pipet.

4. With the pipet held almost vertically, place the tip of the pipet into the diluting fluid and slowly introduce the fluid up to the 11 mark. This gives a dilution of 1:20. Avoid introducing air bubbles into the pipet. Wipe the outside of the pipet with a tissue again.

5. Place the pipet in a horizontal position, holding it between the thumb and the middle finger. Mix the contents well by moving the hand only. Alternatively, a pipet shaker can be used.

6. Change the pipet to a vertical position. Discard the first four drops to remove the diluting fluid in the stem of the pipet, and then wipe off any excess liquid from the outside of the pipet with a tissue.

7. Place the tip of the pipet on the edge of one side of the counting chamber, and allow the mixture to slowly and smoothly seep under the cover slip, until the counting chamber is properly filled. Care must be taken to avoid any of the diluted sample running into the grooved area. Do not move the coverslip during this stage.

8. Repeat the above step with the opposite side of the counting chamber.

9. Allow the counting chamber to stand for about 1 minute to allow the white blood cells to settle before counting.

10. Adjust the microscope as described for the red blood cell count. Using the low power (×10) objective, check to ensure that the white cells are evenly distributed in all four large squares. There should not be more than a ten-cell variation between the four squares.

11. Change to the high power objective (×40) and count the total number of white cells in the upper four large corner squares on the left. To avoid counting the same cells twice, include only those cells lying on the upper and left outside dividing lines of each small square, but not those touching the lower and right margin.

12. Count the cells on the opposite side of the counting chamber, again recording the total number of cells in these four large squares. This total should closely approximate the first count. If the numbers obtained from the first and second count are very different, repeat the procedure from step 1.

13. Add the total white blood cells counted on each side together and divide by 2.0 to obtain the average.

Calculation of the results

The total white blood cell count (10^9/L) can be calculated using the following expression:

$$\frac{\text{Average number of cells counted (N)}}{\text{volume counted (0.4)}} \times \text{dilution} \times 10^6 \text{ per L}$$

If the dilution is 1:20 dilution (step 3), this equation becomes:

$$(N/0.4) \times 20 \times 10^6 \text{ per L}$$

Note that when the cell count is low, all the white cells must be counted in the whole ruled area (= 9 mm^2), or a smaller dilution of blood should be used. For the latter, draw the blood to the 1.0 mark in a white cell pipet, and then dilute with the white cell diluting fluid to the 11.0 mark, giving a dilution of 1:10.

When the cell count is high, a 1:200 dilution is used. This is achieved by drawing the blood up to the 0.5 mark in the white cell pipet and diluting to the 101 mark with the white cell diluting fluid (Brown, 1988).

The total lymphocyte count (10^9/L) can be derived from the percentage of lymphocytes multiplied by the white blood cell count (WBCC) and divided by 100:

$$\text{Total lymphocyte count} = (\% \text{ lymphocytes} \times \text{WBCC})/100$$

Evaluation

Normal ranges for total white blood cell counts for infants, children, and adults are shown in Table 8.9.

In healthy subjects, the average lymphocyte count in peripheral blood is generally above 2.75×10^9/L. In malnutrition, the blood lymphocyte count is reduced. A level between 0.9 to 1.5×10^9/L is said to indicate moderate depletion, whereas below 0.9×10^9/L represents severe depletion (Blackburn et al. 1977). Many other factors, however, can affect the the absolute lymphocyte count, notably stress, sepsis, infection, neoplasia, and steroids. Therefore the specificity and sensitivity of this test is low.

Subject Group	Normal Range
Adults	4–11 ×10^9/L
Infants at birth	10–24 ×10^9/L
Infants at 1 year	6–18 ×10^9/L
Children <10 years	5–14 ×10^9/L

Table 8.9: Normal range for total white blood cell counts. From: Brown BA (1988). Hematology: Principles and Procedures. Lea and Febiger, Philadelphia, pp. 87–92.

References

Blackburn GL, Bistrain BR, Maini BS, Schlamm HT, Smith MF (1977). Nutritional and metabolic assessment of the hospitalized patient. Journal of Parenteral and Enteral Nutrition 1: 11–22.

Brown BA (1988). Hematology: Principles and Procedures. Lea and Febiger, Philadelphia, pp. 87–92.

Chanarin I (ed) (1989). Laboratory Haematology An Account of Laboratory Techniques. Churchill Livingstone, Edinburgh, pp. 11–12.

Chapter 9
Assessment of iron status

Contents

Introduction

The assessment of iron status in population groups is important: iron deficiency is the commonest micronutrient deficiency in both developing and industrialized countries. It is prevalent in infants, young children, and pregnant women. The deficiency may arise from inadequate dietary intakes, poor absorption, excessive loss, or a combination of these factors (Narasinga Rao, 1981).

Three stages characterize the development of iron-deficiency anemia (Cook and Finch, 1979). The first phase is a decrease in iron stores, reflected by a decline in serum/plasma ferritin concentrations. The second phase, iron-deficient erythropoiesis, is characterized by a decrease in serum/plasma iron ($<60\,\mu g/dL$) and an elevation in total iron-binding capacity, resulting in a fall in percentage transferrin saturation ($<15\%$). At the same time, erythrocyte protoporphyrin concentrations will be increased ($>100\,\mu g/dL$), because the supply of iron is no longer adequate for heme synthesis; the hemoglobin and hematocrit remains within the normal range for age and sex. In the third and final stage of iron deficiency, frank microcytic, hypochromic anemia occurs, when decreases in both the hemoglobin concentration and the hematocrit occur, resulting in a low mean cell hemoglobin concentration (MCHC). At this stage, further decreases in serum iron ($<40\,\mu g/dL$) and ferritin ($<10\,\mu g/L$) occur, and increases in erythrocyte protoporphyrin ($>200\,\mu g/dL$) and total iron-binding capacity ($>410\,\mu g/dL$). The presence of hypochromic microcytosis can be confirmed at this stage by using a stained blood film.

To provide the best measure of iron status, several indices should be used simultaneously. The presence of two or more abnormal values generally indicates impaired iron status. The selection of the most appropriate combination depends on the health of the individual(s), and the study objectives. Diagnosis of iron deficiency is particularly difficult in the presence of other conditions which confound the interpretation of the laboratory results. Tests commonly used to confirm the existence of each of the three stages of iron-deficiency anemia are described below.

References

Cook J D, Finch C A (1979). Assessing iron status of a population. American Journal of Clinical Nutrition 32: 2115–2119.

Narasinga Rao B S (1981). Physiology of iron absorption and supplementation. British Medical Bulletin 37: 25–30.

9.1 Serum iron

Principle

The serum iron content reflects the number of atoms of iron bound to the iron transport protein transferrin. Each molecule of transferrin can be bound to one or two atoms of iron, although rarely are both the binding sites occupied.

The colorimetric assay of serum iron described below employs ferrozine as the chromogen (Persijn et al., 1971). At an acid pH and in the presence of a suitable reducing agent (e.g. hydroxylamine hydrochloride), transferrin-bound serum iron dissociates to form ferrous ions. These react with ferrozine to form a magenta-colored complex with an absorption maximum near 560 nm. The difference in color intensity at 560 nm, before and after addition of ferrozine, is proportional to the serum iron concentration.

Reagents

The following reagents can be obtained from the Sigma Chemical Co., St Louis, MO, as a kit for the determination of serum iron, serum unsaturated iron-binding capacity, and total iron-binding capacity. Follow the procedure given by the manufacturer if this differs from that outlined below.

- Iron buffer reagent. Hydroxylamine hydrochloride 1.5% in acetate buffer (pH 4.5) with added surfactant. Store at room temperature.
- UIBC buffer reagent. Contains Tris (hydroxymethyl) aminomethane, 0.5 mol/L, pH 8.1 with added surfactant and preservative. Store at room temperature.
- Iron color reagent. Ferrozine (0.85% wt/vol) in hydroxylamine hydrochloride solution with added stabilizer. Store at room temperature.
- Iron standard solution containing 500 μg/dL (89 μmol/L) iron in hydroxylamine hydrochloride solution. Store at room temperature.
- Sample. Serum is the specimen of choice; plasma obtained using heparin as an anticoagulant may also be used. EDTA interferes with the determination of iron. As soon as blood clots, promptly separate serum to avoid any hemolysis; each milligram of hemoglobin contains 3.4 μg iron. Serum in which there is

severe lipidemia—indicated by the presence of turbidity—may cause errors. Lipids dilute the specimen but do not contain iron. Serum iron reportedly is stable for at least four days stored at room temperature or one week in the refrigerator at 0–5°C.

- Pooled serum sample for assessing precision.
- Serum iron reference material. Serachem Level 1, Fisher Diagnostics, Orangeburg, NY.

Equipment

- Colorimeter or spectrophotometer reading at 560 nm, together with matched cuvets.
- Iron-free glassware; 0.05, 0.5, 1.0, 2.0, and 5.0 mL pipets.
- Water bath 37°C.
- Iron-free distilled deionized water.

Procedure

Blood should be collected using trace-element-free evacuated tubes. Only distilled deionized water should be used.

1. Label test tubes for the blank, standard, reference, pool, and for each test subject.
2. Add 2.5 mL iron buffer reagent to each tube.
3. To blank add 0.5 mL of iron-free water. To standard add 0.5 mL of the iron standard. To reference add 0.5 mL of the serum iron reference material. To pool add 0.5 mL of the pooled serum. For each test subject, add 0.5 mL of serum to the appropriate tube.
4. Mix each test tube well with the vortex mixer.
5. Transfer each sample to a cuvet.
6. Set the wavelength at 560 nm. Zero the spectrophotometer to zero absorbance with the reagent blank.
7. Read and record initial absorbance of the blank, standard, reference, pool, and test samples. Return the samples to the appropriate tubes after reading. This is the initial absorbance ($A_{Initial}$), measured to take into account differences in the turbidity of the sample.

Age (yr)	Percentiles of Serum Iron (µg/dL) by age							Percentiles of Serum Iron (µg/dL) by age						
	5	10	25	50	75	90	95	5	10	25	50	75	90	95
	Male subjects							Female subjects						
3–5	33.1	44.0	62.1	81.0	104.1	134.1	146.1	32.0	44.0	62.0	84.1	106.1	129.1	142.2
6–8	38.0	46.0	65.0	84.0	107.1	125.1	149.1	40.0	51.0	66.1	85.1	106.0	128.1	141.2
9–11	43.0	48.1	65.0	86.1	108.0	129.0	139.2	49.1	60.0	71.0	90.0	115.0	132.1	147.1
12–14	51.0	61.1	74.1	94.1	118.1	139.0	150.1	45.0	57.0	78.1	96.1	118.1	143.0	162.1
15–17	61.0	68.1	85.0	104.1	133.0	159.0	175.0	43.0	48.1	71.0	96.1	122.1	157.1	166.2
18–24	59.0	69.1	87.0	110.1	135.2	164.1	187.1	48.0	56.1	76.1	98.1	128.1	157.1	173.2
25–34	59.0	69.0	86.1	106.1	132.2	158.1	180.1	47.0	59.0	74.0	95.1	124.1	154.1	176.0
35–44	58.0	65.0	78.1	98.1	122.0	144.2	164.1	39.1	51.0	68.1	89.1	115.0	140.2	159.0
45–54	54.1	61.1	78.0	97.1	119.1	143.1	158.0	47.0	56.0	70.1	90.1	113.1	138.1	155.2
55–64	53.1	61.0	76.1	99.0	120.1	143.0	158.1	53.0	60.0	74.1	90.0	111.1	131.2	145.2
65–74	54.0	61.0	76.0	97.0	119.1	143.2	160.1	51.0	59.0	73.1	90.1	108.1	127.0	142.1

Table 9.1: Percentiles of serum iron (µg/dL) by age for males and females of three to seventy-four years. Data are from the U.S. NHANES II (1976–80) survey and were compiled by Fulwood et al. (1982).

8. Add 0.05 mL iron color reagent to each tube. Mix each tube and allow to stand for about ten minutes in a water bath at 37°C.

9. Transfer contents of each tube to a cuvet.

10. Again read and record the absorbance of the blank, standard, reference, pool, and test samples, using the blank to zero the spectrophotometer. This is the final absorbance (A_{Final}).

Calculation of results

If the iron standard contains $500\,\mu g/dL$, the serum iron concentration (µg/dL) of the test sample can be calculated using the following formula:

$$500 \times \left(\frac{\text{Test A}_{Final} - \text{Test A}_{Initial}}{\text{Standard A}_{Final} - \text{Standard A}_{Initial}} \right)$$

Conversion factor to SI units (µmol/L) = ×0.179.

Evaluation

Serum iron (µg/dL) percentiles from the U.S. NHANES II survey for persons three to seventy-four years (all races) are given in Table 9.1.

Iron deficiency results in a fall in serum iron levels. Low serum iron levels also occur in infection, inflammation, and malignancy, arising from defects in the release of iron from the reticuloendothelial cells and the subsequent transport of iron from these stores to transferrin. Together, these defects are termed the 'mucosal block'. When increased erythropoiesis occurs, serum iron may fall below the normal limits, whereas in conditions associated with decreased erythropoiesis,

serum iron levels are normal or slightly above normal. High serum iron levels also occur in conditions such as hemochromatosis, hemolytic anemia, acute liver damage, excessive absorption of iron from the gut, transfusions, and iron therapy.

Natural variation in serum iron concentrations is significant and coefficients of variation may approach 30%. Both diurnal and day-to-day variation occur. In general, serum iron values tend to be elevated in the morning and to be lower in the afternoon and evening (Statland and Winkel, 1977). As a result, measurements of serum iron should preferably be determined on fasting morning blood samples. The analytical coefficient of variation for serum iron may also be high, sometimes approaching 10% if the manual method is used (Dallman, 1984). Copper interferes with the colorimetric method described above, reducing its specificity.

References

Fulwood R, Johnson C L, Bryner J D et al. (1982). Hematological and nutritional reference data for persons 6 months – 74 years of age: United States, 1976–80. Vital and Health Statistics Series 11, No. 32 DHHS Publication No. 83-1682, Washington, DC.

Persijn J P, Slik van der W, Riethorst A (1971). Determination of serum iron and latent iron-binding capacity (LIBC). Clinica Chimica Acta 35: 91–98.

Statland B E, Winkel P (1977). Relationship of day-to-day variation of serum iron concentrations to iron-binding capacity in healthy young women. American Journal of Clinical Pathology 67: 84–90.

9.2   Serum unsaturated iron-binding capacity

Principle

At a slightly alkaline pH, ferrous ions added to a serum specimen bind specifically with transferrin at the unsaturated iron-binding sites. The remaining unbound ferrous ions are complexed with ferrozine to form a magenta-colored compound with an absorption maximum at about 560 nm (Carter, 1971; Persijn et al., 1971). The difference between the amount of unbound iron remaining and the total amount added is equivalent to the quantity bound by transferrin.   This is termed the 'unsaturated iron-binding capacity'. The total iron-binding capacity can then be derived from the sum of serum iron plus the unsaturated iron-binding capacity.

Reagents

The reagents listed below can be obtained from the Sigma Chemical Co., St Louis, MO, as a kit for the determination of serum iron (Section 9.1), serum unsaturated iron-binding capacity, and total iron-binding capacity. Follow the procedure given by the manufacturer if this differs from that outlined below.

- Iron buffer reagent. Contains hydroxylamine hydrochloride 1.5% (wt/vol) in acetate buffer (pH 4.5) with added surfactant. Store at room temperature.
- UIBC buffer reagent. Contains Tris (hydroxymethyl) aminomethane, 0.5 mol/L, pH 8.1 with added surfactant and preservative. Store at room temperature.
- Iron color reagent. Contains ferrozine 0.85% (wt/vol) in hydroxylamine hydrochloride solution with added stabilizer. Store at room temperature.
- Iron standard with 500 µg/dL (89 µmol/L) iron in hydroxylamine hydrochloride solution. Store at room temperature.
- Sample.   Serum is the specimen of choice; plasma obtained using heparin as an anticoagulant may also be used. EDTA interferes with the determination of iron.   As soon as blood clots, promptly separate serum to avoid any hemolysis; each milligram of hemoglobin

contains 3.4 µg iron. Serum in which there is severe lipidemia—indicated by the presence of turbidity—may cause errors. Lipids dilute the specimen but do not contain iron. Serum iron reportedly is stable for at least four days stored at room temperature or one week in the refrigerator at 0–5°C.

- Pooled serum sample for assessing precision.
- Serum iron reference material.   Serachem Level 1, Fisher Diagnostics, Orangeburg, NY.

Equipment

- Colorimeter or spectrophotometer that allows analysis at a transmitted light wavelength of 560 nm, together with matched cuvets for the instrument employed.
- Iron-free glassware and 0.05, 0.5, 1.0, 2.0, and 5.0 mL pipets.
- Water bath 37°C.
- Iron-free distilled deionized water.

Procedure

1. Label test tubes for the blank, standard, reference, pool, and for each test subject.
2. Add 2.0 mL UIBC buffer reagent to each tube.
3. To blank add 1.0 mL of iron-free water.   To standard add 0.5 mL of the iron standard plus 0.5 mL of iron-free water.   To the reference add 0.5 mL of serum reference material plus 0.5 mL of standard.   To pool add 0.5 mL of the pooled serum plus 0.5 mL of standard. For each test subject, add 0.5 mL of serum to the appropriate tube plus 0.5 mL of standard.
4. Mix each test tube well with the vortex mixer.
5. Transfer each sample to a cuvet.
6. Set the wavelength at 560 nm. Zero the spectrophotometer to zero absorbance with the reagent blank.

Age (yr)	Percentiles of TIBC (µg/dL) by age							Percentiles of TIBC (µg/dL) by age						
	5	10	25	50	75	90	95	5	10	25	50	75	90	95
	Male subjects							Female subjects						
3–5	310.0	330.1	355.4	383.4	414.3	443.1	462.0	317.1	326.4	347.4	377.5	404.4	433.3	452.4
6–8	306.2	332.3	353.3	383.4	408.4	431.2	451.4	316.2	328.4	349.4	374.0	411.2	440.4	464.3
9–11	317.4	328.4	354.3	378.5	410.1	438.5	453.0	310.1	322.2	348.4	378.3	408.3	434.2	456.2
12–14	324.3	338.3	364.4	396.4	432.2	460.5	489.2	315.5	333.2	361.0	392.3	428.1	465.3	478.1
15–17	307.5	330.1	358.0	385.5	419.4	452.4	471.4	310.3	328.4	356.5	388.3	424.4	461.3	489.2
18–24	302.2	314.1	341.0	370.2	403.4	435.2	455.1	296.4	318.0	349.0	386.5	430.2	479.4	511.3
25–34	297.3	310.4	331.1	361.2	391.3	426.1	441.2	289.3	305.4	336.1	373.5	421.1	475.3	501.3
35–44	287.0	299.1	324.2	355.4	392.4	428.5	455.0	287.5	306.1	334.2	369.3	406.3	449.1	471.1
45–54	287.4	303.1	330.1	362.2	401.2	430.5	452.4	296.5	308.5	336.3	368.3	411.3	446.4	482.2
55–64	287.2	300.2	325.4	356.3	390.1	426.4	453.4	290.2	303.3	330.2	363.1	394.4	435.1	455.1
65–74	275.2	295.1	315.5	343.5	376.3	409.3	431.2	283.0	299.2	325.4	355.3	389.4	426.4	455.2

Table 9.2: Percentiles of total iron binding capacity (µg/dL) by age for males and females of three to seventy-four years. Data are from the U.S. NHANES II (1976–80) survey and were compiled by Fulwood et al. (1982).

7. Read and record initial absorbance of the blank, standard, reference, pool, and test samples. Return the samples to the appropriate tubes after reading. This is the initial absorbance ($A_{Initial}$), measured to take into account differences in the turbidity of the sample.

8. Add 0.05 mL iron color reagent to each tube. Mix and allow to stand for approximately ten minutes in a water bath at 37°C.

9. Transfer each sample to a cuvet.

10. Again read and record the absorbance of the blank, standard, reference, pool, and test samples, using the blank to zero the spectrophotometer. This is the final absorbance (A_{Final}). Occasionally, the difference between the final absorbance (A_{Final}) and the the initial absorbance may be very small because of the large degree of unsaturation of transferrin with iron. If this occurs, the sample should be diluted (1 part serum and 1 part iron-free water) and the test repeated. The results, calculated using the equation below, must then be multiplied by 2.0.

Calculation of results

If the iron standard contains 500 µg/dL, the serum unsaturated iron-binding capacity (µg/dL) equals:

$$500 - \left(\frac{500 \times (\text{Test A}_{Final} - \text{Test A}_{Initial})}{\text{Standard A}_{Final} - \text{Standard A}_{Initial}} \right)$$

Total iron-binding capacity (TIBC) (µg/dL) = Serum total iron (µg/dL) + serum unsaturated iron-binding capacity (µg/dL). The conversion factor to SI units (µmol/L) = ×0.179.

Evaluation

The total iron-binding capacity (TIBC) is related to the total number of free iron-binding sites on the transport protein transferrin. Normal values for TIBC determined by this method are 250–410 µg/dL. Total iron binding capacity (µg/dL) percentiles from the U.S. NHANES II survey for persons three to seventy-four years (all races) are given in Table 9.2. In iron deficiency, there is an increase in the number of free iron-binding sites. Hence, TIBC is elevated, a trend also observed in women taking oral contraceptive agents (Pilch and Senti, 1984). Levels of TIBC also tend to be above normal in conditions associated with increased erythropoiesis (e.g. hemolysis, polycythemia). Total iron-binding capacity is less subject to biological variation—especially diurnal effects—than serum iron, but is more susceptible to analytical errors (Dallman, 1984).

Serum transferrin saturation measures the iron supply to the erythroid bone marrow. It is derived from serum iron and the total iron-binding capacity. Serum transferrin saturation (as %) equals:

$$\frac{\text{Serum iron (µg/dL)} \times 100\%}{\text{Total iron binding capacity (µg/dL)}}$$

The normal range for transferrin saturation is from 30–40%. Decreased values occur with iron

Age (yr)	Percentiles of Transferrin Saturation (%) by age							Percentiles of Transferrin Saturation (%) by age						
	5	10	25	50	75	90	95	5	10	25	50	75	90	95
	Male subjects							Female subjects						
3–5	10.1	11.9	16.7	21.2	27.8	34.5	39.2	10.9	13.6	16.8	22.6	28.5	34.7	38.7
6–8	11.6	13.1	16.6	21.9	28.1	34.5	39.4	11.7	13.7	17.3	23.0	28.9	34.5	38.2
9–11	11.6	13.2	17.3	22.3	28.7	34.5	38.1	13.4	15.1	18.8	24.8	30.9	36.7	40.8
12–14	12.8	14.9	18.1	23.4	30.1	34.4	39.0	10.9	13.9	19.8	24.5	30.6	36.9	40.9
15–17	16.6	18.1	21.9	27.4	34.3	40.7	45.5	10.9	12.8	18.5	24.7	32.3	40.3	44.8
18–24	15.9	18.0	23.5	29.7	36.6	43.8	49.1	11.6	14.3	19.8	25.7	32.9	40.9	46.0
25–34	16.8	18.6	23.7	29.6	36.2	44.1	48.5	12.1	15.1	19.6	25.6	33.2	41.2	45.7
35–44	15.2	17.6	21.4	27.1	34.1	41.1	46.0	10.9	13.1	18.4	24.6	32.2	39.8	45.3
45–54	14.3	16.7	21.6	27.2	33.6	39.7	44.4	13.3	14.9	18.6	24.3	30.3	36.6	41.2
55–64	14.2	17.0	21.3	27.2	34.1	40.2	44.6	13.9	15.9	20.3	25.2	30.3	37.4	42.6
65–74	15.6	17.6	22.6	28.2	34.9	41.6	47.1	13.9	16.6	20.2	25.3	30.8	36.9	41.5

Table 9.3: Percentiles of transferrin saturation (%) by age for males and females of three to seventy-four years. Data are from the U.S. NHANES II (1976–80) survey and were compiled by Fulwood et al. (1982).

deficiency anemia, arising from a fall in serum iron levels, concomitant with a rise in TIBC. Transferrin saturation tends towards the low end of the normal range in the anemias that occur with infection, rheumatoid arthritis, chronic disease, and neoplasms. Such anemias typically produce both low serum iron and low TIBC because iron cannot be released from the reticulo-endothelial cells and transported to transferrin—termed the 'mucosal block'. Consequently, iron stores are adequate, so that the body does not respond to the fall in serum iron by increasing absorption of iron from the diet. Hence, transferrin synthesis is not increased. In adult subjects, a transferrin saturation below 16% indicates iron-deficient erythropoiesis (Dallman, 1977), provided that infection and inflammation are absent (Cook, 1982).

Age-related differences in normal serum iron (but not TIBC) occur in infants and children, resulting in corresponding changes in the normal levels of transferrin saturation (Dallman et al., 1980). Uncertainties still exist in the extent of these changes. Consequently, cutoff points are not as clearly defined for infants and children as for adults. Pilch and Senti (1984) used cutoff values ranging from <12% to <16% for transferrin saturation in children one to fourteen years of age when assessing iron-deficiency in the U.S. NHANES II survey.

Elevated transferrin saturation values occur in hemochromatosis, thalassemia, and hemosiderosis. In addition, in conditions of decreased erythropoiesis, transferrin saturation may also be high.

In the U.S. NHANES II survey, a transferrin saturation >70% was used as a criterion for detecting iron overload in adults, in conjunction with elevated serum ferritin levels. Transferrin saturation (%) percentiles for U.S. persons three to seventy-four years (all races) are given in Table 9.3.

References

Carter P (1971). Spectrophotometric determination of serum iron at the sub-microgram level with a new reagent (ferrozine). Analytical Biochemistry 40: 450–458.

Cook J D (1982). Clinical evaluation of iron deficiency. Seminars in Hematology 19: 6–18.

Dallman P R (1977). New approaches to screening for iron deficiency. Journal of Pediatrics 90: 678–681.

Dallman P R (1984). Diagnosis of anemia and iron deficiency: analytic and biological variations of laboratory tests. American Journal of Clinical Nutrition 39: 937–941.

Dallman P R, Siimes M A, Stekel A (1980). Iron deficiency in infancy and childhood. American Journal of Clinical Nutrition 33: 86–118.

Fulwood R, Johnson C L, Bryner J D et al. (1982). Hematological and nutritional reference data for persons 6 months – 74 years of age: United States, 1976–80. Vital and Health Statistics Series 11, No. 32 DHHS Publication No. 83-1682, Washington, DC.

Persijn J P, Slik van der W, Riethorst A (1971). Determination of serum iron and latent iron-binding capacity (LIBC). Clinica Chimica Acta 35: 91–98.

Pilch S M, Senti F R (eds) (1984). Assessment of the iron nutritional status of the US population based on data collected in the second National Health and Nutrition Examination Survey, 1976–1980. Life Sciences Research Office, Federation of the American Societies for Experimental Biology, Bethesda, Maryland.

9.3 Serum ferritin

Principle

Ferritin was first identified in human serum by Addison et al. (1972); its function in serum is unknown. Ferritin appears to enter the plasma by secretions from the reticulo-endothelial system (Cook and Skikne, 1982). In most individuals the concentration of serum ferritin parallels the total amount of storage iron, and serum ferritin is the only iron status index that can reflect a deficient, excess, and normal iron status.

Ferritin is assayed using a two-site radio-immunoassay method (Miles et al., 1974). The method is dependent on the competition between native ferritin in the test serum and ferritin labeled with ^{125}I, for a specific binding protein. The latter is normally antiferritin antibodies which are bound to a solid matrix—polyacrylamide beads (ferritin immunobeads).

For the test, each standard and test sample is mixed with ^{125}I-ferritin and the antiferritin antibody, and then incubated. During the one hour incubation, endogenous and labeled ^{125}I-ferritin compete for available binding sites on the antiferritin antibody. Once the binding reaction is completed, the protein bound fraction is washed with saline, and then separated from the unbound, free ^{125}I ferritin and the unlabeled ferritin, by centrifugation. The unbound ferritin is decanted off in the supernatant. The amount of labeled ferritin which is bound to the binding protein (antiferritin antibody) is determined by counting the gamma radiation emitted from the ^{125}I using a gamma counter. A standard curve is constructed of the ferritin concentrations of the standards and their corresponding radioactivity bound to the binding protein (as counts per minute) from which the ferritin concentrations of the test samples can be estimated.

Reagents

The shelf-life of ^{125}I is short. Consequently assay kits should be ordered only when they are required. They can be purchased from Bio-Rad Laboratories, Richmond, CA. Follow the procedure given by the manufacturer if this differs from that outlined below.

- Ferritin standards: blank, 5.0, 10.0, 25.0, 100, 250, 1000, and 2500 ng/mL.

- ^{125}I-Antibody (Ab) to ferritin ($<10\,\mu$Ci). Slowly and carefully reconstitute this by adding distilled deionized water, following the dilution instructions supplied with the tracer. Agitate gently to dissolve. Allow to stand for five minutes. Store at 2–8°C.

- The tracer/immunobead reagent (ferritin bound to polyacrylamide beads) must be prepared within two hours of performing the assay. Mix 100 μL of ^{125}I-Ab to ferritin with 100 μL of ferritin immunobead. 200 μL Tracer/Immunobead reagent is required for each test sample and each standard.

- Normal saline (0.9%).

- Sample—Serum or plasma which has been removed from the red blood cells as soon as is practical. Avoid hemolysis. Samples can be refrigerated if the assay is to be undertaken within seven days after the blood collection. For longer periods, serum/plasma must be frozen at −70°C. Thaw frozen samples and mix before using.

- Pool serum sample for assessing the precision of the determination.

- Serum ferritin reference material. Lyphochek immuno-assay control sera (Anemia, Levels I, II, and III).

Equipment

- Gamma Counter.
- Centrifuge (1500 × g).
- Pipets
  - 50 μL for standards and samples,
  - 200 μL for tracer reagent,
  - 3.0 mL repeating dispenser.
- Graph paper—four-cycle semi-log.
- Polypropylene tubes (12 × 75 mm).
- Vortex mixer.
- Suction apparatus for removing supernatant.

Procedures for handling radioactive material

- Do not smoke or eat while handling radioactive material.

- Do not pipet materials by mouth.

- Use gloves while handling radioactive materials and wash hands thoroughly after use.

- Radioactive spills should be wiped up quickly with some absorbent material. The contaminated absorbent material should then be disposed of in the radioactive waste bin. Then a wipe test should be performed to ensure that all radioactive material has been removed.

Procedure

Note: The standards, pool, reference, and test serums should all be analyzed in duplicate. Allow tracer and standards to come to room temperature before use.

1. Label tubes: Background, blank, 5.0, 10.0, 25.0, 100, 250, 1000, 2500, pool, reference, and tubes for each test subject.

2. Add 50 µL of each standard, pool, reference, and test serums to the respective tubes, commencing with the lowest dilution first.

3. Advise the laboratory supervisor that you are ready for the the Tracer/Immunobead reagent. This should be mixed thoroughly with a stirrer bar to prevent bubble formation, prior to use. To comply with Safety Regulations, a laboratory supervisor may have to supervise the addition of 200 µL of the working tracer to each tube. Set aside the background tube until step 8.

4. Shake the rack of tubes to mix the contents (vortexing is not necessary). Incubate for 30 minutes at 21–30°C (room temperature).

5. Add 3.0 mL saline to all tubes (mixing not necessary at this stage).

6. Centrifuge all the tubes for ten minutes at 1500 × g at 4°C, to pack the solids into the bottom of the tube. Proceed promptly to the next step.

7. Remove the supernatant in each tube using a special suction apparatus.

8. Insert all the tubes (including the background tube) into the gamma counter, noting the order in which the tubes will be counted and the corresponding number on the gamma counter.

9. Count each tube for one minute with the gamma counter.

Calculation of results

1. Record the average counts per minute (CPM) for each of the standards, controls, and test samples.

2. Subtract the mean CPM of the zero standard from the CPM of each standard, control, and test sample, to give the *net* CPM.

3. Plot the net CPM of each of the standards on the Y-axis of four-cycle semilog paper and the corresponding ferritin concentrations (ng/mL) on the X-axis.

4. Read off from the standard curve the ferritin concentrations (ng/mL) of the controls and test samples from their corresponding net CPM.

   Conversion to SI units (µg/L) = ×1.0.

Performance checks

1. The CPM of the zero standard should be less than 6% of the background count. For example:

$$3407/105559 \times 100\% = 3.2\%$$

2. High standard as a percentage of total counts. The CPM of the highest standard (2500 ng/mL) should be greater than 45% of the background count. For example:

$$72513/105559 \times 100\% = 68.7\%$$

3. Reproducibility between assays is determined by analyzing data from the pool serum sample which should be determined with each group of samples.

4. Accuracy of the assay procedure is assessed by analyzing the reference material (Lyphochek) and comparing the results with the certified values.

Age (yr)	Serum Ferritin (ng/mL)	Transferrin Saturation (%)	Erythrocyte Protoporphyrin µg/dL RBC	MCV (fL)
1–2	—	<12	>80	<73
3–4	<10	<14	>75	<75
5–10	<10	<15	>70	<76
11–14	<10	<16	>70	<78
15–74	<12	<16	>70	<80

Table 9.4: Cutoff points used for identifying abnormal values of iron status indices in the analysis of the U.S. NHANES II data. The conversion factors for SI units are: serum ferritin (µg/L) = ×1.0; erythrocyte protoporphyrin (µmol/L) = × 0.0177. From Pilch and Senti (1984).

Age (yrs)	Serum Ferritin Percentiles (ng/mL)						
	5	10	25	50	75	90	95
Children							
3–4		7	9	17	32	39	
5–10	5	8	12	17	25	34	40
Males							
11–14		8	13	17	28	41	
15–19	13	15	21	35	58	80	95
20–44	25	32	54	90	128	181	227
45–64	25	39	66	106	172	255	337
65–74	21	35	60	102	173	290	367
Females							
11–14		8	13	17	28	35	
15–19	3	5	10	20	35	59	69
20–44	7	9	18	30	58	98	118
45–64	5	21	33	62	113	156	193
65–74	8	28	45	73	111	158	231

Table 9.5: Serum ferritin (ng/mL) percentiles for persons one to seventy-four years (all races). Percentiles are for the U.S. NHANES II 'reference population'. Abstracted from the more comprehensive tabulations of Pilch and Senti (1984).

Evaluation

The cutoff values used in the U.S. NHANES II survey for serum ferritin indicative of depletion of iron stores are shown in Table 9.4. Serum ferritin (ng/mL) percentiles for U.S. persons three to seventy-four years (all races) are given in Table 9.5. Percentiles are for the U.S. NHANES II 'reference population' (Pilch and Senti, 1984).

Serum ferritin values fall during iron-deficiency before the characteristic changes in serum iron and TIBC. A low serum ferritin concentration is characteristic only of iron deficiency (Dallman et al., 1980). Elevated serum ferritin values

Age Group	Males	Females
20–44 yr	>200	>150
45–64 yr	>300	>200
65–74 yr	>400	>300

Table 9.6: Cutoff values for serum ferritin (ng/mL) indicative of iron overload in adults. Conversion factor to SI units (µg/L) = ×1.0. From Pilch and Senti (1984).

are useful in diagnosing iron overload disorders. The cutoff values of the U.S. NHANES II survey used as indicative of iron overload in conjunction with transferrin saturation >70%, are shown in Table 9.6. These high levels are not specific to iron overload disorders; they also occur in infection, liver disease, certain neoplastic diseases, and inflammation as shown in Table 9.7 (Dallman, 1977), arising from the 'mucosal block' which results in an increased rate of ferritin synthesis in the reticulo-endothelial system. In acute and chronic liver disease, abnormally high serum ferritin values probably also arise from the release of ferritin from the damaged degenerating liver cells, which contain appreciable amounts of ferritin. Hence, serum ferritin should not be used as an index of iron status in countries where iron deficiency co-exists with infection or inflammation; values may be in the normal range despite

	Age (yr)	Serum Ferritin (µg/L)		
		Both sexes	Males	Females
NHANES II Normal children	3–4	15	14	17
	5–10	19	18	19
	11–14	18	18	18
	15–19	25	35	18
Normal adults	20–44	50	89	28
	45–64	81	110	63
	65–74	83	98	74
Worwood (1979) Iron deficiency anemia	3–14	<10	—	—
	15–74	<12	—	—
Idiopathic hemochromatosis	adults	1000–10,000	—	—
Liver disease	adults	400–3000+	—	—
Inflammation	adults	10–1650	—	—
Acute infections	children	100–510	—	—

Table 9.7: Changes in serum ferritin concentrations with age and disease states. The NHANES II data are from Pilch and Senti (1984), and are the median values and representative of all races.

the presence of iron deficiency. In such cases, alternative indices of iron status, such as red blood cell protoporphyrin, and/or serum iron and total iron-binding capacity, should be used. Changes in serum ferritin concentrations with age and sex are also shown in Table 9.7.

References

Addison G M, Beamish M R, Hayles C N, Hodgkins M, Jacobs A, Llewellyn P (1972). An immunoradiometric assay for ferritin in the serum of normal subjects and patients with iron deficiency and iron overload. Journal of Clinical Pathology 25: 326–329.

Cook J D, Skikne B S (1982). Serum ferritin: a possible model for the assessment of nutrient stores. American Journal of Clinical Nutrition 35: 1180–1185.

Dallman P R (1977). New approaches to screening for iron deficiency. Journal of Pediatrics 90: 678–681.

Dallman P R, Siimes M A, Stekel A (1980). Iron deficiency in infancy and childhood. American Journal of Clinical Nutrition 33: 86–118.

Miles LEM, Lipschitz DA, Bieber CP, Cook JD (1974). Measurement of serum ferritin by a 2-site immunoradiometric assay. Annals of Biochemistry 61: 209–224.

Pilch S M, Senti F R (eds) (1984). Assessment of the iron nutritional status of the US population based on data collected in the second National Health and Nutrition Examination Survey, 1976–1980. Life Sciences Research Office, Federation of the American Societies for Experimental Biology, Bethesda, Maryland.

Worwood M (1979). Serum ferritin. CRC Critical Reviews in Clinical Laboratory Sciences 10: 171–204.

9.4 Erythrocyte protoporphyrin

Principle

Protoporphyrin, a precursor of heme, normally occurs in erythrocytes in low concentrations. In the second stage of iron deficiency, when iron stores are completely exhausted, protoporphyrin IX accumulates in the developing erythrocytes because the supply of iron is not adequate for the synthesis of heme. Consequently, a rise in erythrocyte protoporphyrin concentration is a sensitive indicator of an inadequate iron supply. Erythrocyte protoporphyrin provides the same information as percentage transferrin saturation but is a more stable measurement and responds more gradually to changes in the iron supply to the marrow (Langer et al., 1972). It is also used as an index of chronic lead poisoning in children and adults.

Erythrocyte protoporphyrin can be measured using a simple and inexpensive fluorometric procedure. A hematofluorometer has been designed for field use to determine the zinc chelate of protoporphyrin in erythrocytes by measuring its fluorescence in a thin film of capillary whole blood (Poh Fitzpatrick and Lamola, 1976).

Reagents

- Zinc protoporphyrin red blood cell controls. Low: $35 \mu g \pm 4$ per dL whole blood. Medium: $60 \mu g \pm 6$ per dL whole blood. High: $100 \mu g \pm 10$ per dL whole blood. On special request, a red blood control with values of $200 \mu g$ per dL can be obtained from Aviv Biomedical Inc. Stable at room temperature for 2 weeks; at $2-4°C$ for up to 3 months; and at $-20°C$ for 6 months. Allow to warm to room temperature and then mix gently by inversion. Alternatively use a vortex mixer at a low speed. Remove a $25 \mu L$ aliquot for the assay, reseal the vial and return to the refrigerator.

- Sample—Whole blood, using EDTA or heparin as an anticoagulant. Alternatively, capillary blood collected in a micro hematocrit tube may be used, provided the first drop is discarded. Anticoagulated whole blood can be stored for one day at room temperature or in a refrigerator for one week at 4°C provided no more than about 10% hemolysis has occurred. Frozen blood cannot be used. Blood can be diluted up to three-fold with saline if necessary for the test.

Equipment

- ZP Hematofluorometer (model 206) (available from Aviv Biomedical, Inc., Lakewood, NJ) with 0.15 mm glass cover slips (No. 1).

- Vortex mixer.

Procedure

1. Press the 'ON' button of the Hematofluorometer and insert a blank glass cover slip into the sample holder.

2. Press the 'MEASURE' button and take the reading of the blank glass cover slip. Only use blank cover slips with readings from 000–006.

3. Use a plastic pasteur pipet to place a drop of whole blood (about $20 \mu L$) onto the blank cover slip, spreading it so that it corresponds to the position of the hole.

4. Press the 'MEASURE' button and record reading. Do not subtract blank cover slip reading.

5. Repeat (4) after 10–15 seconds have elapsed and then discard the glass cover slip.

6. For blood controls, deposit a drop of blood (about $35 \mu L$) onto a clean glass cover slip by squeezing bottle. Mix drop of blood with the tip of the bottle. Replace bottle cap.

7. Press the 'MEASURE' button and record reading. Discard glass cover slip.

8. Check blood controls at the beginning and end of each day, or after 50 assays, where applicable. Low, medium, and high control values should be within stated values.

Age (yr)	Percentiles of Erythrocyte Protoporphyrin by age							Percentiles of Erythrocyte Protoporphyrin by age						
	5	10	25	50	75	90	95	5	10	25	50	75	90	95
	Male subjects							Female subjects						
3–5	36.0	40.1	46.1	55.0	65.0	78.1	93.1	37.0	41.0	46.1	55.0	66.0	79.0	97.0
6–8	37.0	41.0	46.0	53.0	62.0	71.0	77.0	35.1	39.0	45.0	54.0	63.1	75.1	83.1
9–11	37.1	41.0	47.0	53.1	62.1	71.1	80.0	36.0	40.0	45.1	53.0	62.1	73.1	80.0
12–14	35.1	37.1	43.0	49.0	57.0	67.0	75.1	37.0	40.0	45.1	53.0	61.0	71.0	76.0
15–17	33.0	36.0	40.0	45.1	52.0	59.0	66.0	37.0	39.0	43.1	50.1	58.0	67.1	79.1
18–24	33.0	36.0	40.0	45.0	51.0	58.0	64.0	37.0	39.0	45.0	51.0	61.0	71.1	80.1
25–34	33.0	35.1	40.0	45.0	51.1	58.0	64.0	37.0	40.0	45.0	52.0	61.0	73.1	84.0
35–44	33.0	36.0	40.0	46.0	52.0	61.0	68.0	37.1	40.0	45.0	52.0	61.0	76.1	92.0
45–54	33.1	36.1	41.0	46.0	54.0	64.1	77.0	37.0	40.0	45.1	52.0	62.0	76.0	93.1
55–64	35.0	37.0	42.0	48.0	57.0	67.1	76.1	35.1	39.0	44.1	52.0	62.0	75.0	89.1
65–74	34.0	37.0	42.0	49.0	58.1	70.0	81.0	37.0	40.0	45.1	54.0	63.0	77.0	88.0

Table 9.8: Percentiles of erythrocyte protoporphyrin (µg/dL RBC) by age for males and females of three to seventy-four years. Data are from the U.S. NHANES II (1976–80) survey and were compiled by Fulwood et al. (1982).

Calculation of results

Zinc protoporphyrin concentrations, expressed as µmol/L RBC's, can be calculated using the following formula, where hematocrit is expressed as the volume fraction of packed red cell:

$$\frac{\text{Zn protoporphyrin in whole blood (µmol/L)}}{\text{Hematocrit (vol. fraction)}}$$

Alternatively zinc protoporphyrin concentrations can be given in µg/dL whole blood: the conversion factor to SI units (µmol/L) = × 0.0177.

Evaluation

The cutoff values for erythrocyte protoporphyrin indicative of abnormal values used in the U.S. NHANES II survey are shown in Table 9.4. In adults, a protoporphyrin level greater than 70 µg/dL (1.24 µmol/L) RBC has been associated with depleted iron stores, and was used as the cutoff point for abnormal values for adults in the U.S. NHANES II survey (Pilch and Senti, 1984). In classical iron deficiency, when microcytic hypochromic anemia occurs, erythrocyte protoporphyrin levels may rise to values ranging from 83 to 457 µg/dL (1.47 to 8.09 µmol/L) RBC. The cutoff points selected for children aged one to fourteen years represent >90th percentile of the U.S. NHANES II reference population data.

Percentiles for erythrocyte protoporphyrin from the U.S. NHANES II survey for persons three to seventy-four years (all races) are given in Table 9.8. However, chronic disease states, such as infection, inflammation, and certain neoplastic diseases, are associated with elevated protoporphyrin levels resulting from the mucosal block defect. Therefore, erythrocyte protoporphyrin values, unlike serum ferritin, cannot be used to differentiate between iron deficiency caused by total body depletion of iron, and that arising from the mucosal block defect: both situations generate elevated erythrocyte protoporphyrin levels. Hence only additional measurements of iron status, such as serum ferritin and total iron-binding capacity, can distinguish these two conditions.

Lead toxicity produces high erythrocyte protoporphyrin levels via interference with heme synthesis, particularly in children up to four years of age.

References

Langer E E, Haining R G, Labbe R F, Jacobs P, Crosby E F, Finch C A (1972). Erythrocyte protoporphyrin. Blood 40: 112–128.

Fulwood R, Johnson C L, Bryner J D et al. (1982). Hematological and nutritional reference data for persons 6 months – 74 years of age: United States, 1976–80. Vital and Health Statistics Series 11, No. 32 DHHS Publication No. 83-1682, Washington, DC.

Pilch S M, Senti F R (eds) (1984). Assessment of the iron nutritional status of the US population based on data collected in the second National Health and Nutrition Examination Survey, 1976–1980. Life Sciences Research Office, Federation of the American Societies for Experimental Biology, Bethesda, Maryland.

Poh Fitzpatrick M, Lamola A A (1976). Direct spectrofluorometry of diluted erythrocytes and plasma: A rapid diagnostic method in primary and secondary porphyrinemias. Journal of Laboratory and Clinical Medicine 87: 362–370.

Chapter 10
Assessment of mineral status

Contents

Introduction

The major mineral components of the body are calcium, phosphorus, and magnesium; all occur in combination with organic and inorganic compounds and as free ions. They have two major roles: structural components in bone and soft tissues, and regulatory agents in body fluids. Trace minerals occur in the body in very small or 'trace' amounts; they generally constitute less than 0.01% of the body mass. Of the trace minerals, ten are essential in humans. They differ in their properties and biological functions; many act primarily by forming metallo-enzymes. Both static and functional tests are used to assess mineral status. Biochemical tests used to assess calcium, copper, and zinc status are included in this chapter.

Calcium is the most abundant mineral in the body, and is stored primarily in the bones. The remainder is involved in enzyme activation, blood coagulation, muscle contractibility, nerve transmission, hormone function and membrane transport. Severe nutritional deficiency of calcium is rare because absorption and urinary excretion of calcium are regulated in response to need.

Nevertheless, inadequate intakes of calcium during early life may limit peak adult bone mass and hence increase the risk of osteoporosis in later life (Spencer et al., 1982). At present, there is no satisfactory routine biochemical method for assessing calcium status. Serum calcium concentrations are assayed in routine clinical laboratories, generally to diagnose pathological rather than nutritional problems. A method based on a fluorometric titration is described in Section 10.1; flame absorption spectrophotometry can also be used.

Copper is an essential trace mineral in humans; it is component of many enzyme systems, including some that catalyze oxido-reduction reactions. Copper deficiency is rare in humans, although the hematological deficiency signs (e.g. neutropenia and hypochromic anemia), which occur first, have been described in premature and/or low birthweight infants and some adults with sickle cell disease receiving prolonged zinc therapy. Most of the reports of copper deficiency in humans have resulted from inadequate dietary intakes of copper, often in association with prolonged diarrhea which prevents reabsorption of copper from the bile. Diseases associated with chronic loss of proteins, such as nephritic syndrome and protein-losing enteropathy, may also cause copper deficiency, as a result of loss of ceruloplasmin and of copper bound to albumin (Mason, 1979).

Most of the clinical manifestations of copper deficiency are explicable in terms of changes in the activities of cuproenzymes. For instance, a reduction in ceruloplasmin, a cuproenzyme found in the α_2-globulin fraction of human serum, impairs the transport of iron to the erythropoietic sites, resulting in hypochromic anemia. Serum ceruloplasmin can be assayed by measuring its enzymatic activity (Sunderman and Nomoto, 1970), or immunochemically by radial immunodiffusion, described in Section 10.2.

Zinc is a constituent of over 200 metallo-enzymes which participate in carbohydrate, lipid, and protein metabolism, and nucleic acid synthesis and degradation. Hence, zinc is essential for many diverse functions including growth and development, reproduction, immune and sensory function, anti-oxidant protection, and the stabilization of membranes (Cousins, 1986).

Marginal zinc deficiency, characterized by slowing of physical growth, poor appetite, and diminished taste acuity, has been described in infants and children in North America and elsewhere, arising, in part, from inadequate intakes and/or poor availability of dietary zinc (Walravens et al., 1983). Other groups susceptible to zinc deficiency include pregnant women (Solomons et al., 1986) and the elderly (Sandstead et al., 1982). Secondary zinc deficiency may occur in the presence of certain disease states such as cystic fibrosis, as well as in renal and liver diseases, and in association with burns and alcoholism (Aggett and Harries, 1979).

No single, specific, and sensitive index of zinc status exists. A combination of static and functional indices is frequently used (Prasad, 1988). Results of animal studies have suggested that certain zinc-metallo-enzymes such as alkaline phosphatase, may be promising as indices of zinc status

(Kirchgessner et al., 1976). The assay of alkaline phosphatase in serum is described in Section 10.3.

References

Aggett P J, Harries J T (1979). Current status of zinc in health and disease states. Archives of Diseases of Childhood 54: 909–917.

Cousins R J (1986). Towards a molecular understanding of zinc metabolism. Clinical Physiology and Biochemistry 4: 20–30.

Kirchgessner M, Roth H P, Weigand E (1976). Biochemical changes in zinc deficiency. In: Prasad A S (ed). Trace Elements in Human Health and Disease. Volume 1. Zinc and Copper. Academic Press, New York, pp. 189–225.

Mason K E (1979). A conspectus of research on copper metabolism and requirements of man. Journal of Nutrition 109: 1979–2066.

Prasad A S (1988). Clinical and diagnostic aspects of human zinc deficiency. In: Prasad A S (ed). Essential and toxic trace elements in human health and disease. Alan R Liss, New York, pp. 3–53.

Sandstead HH, Henriksen LK, Greger JL, Prasad AS, Good RA (1982). Zinc nutriture in the elderly in relation to taste acuity, immune response, and wound healing. American Journal of Clinical Nutrition 36: 1046–1059.

Solomons N W, Helitzer-Allen D L, Villar J (1986). Zinc needs during pregnancy. Clinical Nutrition 5: 63–71.

Spencer H, Kramer L, Osis D (1982). Factors contributing to calcium loss in aging. American Journal of Clinical Nutrition 36: 776–787.

Sunderman F W J r, Nomoto S (1970). Measurement of human serum ceruloplasmin by its ρ-phenylene-diamine oxidase activity. Clinical Chemistry 16: 903–910.

Walravens P A, Krebs N F, Hambidge K M (1983). Linear growth of low income preschool children receiving a zinc supplement. American Journal of Clinical Nutrition 38: 195–201.

10.1 Serum calcium

Principle

This serum calcium method is based on a fluorometric titration using calcein, a fluorescein derivative as the indicator, and EGTA as the titrant (Borle and Briggs, 1968). The EGTA increases the specificity of the determination in the presence of magnesium. The titration is conducted in an instrument called a Calcette (Precision Systems Inc, Natick, MA, 01760). The Calcette consists of a disposable reagent cell containing a measured amount of dry calcein-KCl crystals which are activated by the addition of reagent cell activator. The pH during titration is maintained at above pH 13 to minimize interference. When a sample containing calcium is dispensed into the reagent cell, the amount of fluorescence increases producing extra light on the photocell. This causes EGTA to be added automatically until the fluorescence is quenched. The amount of EGTA added to quench the extra light is indicated by the number of pulses counted by the digital readout. The end point for the photocell is established and verified throughout the procedure by using a series of calcium standards (Alexander, 1971).

Reagents

- Reagent cell activator. This reagent contains potassium hydroxide–50% 1N and 50% denatured absolute ethanol. To reconstitute, pour reagent cell activator into the cell up to the mark (approximately 25 mL). Replace the cap and swirl gently to mix. Remove the cap, wipe off the excess, and set the cell in the cell holder of the Calcette and screw into the optical chamber. Press the button labeled 'sample' to cancel the read light and activate the stirrer. Stir for five minutes.

- EGTA titrant—Ethylene glycol-bis-(β-aminoethyl ether)-N,N^1-tetra-acetic acid. Store in a dark, dry area. Do not refrigerate or expose to sunlight. Do not reuse. The titrant is a degassed solution. Do not pipet. Instead pour contents from the bottle.

- Calcium standard solution. Ca^{++} as calcium carbonate 5.0 mEq/L. Care must be taken

to ensure that the standard solution is not contaminated. Always pour into a clean vial; do not pipet from the bottle; always replace the cap immediately. Always rinse the container which feeds the standard into the Calcette with the calcium standard. Do not return unused solution to the bottle. Store in a dark, dry area; do not refrigerate or expose to sunlight.

- Calcein reagent cells. Each disposable cuvet contains calcein indicator, buffer, stabilizer, and matrix material—100 mg/cell.

- Indicator solution. This is prepared by adding reagent cell activator to the contents of a calcein reagent cell, up to the mark. Replace the cap and mix well. Remove the cap, and wipe any excess from the rim of the cell before placing the cell in the optical chamber of the Calcette. Store in a dark, dry area—do not refrigerate or expose to sunlight.

- Certified reference serum (obtainable from Sigma Diagnostics, Sigma Chemical Co., St Louis, MO).

- Sample—serum or heparinized plasma, separated quickly to avoid prolonged contact with the red blood cells which become permeable to calcium. Anticoagulants such as oxalate, EDTA, or fluoride, which either complex or precipitate calcium, should not be used.

Procedure

The instrument used must be calibrated and adjusted for the determination of serum calcium before use.

1. Wipe the probe tip gently before placing it into the calcium standard solution (10 mg/dL).

2. Press the 'sample' button. The sample light will come on and the 'probe' light will go out. The 'read' light will go out and the digital display will re-set to zero.

3. Remove the standard solution and wipe off probe tip gently.

4. Press the 'titrate' button. The probe will travel into the instrument, 'sample' light will go out and 'titrate' light will come on. Numbers will appear on the read-out. When the end point is reached, 'read' light will come on and the probe will return to the front of the instrument.

5. Record the reading.

6. Repeat steps 1–5. Readings should be between 9.80 and 10.20 for the calcium standard.

7. Mix test serum thoroughly. Repeat steps 1–5 with test serum sample, and record the results.

8. Repeat steps 1–5 with the certified reference serum with a known calcium value.

Evaluation

Serum calcium concentrations in normal healthy adults range from 8.8 to 10.6 mg/dL (2.20 to 2.64 mmol/L). Values decrease with age in men. Females have slightly lower concentrations (8.8 to 10.2 mg/dL; 2.20 to 2.54 mmol/L) than males (9.2 to 10.6 mg/dL; 2.30 to 2.64 mmol/L) associated with the small differences in albumin content and the calcium-reducing effect of estrogens. Serum calcium decreases by 5% to 10% up to the end of the third trimester of pregnancy, after which concentrations rise (Schuette and Linkswiler, 1984).

Serum calcium concentrations cannot be used an an index of calcium status because they are homeostatically controlled and remain remarkably constant under most conditions. If serum calcium concentrations are outside the normal range, pathological rather than nutritional problems should be suspected. In cases of hypoparathyroidism, hypomagnesemia, and acute pancreatitis, serum calcium concentrations are usually low (hypocalcemia). Elevated serum calcium values (hypercalcemia) occur in association with both hyperparathyroidism and sarcoidosis, and when large areas of the body are immobilized. In such cases, calcium from the rapidly atrophying bone is released into the circulating body fluids. Elevated serum calcium levels also occur in cases of vitamin D intoxication.

References

Alexander R L (1971). Evaluation of an automatic calcium titrator. Clinical Chemistry 17: 1171–1175.

Borle A B, Briggs F N (1968). Microdetermination of calcium in biological materials by automatic fluorometric titration. Analytical Chemistry 40: 339–344.

Schuette S A, Linkswiler H M (1984). Calcium. In: Present Knowledge in Nutrition. Fifth edition. The Nutrition Foundation Inc., Washington, D.C., pp. 410–412.

10.2 Ceruloplasmin

Principle

Ceruloplasmin is the major copper-containing protein in the α_2-globulin fraction of human serum. It is a copper transport protein synthesized by the liver, and consists of a single-chain glycoprotein containing eight copper atoms per molecule. Ceruloplasmin can be determined immunochemically by single radial immunodiffusion.

For this technique, specific antibodies for the protein under investigation, are incorporated into an agar-gel layer which contains a series of small wells at spaced intervals. The wells are filled with three concentrations of a specific antigen (i.e. the standard purified protein), a reference serum, and the test serum samples, respectively. The plates are left to stand at room temperature, during which time the antigen diffuses out of the wells, reacts with the antibody incorporated in the agar gel, and eventually forms a diffuse precipitation zone around the well. The zone grows until all the antigen has complexed with the antibody. After 48 hours, the diameter of the precipitation zone is measured. The concentration of the antigen varies directly with the square of the diameter of the precipitation zone (Fuller, 1972).

Reagents

- Physiological saline; 0.9% NaCl.
- Standard human serum manufactured by Behringwerke (Behring Diagnostics)—can be kept frozen.
- Reference serum (Behringwerke AG).
- Undiluted plasma or serum can be used, either fresh or frozen at $-20°$.

Equipment

- Immunodiffusion plates. LC-Partigen plates for ceruloplasmin are available from Behring Diagnostics, Somerville, N.J. 08876. They can be used up to the date of expiry on the label. Once opened, a plate should be used up within a four week period.
- Micropipets 5 µL: Hamilton microliter syringe or Eppendorf pipets.

- Partigen measuring device or magnifying glass (×7).
- Narrow beam lamp to illuminate the precipitin rings against a dark background.
- Linear graph paper.

Procedure

Note: Care must be taken to ensure that the wells do not overflow. The plates should be stored in a horizontal position on a level surface at room temperature throughout the assay procedure.

1. For the standard curve, prepare three different concentrations of the standard human serum with a known ceruloplasmin concentration

    - Dilute one part standard human serum with three parts 0.9% NaCl (i.e. 1:4) giving a concentration of 15.3 mg/dL. Mix with the vortex mixer.
    - Dilute one part standard human serum with one part 0.9% NaCl (i.e. 1:2) giving a concentration of 30.6 mg/dL. Mix with the vortex mixer.
    - Use undiluted standard human serum with a concentration of 61.2 mg/dL.

2. Fill wells 1 to 3 with 5 µL of each of the three standard concentrations, respectively, using a Hamilton syringe, or an Eppendorf micropipet.

3. Fill well 4 with 5 µL of undiluted reference serum.

4. Fill wells 5 and 6 with 5 µL of undiluted test serum, respectively.

5. After loading, allow the plates to stand open for about 10 to 20 minutes, and then close the plates with the plastic lid to protect from drying during the incubation period.

6. Leave the plates to stand in a horizontal position on a level surface at room temperature for 48 hours. This incubation period allows the diffusion to reach the end-point (i.e. all available antigen has combined with the antibody).

7. After 48 hours, measure the diameter of the precipitate rings (to the nearest 0.1 mm) illuminated by the narrow beam lamp against a dark background using a magnifying glass. Alternatively, the Partigen measuring device can be used. When using the latter, place the device so that the precipitin ring touches both sides of the cone at its greatest diameter. Take the measurement at the point of contact between the diameter of the precipitin ring and the markings of the measuring device. Two measurements of each ring should be taken at right angles to each other to minimize errors due to non-circular rings.

Calculation of results

- Using linear graph paper, plot the standard concentrations of the ceruloplasmin (mg/dL) as the abscissa, with the mean diffusion ring diameter squared (mm^2) as the ordinate. The calibration curve should be a straight line which intersects the ordinate at 20 ± 4.5 mm^2.

- Square the diameter of the precipitin ring produced by the test serum, and read off the corresponding concentration of ceruloplasmin in the test serum directly from the standard curve. If the diameters of the rings produced by the test samples lie outside the range of the calibration curve, then the procedure must be repeated using a correspondingly higher or lower concentration of the test serum sample.

- If necessary, multiply the concentration of ceruloplasmin by the appropriate dilution factor, to obtain the correct concentration in the undiluted test serum.

Evaluation

Measurement of serum ceruloplasmin alone is not recommended as an index of copper status in cross-sectional surveys; the concentration of this metalloenzyme in the serum varies markedly among normal healthy individuals (Danks, 1980). Instead, it is preferable to measure serum ceruloplasmin concentrations prior to, and three to four days after, oral supplementation with copper at physiological levels. Following supplementation, serum ceruloplasmin concentrations will be elevated only in those subjects with copper deficiency (Danks, 1980). In patients with decreased ceruloplasmin produced by other causes, serum ceruloplasmin is unchanged after copper supplementation.

Serum ceruloplasmin concentrations are higher than normal during pregnancy and lactation, in women taking oral contraceptive agents, and in association with malignancy, arthritis and inflammatory disease, liver disease, myocardial infarction, and a variety of infectious diseases (Mason, 1979).

References

Danks D M (1980). Copper deficiency in humans. In: Biological Roles of Copper. Ciba Foundation Symposium 79 (New Series). Excerpta Medica, New York, pp. 209–225.

Fuller J B (1972). Selected Topics in Clinical Chemistry. American Society of Clinical Pathologists Commission on Continuing Education, Chicago, Illinois.

Mason K E (1979). A conspectus of research on copper metabolism and requirements of man. Journal of Nutrition 109: 1979–2066.

10.3 Serum alkaline phosphatase

Principle

Alkaline phosphatases are a group of enzymes widely distributed throughout the body. High concentrations are found in bone, the intestinal mucosa, and the kidney, with lower concentrations in the placenta, liver, and leukocytes. The enzymes act by splitting off a terminal phosphate group from an organic phosphate ester. They are zinc-dependent enzymes. Animals fed zinc-deficient diets for 3 to 6 days have markedly reduced serum alkaline phosphatase activity. In human studies, the activity of alkaline phosphatase in serum is reduced in severe zinc deficiency states, but in marginal zinc deficiency, the response has been less consistent (Ruz et al., 1991).

In the procedure which is described below, the substrate p-nitrophenyl phosphate, is hydrolyzed by alkaline phosphatase producing p-nitrophenol and inorganic phosphate. On the addition of alkali, the liberated p-nitrophenol is converted to a yellow complex, which strongly absorbs light at 404 nm. The intensity of the color formed is proportional to the phosphatase activity and can be quantitated colorimetrically (Andersch and Szczypinski, 1947; McComb and Bowers, 1972).

Reagents

The reagents listed below can be obtained from the Sigma Diagnostics, Sigma Chemical Co., St Louis, MO, as a serum alkaline phosphatase kit. Follow the procedure given by the manufacturer if this differs from that outlined below.

- Phosphatase substrate. Dissolve 100 mg disodium p-nitrophenol phosphate in 25 mL distilled deionized water. Store in the dark at below 0°C. Warm to room temperature before opening to avoid condensation.

- Citrate buffer solution—pH 4.8 at 25°C. Contains citrate (90 mmol/L) and chloride (10 mmol/L).

- p-nitrophenol standard (10 μmol/mL). Store in refrigerator at 2–6°C. Do not use if turbid.

- Working p-nitrophenol standard solution. Pipet 0.5 mL of the p-nitrophenol standard solution into a 100 mL volumetric flask. Dilute to 100 mL with 0.02 N NaOH. Mix thoroughly. Discard after 24 hours.

- Tartrate acid buffer solution. L[+]Tartaric acid 0.04 mol/L in citrate buffer (0.09 mol/L) pH 4.8 at 25°C. Chloroform is added as a preservative. Refrigerate at 2–6°C. Do not use if microbial growth is visible.

- Alkaline buffer solution. 2-Amino-2-methyl-1-propanol. 1.5 mol/L, pH 10.3 at 25°C. Store in refrigerator (2–6°C). Do not use if microbial growth is visible.

- Hydrochloric acid—concentrated.

- Sodium hydroxide solution, 0.05 N. Dissolve 2.0 g sodium hydroxide in 1 L deionized water.

- Sodium hydroxide solution, 0.02 N. Dissolve 0.8 g sodium hydroxide in 1 L deionized water.

- Sigma reference serum

- Sample—Serum or heparinized plasma. Anticoagulants such as citrate, oxalate, or EDTA are unsuitable because they inhibit alkaline phosphatase activity.

Equipment

- Colorimeter or spectrophotometer transmitting wavelengths between 400–420 nm.

- Stop-watch and 37°C water bath.

- Pipets: 0.1, 0.5, and 10.0 mL.

Procedure

Alkaline phosphatase is stable in serum for at least 8 days at 20°C, and for longer periods when frozen.

1. Label four test tubes: blank, test 1, test 2, and reference.

2. Add 0.5 mL alkaline buffer solution to each tube along with 0.5 mL substrate solution. Place all tubes in a 37°C water bath for 5 minutes.

3. To the blank add 0.1 mL of distilled-deionized water. To test 1 add 0.1 mL of test 1 serum. To test 2 add 0.1 mL of test 2 serum. To the reference add 0.1 mL of the reference serum. Record the exact time each serum sample was added. Timing is not crucial for the blank.

4. Agitate tubes and replace in the water bath.

5. Exactly fifteen minutes after the addition of each sample, add 10 mL of 0.05 N sodium hydroxide to each tube and mix well by inversion. The alkaline solution of sodium hydroxide stops the reaction and develops the color which is stable for several hours.

6. Set the spectrophotometer wavelength to 404 nm. Zero the spectrophotometer with the reagent blank.

7. Read and record the absorbance of test 1, test 2, and the reference serum samples. Return the solutions to the test tubes.

8. Add four drops concentrated hydrochloric acid to each test and reference sample with a pasteur pipet. The HCl removes the color due to ρ-nitrophenol; the remaining absorbance is produced by the serum. Then read the absorbance of test 1, test 2, and the reference serum again.

Preparation of the standard curve

- Prepare the following tubes listed below in duplicate:

Tube	(ρ-NP) (mL)	NaOH (0.02N) (mL)	Sigma Units/mL
1	1.0	10.0	1.0
2	2.0	9.0	2.0
3	4.0	7.0	4.0
4	6.0	5.0	6.0
5	8.0	3.0	8.0
6	10.0	1.0	10.0

- Mix contents of each tube with a vortex. Transfer tubes to matched cuvets.

- Read absorbance at 404 nm using a cuvet containing 0.02N NaOH to zero the instrument.

- Construct a standard curve. Plot the standard concentration (Sigma Units/mL as the abscissa) against the absorbance.

Calculation of results

Read the activities of alkaline phosphatase in the test serum and the reference serum at steps 7 and 8 directly from the standard curve. Then calculate 'corrected' alkaline phosphatase activity by subtracting units determined at step 8 above from the total units determined at step 7. If

values greater than 10 Sigma Units are obtained, repeat the assay but incubate for only 5 minutes. Then multiply the results by three. If the value is still too high, use less serum and multiply by the appropriate factor. Conversion to SI units (IU/L) = ×16.9.

Evaluation

Adults have serum alkaline phosphatase concentrations of 0.8–3.0 Sigma Units / mL (13–50 IU/L). Children have higher serum alkaline phosphatase concentrations, ranging from 0.8–6.7 Sigma Units per mL (47–112 IU/L) (Schiele et al., 1983).

Some authors have suggested that during longitudinal Zn supplementation studies, the alkaline phosphatase ratio (i.e. post to pretreatment activity) should be used to confirm the presence of mild zinc deficiency (Kasarskis and Schuna, 1980).

The activity of alkaline phosphatase is affected by factors unrelated to zinc status. Low food intake, type of protein consumed, deficiencies of magnesium, manganese, and vitamin D are some of the factors affecting the activity of this enzyme (Chesters and Will, 1978). Low levels are sometimes noted in cases of hypothyroidism, scurvy, celiac disease, and severe chronic nephritis and pernicious anemia. During the third trimester of pregnancy, alkaline phosphatase activity rises.

References

Andersch M A, Szczypinski A J (1947). Use of ρ-nitrophenyl phosphate as the substrate in determination of serum acid phosphatase. American Journal of Clinical Pathology 17: 571–574

Chesters R K, Will M (1978). The assessment of zinc status in an animal from the uptake of Zn by the cells of whole blood in vitro. British Journal of Nutrition 38: 297–306.

Kasarskis E J, Schuna A (1980). Serum alkaline phosphatase after treatment of zinc deficiency in humans. American Journal of Clinical Nutrition 33: 2609–2612.

McComb R B, Bowers G N Jr (1972). A study of optimum buffer conditions for measuring alkaline phosphatase activity in human serum. Clinical Chemistry 18: 97–104.

Ruz M, Cavan K R, Bettger W J, Thompson L U, Berry M, Gibson R S (1991). Development of a dietary model for the study of marginal zinc deficiency in humans. Evaluation of some biochemical and functional indices of zinc status. American Journal of Clinical Nutrition 53: 1–9.

Schiele F, Henry J, Hitz J Petitclerc C, Gueguen R, Siest G 1988. Total bone and liver alkaline phosphatase in plasma: biological variations and reference limits: Clinical Chemistry 29: 634-641.

Chapter 11
Assessment of vitamin status

Contents

Introduction

Clinical deficiency signs for some of the vitamins are not very specific; hence static and functional tests are frequently used to confirm the clinical diagnosis and to detect subclinical deficiency states. Examples of static and functional biochemical tests for assessing riboflavin, pyridoxine, folate, and vitamin C are given in this chapter.

Riboflavin status is conveniently assessed by a functional biochemical test that measures the activity of a flavin adenine dinucleotide (FAD)-dependent enzyme, glutathione reductase, with and without the addition of saturating amounts of the FAD coenzyme *in vitro* (Bamji, 1981). At present, this is the best method for assessing tissue riboflavin status.

The classical signs of riboflavin deficiency, termed ariboflavinosis, are angular stomatitis, cheilosis, and glossitis. Ariboflavinosis usually occurs in association with other vitamin deficiency states, and has been most frequently documented during pregnancy in undernourished populations. In industrialized countries such as North America and the United Kingdom, suboptimal riboflavin status has been reported in vulnerable population groups such as the elderly and pregnant and nonpregnant adolescents of low socio-economic status (Lopez et al., 1980). Several conditions, including alcoholism, diabetes mellitus, liver disease, and gastrointestinal and biliary obstruction, may also precipitate and/or exacerbate riboflavin deficiency (Nichoalds, 1981).

Vitamin B-6 status can be assessed by a variety of methods and the selection of an appropriate index depends on the objectives of the study and the characteristics of the study group. The tryptophan load test is described in this chapter. This is a functional biochemical test which is generally used in clinical settings to provide an indirect measure of tissue vitamin B-6 status.

Vitamin B-6 is widely distributed in foods, so frank dietary deficiencies are very rare. Adults have only a small body pool of this vitamin (20 to 30 mg), which is rapidly depleted when intakes of vitamin B-6 are deficient. In the early stages, pyridoxine deficiency may cause fatigue and headaches. Later, microcytic hypochromic anemia, convulsions, and oral lesions may develop (Sauberlich, 1981). Vulnerable population groups in industrialized counties at risk to suboptimal vitamin B-6 status include the elderly, adolescents, and pregnant and lactating women. Alterations in vitamin B-6 status have also been associated with estrogen therapy, alcohol addiction, uremia, and liver disease, and sometimes with the use of oral contraceptive agents. The drugs isoniazid, cycloserine, penicillamine, and hydrocortisone also interfere with vitamin B-6 metabolism: these must be considered when interpreting biochemical indices of vitamin B-6 status.

Folate status is assessed here by a static biochemical test that measures concentrations of folate in serum and erythrocytes. Such tests are the most frequently used biochemical indices of folate status. Serum folate levels reflect folate balance, fluctuate rapidly with recent changes in folate intakes, and provide no information on the size of tissue folate stores. The latter can be estimated by measuring erythrocyte folate concentrations, which fall in subjects in persistent negative folate balance (Herbert, 1987). Concentrations of folate in erythrocytes, but not serum, also fall in vitamin B-12 deficiency. Consequently, both serum and erythrocyte folate concentrations must be measured to distinguish between folate and vitamin B-12 deficiency.

Deficiencies of both vitamin B-12 and folic acid cause megaloblastic anemia because both vitamins are involved in deoxyribonucleic acid (DNA) synthesis. Interference with DNA synthesis induces the characteristic abnormalities in cell morphology observed in megaloblastic anemia. Large red cell precursors (megaloblasts) in the bone marrow and larger than normal mature red cells (macrocytic cells) in the peripheral blood occur. Macrocytosis can be confirmed by the presence of an elevated mean cell volume (MCV) and mean cell hemoglobin (Section 8.5).

Subclinical folate deficiency is not uncommon in industrialized countries, especially in pregnant and lactating women, and in the presence of certain diseases and drugs (Bailey et al., 1980). In less industrialized countries, megaloblastic anemia resulting from nutritional folate deficiency, may occur in pregnant and lactating women (Coleman, 1977). Deficiency of vitamin B-12 usually results from malabsorption. The latter accounts for >95% of the vitamin B-12 deficiency cases documented in the United States (Herbert, 1984). Nevertheless, nutritional deficiency has been described in persons adhering to diets which exclude animal products (Rose, 1976).

Ascorbic acid concentrations in serum or leukocytes are most frequently used to assess vitamin C status. In persons with chronically low ascorbic acid intakes, serum ascorbic acid concentrations generally reflect body ascorbic acid content and are probably as accurate an index as leukocyte ascorbic acid concentrations (Jacob et al., 1987). Urinary excretion of ascorbic acid is influenced by recent dietary intake. Moreover, the sensitivity and specificity of this index are low and twenty-four-hour urine samples are required. Alternatively, the ascorbic acid saturation test is used.

Clinical deficiency of vitamin C produces scurvy, a rare disease in industrialized countries today. Nevertheless, marginal vitamin C deficiency has been described in selected vulnerable population groups. Excess intakes of vitamin C may produce adverse effects including kidney stones.

References

Bailey L B, Mahan C S, Dimperio D (1980). Folacin and iron status in low-income pregnant adolescents and mature women. American Journal of Clinical Nutrition 33: 1997–2001.

Bamji M S (1981). Laboratory tests for the assessment of vitamin nutritional status. In: Briggs MH (ed). Vitamins in Human Biology and Medicine. CRC Press Inc., Boca Raton, Fl, pp. 1–27.

Coleman N (1977). Folate deficiency in humans. In: Draper HH (ed). Advances in Nutritional Research Volume 1. Plenum Publishing Co., New York, pp. 77–124.

Curry A S, Hewitt J V (1974). Biochemistry of Women: Methods for Clinical Investigation. CRC Press, Cleveland, Ohio, 321–338.

Herbert V (1984). Vitamin B_{12}. In: Present Knowledge in Nutrition. Fifth edition. The Nutrition Foundation Inc, Washington, D.C., pp. 347–364.

Herbert V (1987). Making sense of laboratory tests of folate status: folate requirements to sustain normality. American Journal of Hematology 26: 199–207.

Jacob R A, Skala J H, Omaye S T (1987). Biochemical indices of human vitamin C status. American Journal of Clinical Nutrition 46: 818–826.

Lopez R, Schwartz J V, Cooperman J M (1980). Riboflavin deficiency in an adolescent population in New York City. American Journal of Clinical Nutrition 33: 1283–1286.

Nichoalds G E (1981). Riboflavin. Clinics in Laboratory Medicine 1: 685–698.

Rose M (1976). Vitamin-B-12 deficiency in Asian immigrants. Lancet 2: 681.

Sauberlich H E. (1981). Vitamin B-6 status assessment: past and present. In: Leklem JE, Reynolds RD (eds). Methods in Vitamin B-6 Nutrition. Analysis and Status Assessment. Plenum Press, New York–London, pp. 203–239.

11.1 Erythrocyte glutathione reductase

Principle

Glutathione reductase is a nicotinamide adenine dinucleotide phosphate (NADPH) and flavin adenine dinucleotide (FAD)-dependent enzyme, and is the major flavoprotein in erythrocytes. It catalyses the oxidative cleavage of the disulfide bond of oxidized glutathione (GSSG) to form reduced glutathione (GSH).

$$\underset{\text{oxidized glutathione}}{GSSG + NADPH + H^+} \rightarrow \underset{\text{reduced glutathione}}{2GSH + NADP^+}$$

The principle of the test is outlined below:

- The basal activity of EGR in erythrocytes is measured. This represents the endogenous enzyme activity and is dependent on the amount of the FAD coenzyme in the erythrocytes;

- The enzyme activity with excess FAD coenzyme added *in vitro* is determined. This represents the maximum potential enzyme activity and is referred to as total or 'stimulated' activity;

- The endogenous and stimulated activities are compared to indicate the degree of unsaturation of the enzyme with the FAD-coenzyme;

- The data are expressed in terms of an activity coefficient (AC) or 'percentage stimulation'.

The ratio of stimulated to basal activity is used because: (a) the inter-subject variation in basal erythrocyte enzyme activity measurements is large, and (b) it is assumed that apoenzyme levels are not affected by vitamin deficiencies. In fact, the latter assumption is probably incorrect.

The activity of erythrocyte glutathione reductase (EGR) is measured spectrophotometrically by monitoring the oxidation of NADPH to NADP$^+$ at 340 nm, with and without the presence of added FAD coenzyme. The degree of *in vitro* stimulation of EGR activity depends on the FAD saturation of the apoenzyme, which in turn depends on the availability of riboflavin. In persons with riboflavin deficiency, erythrocyte glutathione reductase activity falls and the *in vitro* stimulation by FAD rises.

Reagents

- Buffer—0.1M K$_2$HPO$_4$ (Potassium phosphate monobasic): Dissolve 16.41 g K$_2$HPO$_4$ and 0.79 g KH$_2$PO$_4$ in 800 mL distilled deionized water. Adjust to pH 7.4 and dilute to 1 L.

- EDTA 0.040 M. Dissolve 0.149 g EDTA in 10 mL distilled deionized water.

- FAD. Dissolve 1.2 mg FAD in 5.0 mL distilled deionized water. Make up daily and keep from light.

- NADPH. Dissolve 16.6 mg NADPH in 10 mL of 1% sodium bicarbonate solution. Make up daily. Keep in a refrigerator.

- Glutathione—23 mg glutathione, oxidized in 5.0 mL distilled deionized water plus 0.04 mL 1N sodium hydroxide (GSSG). Make up daily.

- Sample—Washed red blood cells. 5 mL whole blood should be collected, using EDTA or heparin as an anti-coagulant. After centrifugation, remove the plasma and wash the red blood cells immediately with 0.85% sodium chloride four times. Hemolyzed samples can be kept frozen for up to three months at −25°C without loss of EGR activity.

Equipment

- Spectrophotometer; cuvets.
- Eppendorf pipets.

Procedure

1. Pipet 0.5 mL of washed packed cells into a test-tube containing 9.5 mL distilled water. Mix gently and allow to stand for thirty minutes at 4°C. Centrifuge and collect the supernatant. (The latter can be frozen at −70°C for up to two weeks).

2. Dilute the hemolysate 1 : 1 with distilled deionized water.

3. Add the solutions listed to four cuvets:

| | with FAD | | without FAD | |
	Blank	Test	Blank	Test
Buffer	1.8 mL	1.8 mL	1.8 mL	1.8 mL
EDTA	0.3 mL	0.3 mL	0.3 mL	0.3 mL
FAD	0.1 mL	0.1 mL	-	-
Water	-	-	0.1 mL	0.1 mL
Hemolysate	0.15 mL	0.15 mL	0.15 mL	0.15 mL

4. Mix the contents of each cuvet with a pasteur pipet. Be careful not to scratch the optical surfaces if quartz glass cuvets are used. Then incubate all tubes for ten minutes in a water bath at 37°C.

5. Add GSSG and distilled deionized water to each tube as shown below:

| | with FAD | | without FAD | |
	Blank	Test	Blank	Test
GSSG	-	0.3 mL	-	0.3 mL
Water	0.3 mL	-	0.3 mL	-

6. Incubate tubes again for ten minutes in a water bath at 37°C.

7. Add 0.2 mL NADPH to each tube, mix well, and record the initial absorbance of each tube (including the blanks) at 340 nm. (Note: Do not attempt to zero the instrument with the blank)

8. For each tube, record the absorbance readings at 60 second intervals for fifteen minutes.

9. Subtract the absorbance readings for the blanks from each of the test absorbance readings with and without FAD. (Normally the readings for the blank should be zero).

Calculation of results

Calculate the activity coefficient (AC) as the ratio of change of the enzyme activity in the presence or absence of FAD.

$$\text{EGR AC} = \frac{\text{Enzyme activity (+FAD)}}{\text{Basal enzyme activity (−FAD)}}$$
$$= \frac{\text{Abs. at 0 min. − abs. at 15 min. (+FAD)}}{\text{Abs. at 0 min. − abs. at 15 min. (−FAD)}}$$

The percentage stimulation is:

$$(\text{Activity coefficient} \times 100) - 100$$

Evaluation

The EGR AC appears to be relatively independent of gender, and a single interpretive criterion for acceptable (<1.2), low (1.2–1.4), or deficient (>1.4) states is used (McCormick, 1985). It is important to note that the extent to which the EGR AC is elevated above 1.4, does not necessarily indicate the degree of riboflavin deficiency. Consistent correlations between EGR AC values and clinical signs of riboflavin deficiency have not been observed (Bates et al., 1981). Furthermore, the guidelines are tentative, as several factors are known to affect EGR AC values. For example, a trend toward lower EGR ACs with increasing age has been noted (Garry et al., 1982). If this trend is more firmly established, specific guidelines for EGR AC values for the elderly may be required. In addition, the concentration of FAD used in the assay to stimulate EGR (Rutishauser et al., 1979), and probably, the age of erythrocytes (Powers and Thurnham, 1981) affects the EGR AC values obtained.

The EGR AC test is not appropriate for assessing the riboflavin status of subjects with glucose-6-phosphate dehydrogenase deficiency, or a pyridoxine deficiency (Prentice et al., 1981). Increased avidity of the EGR for FAD occurs in glucose-6-phosphate dehydrogenase deficiency, resulting in ACs within the normal range, even in the presence of clinical signs of riboflavin deficiency (Thurnham, 1972). Pyridoxine deficiency also interferes with the EGR AC test, resulting in a decreased erythrocyte glutathione reductase activity but no change in the activity coefficient, probably as a result of a decrease in apoenzyme. No comparable effects have been observed for other vitamin deficiencies (Sharda and Bamji, 1972). Increased erythrocyte glutathione reductase activity has been documented in persons with iron deficiency anemia (Ramachandran and Iyer, 1974), and in patients with severe uremia and cirrhosis of the liver.

References

Bates C J, Prentice A M, Paul A A, Sutcliffe B A, Watkinson M, Whitehead R G (1981). Riboflavin status in Gambian pregnant and lactating women and its implications for Recommending Dietary Allowances. American Journal of Clinical Nutrition 34: 928–935.

Garry P J, Goodwin J S, Hunt W C (1982). Nutritional status in a healthy elderly population: riboflavin. American Journal of Clinical Nutrition 36: 902–909.

McCormick D M (1985). Vitamins. In: Textbook of Clinical Chemistry. WB Saunders, Philadelphia.

Powers H J, Thurnham D I (1981). Riboflavin deficiency in man: effects on haemoglobin and reduced glutathione in erythrocytes of different ages. British Journal of Nutrition 46: 257–266.

Prentice A M, Bates C J, Prentice A, Welch S G, Williams K, McGregor IA (1981). The influence of G-6-PD activity on the response of erythrocyte glutathione reductase to riboflavin deficiency. International Journal for Vitamin and Nutritional Research 51: 211–215.

Ramachandran M, Iyer G Y (1974). Erythrocyte glutathione reductase in iron deficiency anemia. Clinica Chimica Acta 52: 225–229.

Rutishauser I H, Bates C J, Paul A A, Black A E, Mandel A R, Patnaik B K (1979). Long term vitamin status and dietary intake of healthy elderly subjects. I. Riboflavin. British Journal of Nutrition 42: 33–42.

Sharda D, Bamji M S (1972). Erythrocyte glutathione reductase activity and riboflavin concentration in experimental deficiency of some water soluble vitamins. International Journal for Vitamin and Nutrition Research 42: 43–49.

Thurnham D I (1972). Red cell enzyme tests of vitamin status: do marginal deficiencies have any physiological significance? Proceedings of the Nutrition Society 40: 155–163.

11.2 L-Tryptophan load test

Principle

Vitamin B-6, as pyridoxal phosphate, is a coenzyme for kynureninase and kynurenine aminotransferase in the tryptophan-niacin pathway. Normally, these enzymes catalyze the conversion of kynurenine and 3-hydroxykynurenine to anthranilic acid and 3-hydroxyanthranilic acid, respectively. In vitamin B-6 deficiency, therefore, kynurenic acid formed from tryptophan metabolism is converted via hydroxykynurenine to xanthurenic acid which accumulates and is excreted in the urine, especially if preceded by an oral loading dose of tryptophan (Brown, 1981).

The L-isomer of tryptophan is used for the loading dose, as the D-isomeric form is not metabolized via the tryptophan-niacin pathway. A loading dose of 2 g of L-tryptophan is sufficient to cause an increased urinary excretion of metabolites of the kynurenine pathway for adults. Of the metabolites excreted, xanthurenic acid is the most frequently determined after a tryptophan load because it is the most easily measured. Ferric salts react with xanthurenic acid to form a complex with an intense green colour which can be quantitated colorimetrically.

Reagents

- 2 g L-Tryptophan dissolved in 200 mL orange juice. To be taken at breakfast.

- Tris Buffer. 30.3 g Tris and 26.0 g maleic acid in 250 mL distilled deionized water. Add 2.0 g Norit (charcoal) to above. Shake well and filter. Add 242 mL 1N sodium hydroxide to 200 mL filtrate. Adjust to pH 7.8 and use as diluent for xanthurenic acid stock solution.

- Xanthurenic acid, stock standard solution (500 μg/mL). Dissolve 50 mg xanthurenic acid in 100 mL of Tris buffer. When stored in the frozen state, solution is stable for two to three months.

- Xanthurenic acid, working standard solution (100 μg/mL). Pipet 10 mL xanthurenic acid standard solution into a 50 mL volumetric flask. Dilute to 50 mL with Tris buffer. Prepare daily.

- Ferric ammonium sulfate solution: dissolve 1.7 g $FeNH_4(SO_4)_2.12H_2O$ in 100 mL distilled deionized water.

- Two twenty-four-hour urine samples. One twenty-four-hour preload basal urine collection; one twenty-four-hour postload urine collection. Acidify to pH 3–4 with 2–3 drops concentrated HCl to reduce bacterial growth and to stabilize the metabolites. Measure total volume and freeze an aliquot of each urine sample at −15°C. Tryptophan metabolites are stable for two to three months, if frozen. Then adjust the pH of the urine to between 7.3–7.5 with phosphate buffer. Filter urine before use.

Equipment

- Spectrophotometer.
- Large test tubes.
- Funnel, filter paper, flask.
- Pipets—100 μL, 1 mL, 5 mL.

Procedure

1. Ask the subject to collect a twenty-four-hour preload basal urine sample following the instructions given in Section 7.4.

2. Give the subject, on the morning of the test, a 2 g L-tryptophan suspended in milk or orange juice at breakfast. This avoids side effects such as somnolence and nausea.

3. Instruct the subject to start collecting a second twenty-four-hour urine sample immediately after the load. Continue collecting urine throughout the following twenty-four-hours, retaining the urine sample voided at the same time on the morning of the next day.

4. Label three test tubes: blank 1 (preload), recovery 1 (preload), test 1 (preload).

5. Label three test tubes: blank 2 (postload), recovery 2 (postload), test 2 (postload).

6. To each recovery tube add 1 mL xanthurenic acid working standard (100 μg/mL).

7. To each test, add 1 mL distilled deionized water.

8. To each recovery and test tube add 4 mL filtered urine.

9. To each blank, add 5 mL distilled water, and then a further 5 mL distilled water to ALL tubes.

10. Add 0.1 mL (100 μL) 1.7% ferric ammonium sulfate solution to all tubes. This compound forms a green colored iron-xanthurenic acid complex in the sample.

11. Mix all tubes thoroughly with gentle agitation and leave for five minutes for color to develop, before transferring to matched cuvets.

12. Set wavelength at 610 nm. Adjust the spectrophotometer with one of the blanks to zero absorbance.

13. Read the absorbance of the tests and recovery tubes.

Preparation of standard curve

- Prepare the following tubes in duplicate:

Tube number	Xanthurenic acid stock solution	Water	Concentration (μg/mL)
Blank	0	1.00 mL	0
1	0.05 mL	0.95 mL	25
2	0.10 mL	0.90 mL	50
3	0.15 mL	0.85 mL	75
4	0.20 mL	0.80 mL	100
5	0.30 mL	0.70 mL	150
6	0.40 mL	0.60 mL	200

- To all tubes add a further 9.0 mL distilled deionized water. Mix.

- To all tubes add 0.1 mL 1.7% ferric ammonium sulfate solution, mix and leave for five minutes for color to develop before transferring to matched cuvets.

- Use the blank to zero the instrument and then read the absorbance at 610 nm within 10 minutes of developing the color.

- Construct a standard curve. Plot the standard concentration μg/mL xanthurenic acid as the abscissa, against the absorbance as the ordinate on regular graph paper.

Calculation of results

- Read the xanthurenic acid concentrations of the basal and post load urine samples and the recoveries directly from the calibration curve.

- Divide result by 1000 and multiply the above result by the total twenty-four-hour urine volume (in mL). This gives the xanthurenic acid excretion for the basal and post load urine samples in milligrams per 24 hours.

- Subtract the basal value from the post load value and divide by 4.0 to obtain the net xanthurenic acid excreted post load (mg/24 hours).

Evaluation

Tentative guidelines for the excretion of xanthurenic acid after a 2 g L-tryptophan load are: >50 mg/24 hours (marginal or inadequate vitamin B-6 status); <25 mg/24 hours (acceptable) (Sauberlich et al., 1974).

Protein intake, exercise, lean body mass, and the size of the tryptophan loading dose affect the subsequent urinary excretion of xanthurenic acid. The tryptophan load test is also not appropriate for pregnant subjects and women taking oral contraceptive agents. Certain drugs (e.g. hydrocortisone) also interfere with the tryptophan load test by increasing urinary kynurenine excretion. Some drugs also interfere with the colorimetric analytical procedures (e.g. sulfonamides and para-aminosalicylic acid). Cancer patients also have increased urinary excretion of xanthurenic acid and other metabolites of tryptophan after a tryptophan load.

References

Brown R R (1981). The tryptophan load test as an index of vitamin B₆ nutrition. In: Leklem JE, Reynolds RD (eds). Methods in Vitamin B-6 Nutrition. Analysis and Status Assessment. Plenum Press, New York–London, pp. 321–340.

Rosen F, Lowy R S, Sprince H (1951). A rapid assay for xanthurenic acid in urine. Proceedings of the Society of Experimental Biology and Medicine 77: 399–401.

Sauberlich H E, Dowdy R P, Skala J H (1974). Laboratory Tests for the Assessment of Nutritional Status. CRC Press Inc, Cleveland, Ohio.

11.3 Folate in plasma and red blood cells

Principle

'Folate' is the term used as a generic descriptor for folic acid (pteroylmonoglutamic acid) and related compounds which exhibit the biological activity of folic acid.

A method based on a radio-immunoassay (RIA) is often used to analyze plasma and red blood cell folate concentrations; it is fast and results correlate well with the more traditional microbiological method. The RIA for folate is dependent on the competition between native folates in the plasma or red cell hemolysate and a radioactive folate derivative (^{125}I-folate), for a high affinity folate binder. The latter is a porcine folate binding protein (Kamen and Caston, 1974).

For the test, each standard and sample is mixed with ^{125}I-folate in a solution containing dithiothreitol (DTT) and cyanide. The mixture is boiled to denature endogenous folate binding proteins. The DTT serves to prevent oxidation of folate during boiling. The mixture is cooled and the antibody (i.e. porcine folate binding protein) is added. During a one hour incubation, endogenous unlabeled and labeled folate compete for available binding sites on the porcine folate binding protein. The final step consists of the separation of the bound fraction from the unbound fraction by centrifugation. After this step, the porcine folate binding protein-folate complexes form a pellet in the bottom of the tubes and the unbound folate is decanted off in the supernatant. The amount of labeled folate which is bound to the porcine folate binding protein (folate antibody) is determined by counting the gamma irradiation emitted from the ^{125}I using a gamma counter. A standard curve is constructed of the folate concentrations of the standards and their corresponding radioactivity bound to the binding protein (as counts per minute) from which the folate concentrations of the test samples can be estimated (Dawson et al., 1980).

Note that red blood cells contain some pteroylpolyglutamates. These polyglutamate chains must be cleaved to form pteroylmonoglutamate before analyses to avoid underestimating the folate concentration of red blood cells.

Reagents and sample preparation

The shelf-life of ^{125}I is short. Consequently, kits should be ordered only when they are required. The reagents, standards, and reference serum mentioned below are available from Bio-Rad Laboratories, Hercules, California 94547. Follow the procedure given by the manufacturer if this differs from that outlined below.

- Folate standards (1, 2.5, 5, 10, and 25 ng/mL) Store at 2–8°C.

- Folate zero standard. Contains 4 mL folate-free HSA base and sodium azide (<0.5%). Store at 2–8°C.

- Microbead Reagent. Contains 10.5 mL of affinity purified porcine intrinsic factor and folate binding proteins covalently coupled to polymer beads in phosphate buffer with sodium azide (<0.5%). Store at 2–8°C.

- Blank Reagent. Contains 3 mL of polymer beads in phosphate buffer with sodium azide (<0.5%). Store at 2–8°C.

- Folate Tracer. Contains 100 mL ^{125}I labeled folate (<8 μCi) in 0.05M borate buffer with 10 μg/mL potassium cyanide. Store at 2–8°C.

- Working Tracer Reagent—Reconstitute the DTT with 10 mL distilled deionized water. Agitate gently to dissolve. Allow to stand for five minutes, and then transfer into the folate tracer bottle. Mix by inversion. Stable for thirty days when stored at 2–8°C.

- Ascorbic acid solution 0.4%. (0.2 g/50 mL H$_2$O). Prepare fresh daily.

- Red Cell Folate Diluent—Reconstitute vial labeled whole blood diluent by adding 5 mL distilled water to each vial. Allow to stand for thirty minutes. Aliquots of the diluent can be frozen for one month at −20°C.

- Reference serum; e.g. Lyphochek (Bio-Rad).

- Sample serum. Let whole blood, without additives, stand to coagulate for at least 90 minutes. Centrifuge in a refrigerated centrifuge (2000 rpm, 4°C) for twenty minutes. Separate the serum into tubes containing a known quantity of ascorbic acid such that plasma samples contain 1% ascorbic acid. Mix well. Samples should be frozen within 2–3 hours after blood collection at $-70°C$. Serum must not be preserved with ascorbic acid when determining vitamin B-12.

- Sample—Whole blood hemolysate for red blood cell folate assay. Dilute 0.1 mL of whole EDTA anticoagulated blood with 1.0 mL of freshly prepared ascorbic acid solution to lyse the red blood cells. Invert gently twice. Freeze immediately at $-70°C$ unless the assay is performed within ten days; the hemolysate is stable for this long if stored at $-20°C$.

- Determine the hematocrit on an aliquot of the whole blood.

Equipment

- Gamma Counter.
- Centrifuge $1500 \times g$.
- Water bath at $100°C$ and ice bath.
- Pipets—100, $200\,\mu L$; 1 mL.
- Log-log graph paper and aluminum foil.
- Glass test tubes ($12 \times 75\,mm$).
- Vortex mixer.

Procedures for handling radioactive material

- Do not smoke or eat while handling radioactive material.
- Do not pipet materials by mouth.
- Use gloves while handling radioactive materials and wash hands thoroughly after use.
- Radioactive spills should be wiped up quickly with some absorbent material. The contaminated absorbent material should then be disposed of in the radioactive waste bin. Then a wipe test should be performed.

Procedure

Note: The standards and tests should be analyzed in duplicate.

1. Plug in water bath and bring water to boiling point. This may take some time!
2. Allow all reagents and materials from the radio-immunoassay kit to come to room temperature before use.

3. If necessary, thaw blood samples in a dark location. Keep samples on ice after thawing.

4. Label tubes: total counts, blank, zero standard (S), 1 S, 2.5 S, 5 S, 10 S, 25 S, reference (R), test sample plasma (P), test sample hemolysate (RBC).

5. Add $100\,\mu L$ of thawed RBC hemolysate to the appropriately labeled tubes (i.e. RBC); add $100\,\mu L$ of the red cell folate diluent to the same tube.

6. Add $200\,\mu L$ of each standard, reference or sample to the respective tubes, commencing with the lowest dilution standard first. Add $200\,\mu L$ of zero standard to the blank tube.

7. Advise the laboratory supervisor that you are ready for the working tracer (i.e. ^{125}I-folate). To comply with Safety Regulations, the laboratory supervisor should supervise the addition of 1 mL of the working tracer to each tube (including the blank). Mix each tube with the vortex mixer.

8. Add 1 mL working tracer to total counts tube. Set aside total counts tube until step No. 13

9. Cover the test tube rack containing the tubes with aluminum foil and place in the boiling water bath for twenty minutes. (Ensure that the water does not flood the samples).

10. Cool samples in an ice bath (ice cubes in a sink of cold water works well) until they are at room temperature.

11. Add $100\,\mu L$ of thoroughly mixed microbead reagent to all tubes except blank tubes. Add $100\,\mu L$ blank reagent to the blank tubes. Mix tubes with a vortex mixer.

12. Incubate tubes at room temperature for one hour and then centrifuge for ten minutes at $1500 \times g$ at $4°C$ and then immediately remove the supernatant using a suction apparatus.

13. Place all tubes in a gamma counter, including the total counts tube, noting the order in which the tubes will be counted and the corresponding number on the gamma counter. Then count each tube for one minute.

Calculation of results

1. Record the average counts per minute (CPM) for each standard, reference, and test sample.

2. Subtract the mean CPM of the blank from the CPM of each standard, reference, and test sample, to give the average corrected CPM.

3. Divide the average corrected CPM of the standards and samples by the average corrected CPM of the zero standard. This gives the percent of bound labeled folate associated with each standard and sample.

$$\%B/B_0 = \frac{\text{Average corrected CPM standard or sample}}{\text{Average corrected CPM zero standard}}$$

4. Plot $\%B/B_0$ for each standard on the Y-axis on log-log paper and the appropriate folate concentration (ng/mL) on the X-axis.

5. Read off from the standard curve the folate concentrations (ng/mL) of the reference and test samples from their corresponding $\%B/B_0$.

6. Calculate the red blood cell folate concentration from the following equation:

$$\text{ng/mL RBCF} = \frac{\text{WBF} - (\text{SF} \times (1 - \text{HCT}))}{\text{HCT}}$$

Where RBCF = red blood cell folate concentration; WBF = whole blood folate concentration; SF = serum folate concentration; and HCT = fractional hematocrit. For example: if the folate concentration in the whole blood, read from the standard curve = 6.0 ng/mL, and the serum folate concentration = 5.0 ng/mL, and the hematocrit = 0.45, then

$$\text{WBF} = 6.0 \times 22 = 132$$

$$\text{RBCF} = \frac{132 - (5.0 \times (1 - 0.45))}{0.45} = 287.2 \, \text{ng/mL}$$

The conversion factor to SI Units (nmol/L) = ×2.266

Evaluation

The serum folate cutoff point usually used as an indicator of low serum folate concentrations is <3 ng/mL (<6.8 nmol/L) (Herbert, 1967; Senti and Pilch, 1985). Such low levels are indicative of negative folate balance, but not necessarily folate depletion, unless the negative balance persists for at least one month. Then folate stores become gradually reduced, resulting in a state of folate depletion, characterized by a fall in erythrocyte and liver folate concentrations (Herbert, 1987a,b). Abnormal hematological changes do not occur

until after three to four months of folate deprivation. Most individuals with megaloblastic changes resulting from folate deficiency have low serum folate levels, but exceptions do occur. In vitamin B-12 deficiency uncomplicated by folate deficiency, serum folate levels are normal or raised.

Several non-nutritional factors affect serum folate concentrations. Age-related trends in serum folate levels were documented in the NHANES II survey. Alcohol ingestion results in an acute drop in serum folate levels, because reabsorption of folate is impaired by alcohol (Hillman et al., 1977). Hemolysis may produce misleadingly elevated serum folate values as the folate content of erythrocytes is much higher than plasma. Raised serum folate values have also been reported in patients with stagnant-loop syndrome, acute renal failure, and with active liver damage. Some investigators (Martinez and Roe, 1977) have reported low serum folate values in women taking oral contraceptives. Smoking lowers serum folate concentrations via its enhancing effect on erythropoiesis, which, in turn, increases folate requirements. In the NHANES II survey, significantly more women smokers had low serum folate concentrations (<3.0 ng/mL; <6.8 nmol/L) compared to nonsmoking women (Senti and Pilch, 1985).

Erythrocyte folate values in the NHANES II survey ranging from 140 to 160 ng/mL (322 to 368 nmol/L) were assumed to be low and suggestive of an individual at risk, whereas an erythrocyte concentration below a cutoff point of 140 ng/ml (322 nmol/L) was selected as indicative of a deficiency; a summary appears in Table 11.1. Herbert (1987b,c) suggested that concentrations of less than 160 ng/mL (368 nmol/L) indicate a state of folate depletion, at which stage there is no evidence of biochemical or clinical functional deficit. Concentrations below a cutoff point of less than 120 ng/mL (280 nmol/L) indicate the second

Folate Measurement	Deficient	Borderline	Acceptable
Serum (ng/mL)	<3.0	3.0–6.0	>6.0
Erythrocyte (ng/mL)	<140	140–160	>160

Table 11.1: Guidelines for the interpretation of folate concentrations. Conversion factor to nmol/L = ×2.266. Modified from Wagner C (1984). Folic acid. In: Present Knowledge in Nutrition. Fifth edition. The Nutrition Foundation Inc., with permission.

stage in the development of folate deficiency, termed 'folate-deficient erythropoiesis', sometimes referred to as 'subclinical' deficiency. At this stage, biochemical function is affected, as indicated by an abnormal deoxyuridine (dU) suppression test and hypersegmented neutrophils, first in the bone marrow, and then in the peripheral blood. Folate-deficiency anemia, the third stage of folate depletion, only occurs when erythrocyte folate concentrations fall to less than 100 ng/mL (227 nmol/L), at which time liver folate concentrations are often below 1 µg/g (2.3 nmol/g). This stage is characterized by the appearance of macro-ovalocytic erythrocytes and a hemoglobin level below 13 g/dL (130 g/L) in men and below 12 g/dL (120 g/L) in women (Herbert, 1987c). Nearly all persons with folate-deficiency anemia have *low* erythrocyte (and serum) folate concentrations.

Low erythrocyte folate concentrations are not specific for folate deficiency. Low concentrations also occur in vitamin B-12 deficiency (Hoffbrand et al., 1966), although serum folate levels are normal or even raised. Hence to identify folate deficiency, both erythrocyte folate and serum vitamin B-12 concentrations should be measured. Vitamin B-12 deficiency produces secondary folate deficiency because vitamin B-12 is involved in the transport and storage of folate in cells (Herbert, 1964).

The interpretation of erythrocyte folate values is also confounded by the presence of other disease states. If patients have a raised reticulocyte count (e.g. when hemorrhage or hemolytic anemia is present), erythrocyte folate concentrations increase because reticulocytes tend to have a higher folate concentration than older cells (Hoffbrand et al., 1966). Erythrocyte (and serum) folate values may also increase in iron deficiency (Omer et al., 1970), although the magnitude of this effect, and the reason, is unknown. In such cases, a hidden folate deficiency may be present, as indicated by an abnormal deoxyuridine suppression test and hypersegmentation in the peripheral blood (Herbert, 1987b).

Age-related trends in erythrocyte folate levels, comparable to those noted for serum folate, were observed in the NHANES II survey (Senti and Pilch, 1985). Median erythrocyte folate concentrations were relatively high for infants and young children, but declined in later childhood and adolescence. In females, pregnancy, oral contraceptive use, parity, and smoking tended to be associated with lower erythrocyte folate concentrations.

References

Dawson D W, Delamore I W, Fish D I, Flaherty T A, Gowenlock A H, Hunt L P, Hyde K, MacIver J E, Thornton J A, Waters H M (1980). An evaluation of commercial radioisotope methods for the determination of folate and vitamin B-12. Journal of Clinical Pathology 33: 234–242.

Herbert V (1964). Studies of folate deficiency in man. Proceedings of the Royal Society of Medicine 57: 377–384.

Herbert V (1967). Biochemical and hematological lesions in folic acid deficiency. American Journal of Clinical Nutrition 20: 562–568.

Herbert V (1987a). Recommended dietary intakes (RDI) of folate in humans. American Journal of Clinical Nutrition 45: 661-670.

Herbert V (1987b). Making sense of laboratory tests of folate status: folate requirements to sustain normality. American Journal of Hematology 26: 199–207.

Herbert V (1987c). The 1986 Herman Award Lecture. Nutrition Science as a continually unfolding story: the folate and vitamin B-12 paradigm. American Journal of Clinical Nutrition 46: 387–402.

Hillman R S, McGuffin R, Campbell C (1977). Alcohol interference with the folate enterohepatic cycle. Transactions of the Association of American Physicians 90: 145–156.

Hoffbrand A V, Newcombe B F A, Mollin D L (1966). Method of assay of red cell folate activity and the value of the assay as a test for folate deficiency. Journal of Clinical Pathology 19: 17–28.

Kamen B A, Caston D (1974). Direct radiochemical assay for serum folate: competition between ^{3}H-folic acid and 5-methyltetrahydrofolic acid for a folate binder. Journal of Laboratory and Clinical Medicine 83: 164–174.

Martinez O B, Roe D A (1977). Effect of oral contraceptives on blood folate levels in pregnancy. American Journal of Obstetrics and Gynecology 128: 255–261.

Omer A, Finlayson N D C, Shearman D J C, Samson R R, Girdwood R H (1970). Plasma and erythrocyte folate in iron deficiency and folate deficiency. Blood 35: 821–828.

Senti F R, Pilch S M (1985). Assessment of the folate nutritional status of the U.S population based on data collected in the second National Health and Nutrition Examination Survey 1976–1980. Life Sciences Research Office, Federation of American Societies for Experimental Biology, Bethesda, Maryland.

Wagner C (1984). Folic acid. In: Present Knowledge in Nutrition. Fifth edition. The Nutrition Foundation Inc., Washington, D.C., pp. 332–346.

11.4 Ascorbic acid in serum and urine

Principle

Serum ascorbic acid concentrations are the most frequently used and practical index of vitamin C status in humans. Levels are influenced by any recent intake of the vitamin, especially when intakes are high, making fasting blood samples essential (Omaye et al., 1979).

Urine is the major excretory route for absorbed ascorbic acid and its metabolites, levels reflecting recent dietary intake. When intakes are greater than 1 g/day, ascorbic acid is excreted largely in its unmetabolized form whereas at low intakes (i.e. < 100 mg/day), oxalate is the major urinary metabolite.

Several methods are available for measuring vitamin C in the reduced form or as total ascorbic acid (Pelletier, 1985). For all methods, metaphosphoric acid or trichloroacetic acid is used to precipitate the protein in the samples and to stabilize the ascorbic acid. Described below is the 2,6-dichloroindophenol method, in which ascorbic acid is first oxidized to dehydro-ascorbic acid by the action of 2,6-dichloro-phenolindophenol. The dehydroascorbic acid is then hydrolyzed to diketogluconic acid, which, when dissolved in sulfuric acid and treated with 2,4-dinitrophenylhydrazine, forms an osazone. The osazone forms a stable reddish-brown product that can be measured photometrically at 500 nm.

Reagents

- Trichloroacetic acid (TCA) 5% solution. Dissolve 5 g TCA crystals in 100 mL water. Store in the refrigerator at 0–5°C.

- 2,6-Dichlorophenolindophenol solution. Dissolve 100 mg 2,6-dichlorophenolindophenol, Na salt in 40 mL hot distilled deionized water, and then make up to 50 mL. Replenish if solution turns purple.

- Sulfuric acid 9N. Add carefully 25 mL concentrated sulfuric acid to 75 mL water, stirring constantly.

- 2,4-Dinitro-phenyl-hydrazine (DNP)-thiourea reagent. Dissolve 2.0 g DNP and 1 g thiourea

in 100 mL 9N sulfuric acid. Filter when necessary. If excessive precipitate develops, replenish.

- Sulfuric acid 85% (v/v). Carefully add 85 mL concentrated sulfuric acid to 13 mL water, stirring constantly.

- Ascorbic acid 50 mg/dL. Dissolve 50 mg ascorbic acid in 5% TCA and make up to 100 mL with 5% TCA. Refrigerate.

- Ascorbic acid working standard. Dilute 1 mL stock solution to 100 mL with 5% TCA, to give working concentration of 5 mg/dL. Prepare fresh daily.

- Serum/plasma from fasting blood samples— Add 6.0 mL 5% TCA to 2.0 mL serum/plasma in a centrifuge tube. Mix with the vortex mixer and then centrifuge. Use the protein-free supernatant for assay.

- Urine sample—Collect a twenty-four-hour sample. Dilute 1.0 mL with 19 mL 5% TCA in a centrifuge tube. Mix with the vortex mixer and then centrifuge, if necessary. Use the protein-free supernatant for assay.

Equipment

- Spectrophotometer.
- Centrifuge tubes; test tubes.
- Water bath at 60°C.
- Pipets—2.0 mL, 1 mL, 100 μL, 0.5 mL, 5.0 mL.
- Ice bath.

Procedure

1. Label four test tubes: test blank, test, standard, standard blank.

2. To the test blank and test tubes, add 2 mL supernatant.

3. To the standard add 2 mL working ascorbic acid solution and to the standard blank tubes add 2 mL 5% TCA.

4. To all tubes add 0.1 mL indophenol reagent. Mix tubes with a vortex.

Age (yr)	Percentiles of serum vitamin C (mg/dL) by age							Percentiles of serum vitamin C (mg/dL) by age						
	5	10	25	50	75	90	95	5	10	25	50	75	90	95
	Male subjects							Female subjects						
3–5	0.7	0.9	1.3	1.8	1.8	2.2	2.4	0.7	0.9	1.2	1.5	1.8	2.1	2.4
6–8	0.6	0.9	1.2	1.4	1.7	2.1	2.3	0.6	0.9	1.2	1.5	1.7	2.0	2.2
9–11	0.6	0.8	1.1	1.4	1.6	1.9	2.1	0.6	0.7	1.1	1.4	1.7	1.8	2.1
12–14	0.4	0.6	0.9	1.2	1.5	1.8	2.0	0.4	0.8	0.9	1.3	1.5	1.8	1.9
15–17	0.4	0.4	0.7	1.1	1.4	1.6	1.8	0.3	0.4	0.7	1.1	1.4	1.8	1.9
18–24	0.3	0.4	0.8	1.0	1.3	1.6	1.7	0.3	0.4	0.7	1.1	1.4	1.8	1.9
25–34	0.2	0.3	0.5	0.9	1.2	1.5	1.7	0.3	0.4	0.7	1.1	1.4	1.7	1.9
35–44	0.2	0.3	0.5	0.9	1.2	1.5	1.8	0.3	0.3	0.8	1.1	1.4	1.8	1.8
45–54	0.2	0.3	0.5	0.9	1.3	1.8	2.0	0.3	0.4	0.7	1.2	1.4	1.7	1.8
55–64	0.2	0.3	0.5	0.9	1.3	1.5	1.7	0.3	0.4	0.9	1.3	1.8	1.9	2.0
65–74	0.2	0.3	0.6	1.1	1.4	1.7	1.9	0.4	0.5	0.9	1.3	1.6	1.9	2.1

Table 11.2: Percentiles of serum vitamin C (mg/dL) by age for males and females of three to seventy-four years. Data are from the U.S. NHANES II (1976–80) survey and were compiled by Fulwood et al. (1982).

5. To the test and standard tubes, add 0.5 mL DNP-thiourea. Do not add to the blanks.

6. Place all tubes in a 60°C water bath for one hour. Then cool tubes in an ice bath.

7. To the test blank and standard blank tubes, add 0.5 mL DNP-thiourea.

8. Add 2.5 mL 85% sulfuric acid slowly to all tubes in the ice bath.

9. Set the spectrophotometer wavelength to 500 nm. Zero the spectrophotometer with the standard-blank, and read the absorbance of the standard.

10. Zero the spectrophotometer with the test-blank, and read the absorbance of the test samples.

Calculation of results

If the ascorbic acid standard contains 0.5 mg/dL, the serum ascorbic acid (mg/dL) is given by

$$\frac{2.0 \times \text{Abs}_T}{\text{Abs}_S}$$

If the ascorbic acid standard contains 0.5 mg/dL, the urine ascorbic acid (mg/24 hr sample) is given by

$$\frac{\text{Abs}_T \times 0.1 \times \text{total volume 24-hour urine (mL)}}{\text{Abs}_S}$$

where Abs_T = absorbance of the test sample and Abs_S = absorbance of the standard.

Evaluation

Interpretive criteria for serum ascorbic acid concentrations (mg/dL) are: >0.3 acceptable (low risk), 0.2–0.3 low (medium risk), and <0.2 deficient (high risk) (Sauberlich 1981). Levels are influenced by any recent intake of the vitamin, especially when intakes are high, making fasting blood samples essential (Omaye et al., 1979). Serum ascorbic acid concentrations increase with dietary intakes until a serum concentration of approximately 1.4 mg/dL (79.5 μmol/L) is reached. Serum concentrations rarely exceed this threshold concentration, despite very large doses, because the renal clearance of the vitamin rises sharply with daily intakes greater than 100 mg (Friedman et al., 1940). Consequently, serum ascorbic acid levels cannot be used to identify person regularly consuming excessive amounts of vitamin C. In persons consuming chronically low ascorbic acid intakes, however, serum ascorbic acid concentrations probably reflect body ascorbic acid content and are probably as accurate an index as leukocyte ascorbic acid concentrations (Jacob et al., 1987).

Serum ascorbic acid levels are lowered by several non-nutritional factors, some of which do not relate to changes in body stores of ascorbic acid. These factors include acute stress, imposed by cold or elevated temperatures, surgery, and trauma, oral contraceptive agents, chronic inflammatory diseases, acute and chronic infection (e.g. tuberculosis and rheumatic fever) and probably cigarette smoking (Sauberlich et al., 1974). Women appear to have higher plasma ascorbic acid levels than men on similar intakes of vitamin C, suggesting physiological differences in the metabolism or retention of vitamin C (VanderJagt et al., 1987). Such sex differences are not apparent before adolescence. In contrast, women using oral contraceptive agents have lower serum vitamin C levels than nonusers (Rivers, 1975). Reasons for these differences are unclear.

Urinary excretion of ascorbic acid is not a very sensitive index of ascorbic acid status; differences between persons with adequate or deficient intakes of ascorbic acid are small (Jacob et al., 1987). Specificity is also low. Drugs such as aminopyrine, aspirin, barbiturates, hydantoins, and paraldehyde increase urinary ascorbic acid excretion (Sauberlich, 1981). An additional disadvantage of this test as an index of vitamin C status in humans is the requirement for twenty-four-hour urine specimens. Measurement of urinary ascorbic acid after an oral dose of ascorbic acid (0.50 to 2.0 g of ascorbic acid per day) in divided doses for four consecutive days is sometimes used as an alternative method for assessing tissue ascorbic acid levels. Recovery of the test dose in the urine should be between 60% and 80% for subjects with normal tissue saturation of ascorbic acid (Sauberlich et al., 1974).

References

Friedman G L, Sherry S, Ralli E P (1940). Mechanism of excretion of vitamin C by the human kidney at low and normal plasma levels of ascorbic acid. Journal of Clinical Investigation 19: 685–689.

Fulwood R, Johnson C L, Bryner J D et al. (1982). Hematological and nutritional reference data for persons 6 months – 74 years of age: United States, 1976–80. Vital and Health Statistics Series 11, No. 32 DHHS Publication No. 83-1682, Washington, DC.

Jacob R A, Skala J H, Omaye S T (1987). Biochemical indices of human vitamin C status. American Journal of Clinical Nutrition 46: 818–826, 1987.

Omaye S T, Turnbull J D, Sauberlich H E (1979). Selected methods for the determination of ascorbic acid in animal cells, tissues, and fluids. Methods in Enzymology 62: 3–11.

Pelletier O (1985). Vitamin C (L-ascorbic acid and dehydro-L-ascorbic acids). In: Augustin J, Klein B P, Becker D, Venugopal P B (eds). Methods of Vitamin Assay. Fourth edition. John Wiley and Sons Inc., New York, pp. 303–347.

Rivers J M (1975). Oral contraceptives and ascorbic acid. American Journal of Clinical Nutrition 28: 550–554.

Sauberlich H E (1981). Ascorbic acid (vitamin C). In: Labbé R F (ed). Symposium on Laboratory Assessment of Nutritional Status. Clinics in Laboratory Medicine 1: 673–684.

Sauberlich H E, Dowdy R P, Skala J H (1974). Laboratory Tests for the Assessment of Nutritional Status. CRC Press Inc., Cleveland, Ohio, pp. 13–22.

Sauberlich H E, Green M D, Omaye S T (1982). Determination of ascorbic acid and dehydroascorbic acid. In: Seib P A, Tolbert B M (eds). Ascorbic Acid: Chemistry, Metabolism, and Uses. Advances in Chemistry Series, No. 200. American Chemical Society, Washington, D.C.

VanderJagt D J, Garry P J, Bhagavan H N (1987). Ascorbic acid intake and plasma levels in healthy elderly people. American Journal of Clinical Nutrition 46: 290–294.

Chapter 12
Assessment of lipid status

Contents

Introduction

The assessment of blood lipids in human nutrition has become increasingly important as their association with coronary heart disease (CHD) risk has become clearer. Lipoproteins are the important carriers of lipids in the blood. Four classes of lipoproteins exist: chylomicrons, very low density (VLD) lipoproteins, low density lipoproteins (LDL), and high density lipoproteins (HDL). All contain varying amounts of cholesterol, and hence contribute to the total blood cholesterol level. Generally, lipoproteins are measured in the blood as the cholesterol fraction (e.g. HDL cholesterol). A high serum cholesterol may arise from an increase in at least one of these lipoproteins.

Evidence from experimental, clinical, and epidemiological studies suggests that it is the level of the LDL fraction in the blood which is most closely linked to the process of atherosclerosis, and therefore for most of the CHD risk associated with elevated serum total cholesterol (Gordon et al., 1977). In contrast, the HDL fraction in serum is said to be protective against CHD. As a result,

the serum lipid profile most strongly linked to the development of atherosclerosis is a high level of both total cholesterol and LDL cholesterol in the serum, a low level of HDL cholesterol, and a high ratio of total cholesterol to HDL cholesterol.

The VLDL fraction consists mainly of triglycerides. The role of triglycerides in the process of atherosclerosis is not yet clear. Nevertheless, elevated serum triglyceride levels are useful for identifying persons with increased CHD risk. These individuals may have diseases such as diabetes mellitus, chronic renal disease, and certain primary lipidemias, all of which are associated with increased risk for cardiovascular disease. Alternatively, abnormally high triglyceride levels may be a marker of certain lipoprotein abnormalities (e.g. low HDL cholesterol).

The tests described here were recommended by the Panellists of the Canadian Consensus Conference on Cholesterol (1988) as a minimum to determine lipid risk factors for coronary heart disease.

References

Gordon T, Castelli W, Hjortland M C, Kannel W B, Dawber T R (1977). High density lipoproteins as a protective factor against coronary heart disease: the Framingham Study. American Journal of Medicine 62: 707–714.

Panellists of the Canadian Consensus Conference on Cholesterol. (1988). Final Report. The Canadian Consensus Conference on the prevention of heart and vascular disease by altering serum cholesterol and lipoprotein risk factors. Canadian Medical Association Journal 139 (supplement) 1–8.

12.1   Serum cholesterol

Principle

Cholesterol is an important precursor for the synthesis of bile acids and steroid-hormones, and for the structure of membranes and nervous tissues. An elevated level of total cholesterol in the serum, however, is one of the risk factors associated with the development of coronary heart disease. Consequently, serum cholesterol is used to screen for patients with increased risk of coronary heart disease.

Serum cholesterol is frequently assayed using an enzymatic method in which all the cholesterol esters present in serum are split quantitatively into free cholesterol and fatty acids by cholesterol esterase. In the presence of oxygen, free cholesterol is oxidized by cholesterol oxidase to Δ^4-cholesterone and hydrogen peroxide. The hydrogen peroxide then reacts in the presence of peroxidase with phenol and 4-amino-phenazone to form a quinoneimino dye. The intensity of the color formed is proportional to the cholesterol concentration and can be measured photometrically as an increase in the absorbance at 500 nm (Allain et al., 1974).

$$\text{cholesterol ester} + H_2O \rightarrow \text{cholesterol} + RCOOH$$

$$\text{cholesterol} + O_2 \rightarrow \Delta^4\text{-cholesterone} + H_2O_2$$

$$2H_2O_2 + \text{4-aminophenazone} + \text{phenol} \rightarrow$$
$$\text{4-}(\rho\text{-benzoquinone-mono imino)-phenazone} + H_2O$$

Reagents

The reagents listed below can be obtained as part of a kit from Boehringer Mannheim GmbH for the determination of serum and HDL cholesterol. Follow the procedure given by the manufacturer if this differs from that outlined below.

- Cholesterol reagent. Reconstitute by adding distilled or deionized water up to the mark (approximately 32 mL). This reagent contains:
  - Tris buffer (100 mmol/L, pH 7.7)
  - Magnesium aspartate (50 mmol/L)
  - 4-aminoantipyrine (4-aminophenazone) (1 mmol/L)
  - Phenol (6 mmol/L)

  - 3,4-dichlorophenol (4 mmol/L)
  - Hydroxypolyethoxy-n-alkane (0.3%)
  - Sodium cholate (10 mmol/L)
  - Cholesterol esterase (25°C, ≥ 400 U/L)
  - cholesterol oxidase (25°C, ≥ 250 U/L)
  - peroxidase (25°C, ≥ 200 U/L)
  - nonreactive stabilizers.

  This solution is stable for 4 weeks if stored in a refrigerator at 2–8°C or for seven days at 15–25°C (room temperature).

- Certified reference serum: Precinorm L. Boehringer Mannheim GmbH.

- Standard cholesterol solutions.

- Sample — Serum or heparinized/EDTA plasma, preferably from a fasting blood sample. Stable for up to six days at 4°C.

Equipment

- Spectrophotometer.
- Water bath at 37°C.
- Micro-pipets 20 μL.
- 2 mL pipets.
- Test tubes

Procedure

1. Label four test tubes: blank, reference, test 1, and test 2.

2. To the blank add 20 μL of distilled water. To the reference tube add 20 μL of the reference serum. To test 1 add 20 μL of test serum 1. To test 2 add 20 μL of test serum 2.

3. Add 2.0 mL of the cholesterol reagent solution to each of the four tubes. Mix each test tube well and allow to stand for 5 minutes in a water bath at 37°C. The color developed at this time is stable for up to 2 hours.

4. Set wavelength at 500 nm. Zero the spectrophotometer with the reagent blank.

5. Read and record absorbance of the reference, test 1, and test 2 samples.

Age Group (years)	Total cholesterol	
	Male	Female
5–9	159	163
	130–191	134–195
10–19	150	156
	124–187	129–190
20–29	172	164
	137–216	133–206
30–39	194	177
	153–244	143–219
40–49	207	195
	166–254	158–241
50–59	211	222
	168–262	178–275
>60	208	228
	168–256	183–279

Table 12.1: Reference values for plasma total cholesterol. The values quoted are the 50th percentile and the range from the 10th to the 90th percentiles. From Lipid Research Clinics Population Studies Data Book, 1980.

Calculation of results

The concentration (C) of cholesterol in the sample at a wavelength of 500 nm is:

$$C = 575 \times A_T \ (mg/dL)$$

where A_T = absorbance of the test sample. Note that if the values exceed 1000 mg/dL (25.9 mmol/L), dilute 0.1 mL of the sample with 0.2 mL 0.9% NaCl. Multiply the new result × 3.0 to correct for this additional dilution. Conversion to SI units (mmol/L) = ×0.02586.

Evaluation

The serum cholesterol concentration gradually increases in men 20 to 50 years of age. Values are slightly lower in women than men until menopause, after which values are higher than in men.

The intra-individual variation in serum cholesterol values is large, making a single determination of serum cholesterol in an individual of limited use. Fasting blood samples should be used for serum cholesterol determinations; values can alter by as much as 20% depending on the fatty acid composition and cholesterol content of the diet in the previous 10 to 14 day period (Demacker et al., 1982).

Table 12.1 presents the reference values for plasma total cholesterol from the the U.S. Lipid Research Clinics Population Studies Data Book (1980). Recommendations of the Task Force on the Use and Provision of Medical Services (1989) are summarized below:

- No treatment is indicated when the total serum cholesterol <5.2 mmol/L.

- Efforts should be made to reduce total serum cholesterol when it is >7.75 mmol/L.

- For total serum cholesterol ranging from 5.2–6.2 mmol/L, there is a gradual increase in risk of coronary heart disease, but the relative risk gradient remains small. Relative risk increases in the range 6.2–7.75 mmol/L.

References

Allain C C, Poon L S, Chan C S G, Richmond W, Fu P (1974). Enzymatic determination of total serum cholesterol. Clinical Chemistry 20: 470–475.

Demacker P C M, Schade R W B, Jansen R T P, Van't Lr A (1982). Intra-individual variation of serum cholesterol, triglycerides and high density lipoprotein cholesterol in normal humans. Atherosclerosis 45: 259–266.

Lipid Research Clinics Population Studies Data Book, The prevalence study, Washington D.C., Department of Health and Human Studies, July, 1980, pp. 28–81. NIH publication #80-1527.

The Task Force on the Use and Provision of Medical Services (1989). Detection and management of asymptomatic hypercholesterolemia. Ontario Ministry of Health and the Ontario Medical Association.

12.2 Serum HDL cholesterol

Principle

The concentration of HDL cholesterol is associated inversely to the risk of cardiovascular disease. The range of HDL cholesterol in the serum is narrow and the precision of the assay poor compared to that for total serum cholesterol.

The addition of phosphotungstic acid and magnesium ions precipitates chylomicrons, very low-density lipoproteins (VLDL), and low-density lipoproteins (LDL) in the sample. The sample is then centrifuged; only the high-density lipoproteins (HDL) remain in the supernatant (Friedewald et al., 1972). The cholesterol content of the supernatant is then determined enzymatically following the procedure outlined in Section 12.1.

Reagents

The reagents listed below can be obtained as part of a kit from Boehringer Mannheim GmbH for the determination of serum and HDL cholesterol. Follow the procedure given by the manufacturer if this differs from that outlined below.

- Cholesterol reagent (see Section 12.1)

- Phosphotungstic acid 0.55 mmol/L; magnesium chloride 25 mmol/L. For the micro-assay, dilute this precipitant 1:4 with distilled water.

- Certified reference serum: Precinorm L. Boehringer Mannheim GmbH.

- Sample — Serum or heparinized/EDTA plasma, preferably from a fasting blood sample. Stable for up to six days at 4°C.

Equipment

- Spectrophotometer.

- Water bath at 37°.

- Micro-pipets (200 μL) and 2 mL pipets.

- Test tubes

Procedure

1. Label three test tubes: reference, test 1, and test 2.

2. To the reference tube add 200 μL of the reference serum. To test 1 add 200 μL of test 1 serum. To test 2 add 200 μL of test 2 serum.

3. Add 500 μL of the diluted precipitant to each of the three tubes. Mix each test tube well and allow to stand for ten minutes at room temperature.

4. Centrifuge all the tubes for ten minutes at 4000 rpm or more, or for two minutes at 12,000 rpm.

5. After centrifugation, separate the clear supernatant within two hours. The supernatant can be stored up to five days at 2–25°C. Note the supernatant must be clear. If the sample has a high triglyceride content (above 1000 mg/dL), lipoprotein precipitation may be incomplete (cloudy supernatant), or part of the precipitate may float on the surface. In these cases, the test sample must be diluted 1:1 with 0.9% NaCl solution and steps 3–5 repeated. In these circumstances, the result of the cholesterol assay for this sample must be multiplied by 2.0.

6. To determine the cholesterol content of the supernatant, label four test tubes: blank, reference, test 1, and test 2.

7. To the blank add 200 μL of distilled water. To the reference add 200 μL of the reference supernatant. Add 200 μL of the test 1 supernatant to test 1. To test 2 add 200 μL of the test 2 supernatant.

8. Add 2.0 mL of the cholesterol reagent solution to each of the four test tubes. Mix each test tube well and allow to stand for ten minutes at 20–25°C or for 5 minutes at 37°C. The color developed at this time is stable for up to two hours.

9. Set the wavelength at 500 nm. Zero the spectrophotometer with the reagent blank.

10. Read and record the absorbance of the reference, test 1, and test 2.

Age Group	HDL		LDL	
(years)	Male	Female	Male	Female
5–9	54	52	90	98
	42–70	38–67	69–117	73–125
10–19	51	52	93	94
	37–65	39–66	70–123	70–126
20–29	45	52	108	100
	32–58	39–71	74–148	68–138
30–39	44	53	127	112
	32–59	39–72	90–171	79–152
40–49	44	55	138	123
	32–59	39–78	102–180	89–169
50–59	45	58	144	143
	31–61	39–80	103–188	102–198
>60	49	60	144	151
	33–71	39–82	103–190	106–199

Table 12.2: Reference values for plasma HDL and LDL cholesterol. The values quoted are the 50th percentile and the range from the 10th to the 90th percentiles. From Lipid Research Clinics Population Studies Data Book, 1980.

Calculation of HDL cholesterol

The concentration of HDL cholesterol (C) in the sample at a wavelength of 500 nm is:

$$C = 219.2 \times A_{test} \; (mg/dL)$$

where A_{test} is the absorbance of the test sample. Conversion to SI units (mmol/L) = ×0.02586.

Calculation of LDL cholesterol

When all concentrations are given in mg/dL, the LDL cholesterol equals:

$$\text{total chol.} - (\text{triglyc.}/5.0) - \text{HDL chol.} \, (mg/dL)$$

In SI units (mmol/L):

$$\text{total chol.} - (\text{triglyc.}/2.2) - \text{HDL chol.} \, (mmol/L)$$

The factor (serum triglycerides/5.0) is a correction for the average cholesterol concentration in serum of very low density lipoproteins. The values obtained are reliable provided that:

- no chylomicrons are present in the sample;
- the concentration of triglycerides does not exceed 400 mg/dL;
- and the sample does not show signs of type III hyperlipoproteinemia.

Evaluation

HDL cholesterol concentrations in serum are 15–20% higher in women than in men, for subjects more than twenty years of age. Other factors associated with high serum HDL concentrations include estrogen use, exercise, moderate alcohol consumption, and weight loss. Cigarette smoking and obesity have been associated with lower levels (Heiss et al., 1980)

LDL cholesterol concentrations in serum in industrialized countries increase three to fourfold by adulthood. The serum LDL cholesterol concentration is lower in women than men until after aged 50 years, when it gradually increases. A low LDL cholesterol concentration lowers the risk of coronary artery disease. Low density lipoprotein levels are also influenced by risk factors such as diabetes, cigarette smoking, and obesity (Schwarz et al., 1982).

Reference values for HDL and LDL cholesterol compiled from the Lipid Research Clinics Population Studies Data Book (1980) are shown in Table 12.2. The Task Force on the Use and Provision of Medical Services (1989) has proposed that a serum HDL cholesterol level of <35 mg/dL (0.9 mmol/L) is an additional risk factor in the development of coronary artery disease.

LDL/HDL ratios are said to be the strongest determinants of coronary heart disease risk by some investigators (Gordon et al., 1989). If the ratio is >3.5, diet therapy is suggested to reduce an elevated plasma LDL cholesterol level (Grundy et al., 1989).

References

Friedewald W T, Levy R I, Fredrickson D S (1972). Estimation of the concentration of low-density lipoprotein cholesterol in plasma, without use of the preparative ultracentrifuge. Clinical Chemistry 18: 499–502.

Gordon D J, Probstfield J L, Garrison R J (1989). High-density lipoprotein cholesterol and cardiovascular disease. Four prospective American studies. Circulation 79: 8–15.

Grundy SM, Goodman DeWS, Rifkind BM, Cleeman JI (1989). The place of HDL in cholesterol management. A perspective from the National Cholesterol Education Program. Archives Internal Medicine 149: 505–510.

Heiss G, Johnson N J, Reiland S, Davis C E, Taylor H A (1989). The epidemiology of plasma high density lipoprotein cholesterol levels. The Lipid Research Clinics Program Prevalence Study Summary. Circulation 62 (supplement 4): 116–136.

Lipid Research Clinics Population Studies Data Book, The prevalence study, Washington D.C., Department of Health and Human Studies, July, 1980, pp. 28–81. NIH publication #80-1527.

Schwarz W, Trost DC, Reiland SL, Rifkind BM, Heiss G (1982). Correlates of low density lipoprotein cholesterol: associations with physical, chemical, dietary, and behavioral characteristics. The Lipid Research Clinics Program Prevalence Study. Arteriosclerosis 2: 513–522.

The Task Force on the Use and Provision of Medical Services (1989). Detection and management of asymptomatic hypercholesterolemia. Ontario Ministry of Health and the Ontario Medical Association.

12.3 Serum triglycerides

Principle

Serum triglycerides concentrations are used to identify different forms of hyperlipidemia. Elevated serum triglyceride concentrations are also one of the risk factors in coronary heart disease.

Serum triglyceride concentrations can be determined by a series of coupled enzymatic reactions. In the assay described below, the triglycerides are first hydrolyzed into free glycerol and free fatty acids by a mixture of lipase and an esterase (Wahlefeld, 1974). The free glycerol is then determined enzymatically by the following equations:

$$\text{triglycerides} + 3H_2O \rightarrow \text{glycerol} + 3RCOOH$$

$$\text{glycerol} + ATP \rightarrow \text{glycerol-3-phosphate} + ADP$$

$$\text{glycerol-3-phosphate} + O_2 \rightarrow$$
$$\text{dihdroxyacetone phosphate} + H_2O_2$$

$$H_2O_2 + \text{4-aminophenazone} + \text{4-chlorophenol} \rightarrow$$
$$\text{4-(ρ-benzoquinone-mono imino)-phenazone} + H_2O + HCl$$

The intensity of the color produced is proportional to the glycerol concentration and can be measured as an increase in absorbance at 500 nm.

Reagents

The reagents listed below can be obtained as part of a kit from Boehringer Mannheim GmbH for the determination of serum triglycerides. Follow the procedure given by the manufacturer if this differs from that outlined below.

- Buffer solution. No preparation required. Stable until expiration date when stored at 2–8°C. Do not swallow or inhale vapors from the buffer which contains:
    - Tris buffer (0.15 mol/L, pH 7.6)
    - Magnesium sulfate (17.5 mmol/L)
    - EDTA, disodium salt (10 mmol/L)
    - 4-chlorophenol (3.5 mmol/L)
    - Sodium cholate (0.15%)
    - Potassium hexacyanoferrate (II) (6 μmol/L)
    - Hydroxypolyethoxy-n-alkanes (0.12%)

- Enzyme lyophilisate containing:
    - ATP (≥ 0.5 mmol/L)
    - 4-aminophenazone (0.35 mmol/L)
    - Lipase (≥ 3 U/mL)
    - Glycerol phosphate oxidase (≥ 2.5U/mL)
    - Glycerol kinase (≥ 0.2 U/mL)
    - Peroxidase (≥ 0.15 U/mL)

- Reagent solution. Combine the buffer solution with the enzyme lyophilisate, following the manufacturers instructions.

Equipment

- Micropipet: 20 μL.
- Waterbath at 37°C.
- Spectrophotometer.

Procedure

1. Pipet 2.0 mL of the reagent solution and add 20 μL of test serum.

2. Mix and incubate at 20–25°C for ten minutes.

3. Set the wavelength at 500 nm. Zero the spectrophotometer with the working solution as a blank.

4. Read the absorbance.

Calculation of triglycerides

The concentration (C) of triglycerides in the sample at a wavelength of 500 nm is:

$$C = 760 \times A_T \ (\text{mg/dL})$$

where A_T = absorbance of the test sample. Note that if the values exceed 1000 mg/dL (11.4 mmol/L), dilute 0.1 mL of the sample with 0.5 mL 0.9% NaCl. Multiply the new result × 6.0 to correct for this additional dilution. Conversion to SI units (mmol/L) = ×0.0113

Evaluation

Serum triglyceride concentrations are low in newborns, rising to the adult level by the third day of life. Values for adults increase gradually after the third decade. The range for healthy North American adults and children is 35 to 200 mg/dL (0.40 to 2.26 mmol/L).

Adult females tend to have higher serum triglyceride concentrations than males. Women 55 years and over with plasma triglyceride levels >205 mg/dL may be at risk of hypertriglyceridemia. Intra-individual variation in serum triglyceride concentrations may range from 12.9% to 40% (Demacker et al., 1982), of which 60% is biological fluctuation and the remainder analytical variation. Patients with diabetes mellitus, chronic renal disease, and certain primary hyperlipidemias have high serum triglyceride levels.

References

Demacker P C M, Schade R W B, Jansen R T P, Van't Laar A (1982). Intra-individual variation of serum cholesterol, triglycerides and high density lipoprotein cholesterol in normal humans. Atherosclerosis 45: 259–266.

Wahlefeld A W (1974). Triglyceride determination after enzymatic hydrolysis. In: Bergmeyer HU (ed). Methods of Enzymatic Analysis. 2nd ed. Academic Press, New York, pp. 1831.

Glossary

Accuracy describes the extent to which the measurement is close to the true value. To ensure accuracy, measurements must have a high precision and be free from systematic bias. The accuracy of an analytical method is assessed by the difference between the reported and the true content of the nutrient/metabolite present in a certified reference material.

Activity coefficient is a term used to express enzyme activity in red blood cells. It represents the ratio of enzyme activity with and without added coenzyme.

Analytical errors of a random nature may occur during any analytical procedure. For example, such errors made during the assay of the nutrient content of a food may lead to inaccuracies in food composition data tables.

Analytical sensitivity refers to the smallest amount that can be measured by an analytical method and distinguished from zero.

Analytical specificity describes the ability of an analytical method to measure only the substance of interest. Specific methods do not generate false-positive results and have few or no interferences.

Anthropometer is a portable instrument used to measure standing height of persons at least two years of age. Recurved branches can be inserted in some models to measure other parameters (e.g. chest depth and cranial width).

Antibody is an immunoglobulin produced by the plasma cells of a host in response to the introduction of a foreign macromolecule such as a protein.

Antigen is a foreign molecule that initiates an immune response from the host or that combines with an antibody specific for it.

Biochemical marker refers to any biochemical index in an easily accessible sample that gives a predictive response to a given dietary component.

Body mass indices measure body weight in relation to height, but cannot distinguish between excessive weight produced by adiposity, muscularity, or edema.

Certified reference materials are used to test the accuracy of an analytical method by comparing analyzed values with the certified values supplied by the manufacturer.

Chromatography separates components in a solution by differences in migration rate as the solution mixture (mobile phase) is passed over or through a stationary phase.

Coefficient of variation (CV) expresses the standard deviation as a percentage of the mean value. It is the normal method of comparing the precision of an analytical method at differing concentration levels.

Colorimeter isolates specific wavelengths of light with interchangeable filters for the visible portions of the spectrum (i.e. 380–750 nm).

Cutoff points are based on the relationship between nutritional assessment indices and functional impairment and/or clinical signs of deficiency. They are used to establish the prevalence of malnutrition within a population or to identify and classify malnourished individuals.

Dilutions are generally expressed as a ratio of the original volume to the total final volume. For example, if 1 mL of serum is diluted to 5 mL, the dilution is described as 1:5 dilution. The concentration of the substance in the diluted solution is calculated using the formula: $V_1 C_1 = V_2 C_2$ as long as the same units of volume and concentrations are used for both the original and the final solutions.

Distance growth curves are based on cross-sectional reference growth data of stature, weight, or head circumference, tabulated against age and/or stature. The data allow comparison of the stature or weight attained by an individual with data for a reference population. The curves are only suitable for making comparisons with data obtained during cross-sectional surveys.

False negatives occur when malnourished persons are classified as 'well'.

False positives occur when well-nourished persons are classified as 'ill'.

Fat-free mass consists of the skeletal muscle, nonskeletal muscle, soft lean tissues, and the skeleton. As the body muscle is composed largely of protein, the assessment of body muscle can provide an index of the protein reserves of the body.

Flat slope syndrome occurs in twenty-four-hour recalls from the tendency for low food intakes to be overestimated and high food intakes to be underestimated.

Fluorometry is used to measure molecules that fluoresce, or emit light after exposure to light of a certain wavelength. Light is emitted in a short time (10^{-9} to 10^{-6} s) and is of lower energy (longer wavelength) than the light absorbed. The intensity of the fluorescence varies directly as the concentration of the solute. This method is used to determine erythrocyte protoporphyrin.

Frankfurt plane is a conceptual plane which passes through the external auditory meatus (the small flap of skin on the forward edge of the ear) and the tops of the lower bone of the eye sockets immediately below the eye. The head must be in the Frankfurt plane for the measurements of length, stature, and head circumference.

Functional laboratory tests measure the functional consequences of a specific nutrient deficiency.

Graduated food models assist in quantifying portions of foods consumed in recall dietary methods. They consist of a collection of papier-maché, plastic, wooden, or hardboard shapes of various volumes or surface areas, together with a series of thickness indicators, which are used to assess the overall size and thickness of foods.

Gram equivalent weight of a substance is defined as the weight of that substance that can combine with, or displace, 1.008 g hydrogen.

Growth velocity curves provide information on the rate of change of growth measurements with age. This rate of change, in variables such as weight and height, is generally termed the 'growth velocity'. Growth velocity curves are derived from longitudinal data.

Indices are constructed from two or more measurements and are simple numerical ratios such as weight/(height)^2, or combinations such as weight for age, height for age, and weight for height.

Infantometer is designed for postneonatal growth studies and measures recumbent length on infants and children less than two years of age.

Inter-subject variation describes the extent to which a particular parameter varies between subjects within a sample population.

Interviewer bias occurs if different interviewers probe for information to varying degrees, intentionally omit certain questions and/or recall responses incorrectly.

Intra-subject variation describes the extent to which a particular parameter varies within one subject over time.

Load test involves administering a loading dose of the nutrient or an associated compound, after which a timed urine sample is collected. The urinary excretion of the nutrient or metabolite is then determined. In a deficiency state, excretion of the nutrient or metabolite will be low because net retention is high.

Mean value ($\bar{x}$) is the average value for a particular variable ($\Sigma x/n$).

Median value is that value of the variable, in an ordered list of values, that has an equal number of items on either side of it; i.e. the middle value.

Molar solutions contain one mole of solute per liter of solution.

Mole of any pure compound is the molecular weight of the compound expressed in grams.

Normal solution contains one gram equivalent of solute per liter of solution.

Normality is defined as the number of equivalents of solute present per liter of solution.

Peak height velocity refers to the period of maximum height velocity.

Percent Solutions weight/volume (w/v): A solution containing 5 g NaCl dissolved in water and diluted to a final volume of 100 mL of solution is equivalent to 5% (w/v) solution.

Percentile refers to the position of the measurement value in relation to all (or 100%) of the measurements for the reference population, ranked in order of magnitude.

Phase-difference effect refers to the timing of the adolescent growth spurt at markedly different ages in different children.

Plasma is the clear, yellow fluid obtained when blood is taken into a tube containing an anticoagulant and centrifuged. It contains the protein fibrinogen.

Precision measures the degree to which repeated measurements of the same variable give the same value. It is a function of the random measurement error of a specific method. Repeated measurements on a single sample (e.g. a pooled serum sample), or individual, can be used to assess precision. The coefficient of variation (CV) is a quantitative measure of precision. The precision of a method varies inversely with the CV: the lower the CV, the greater the precision.

Predictive value can be defined as the likelihood that an index correctly predicts the presence or absence of malnutrition or disease. Numerically, the predictive value of a test is the proportion of all tests that are true (the sum of the true positives and true negatives divided by the total number of tests).

Prevalence is a measure of the number of persons with malnutrition or disease at a given time. Numerically, the prevalence is the proportion of individuals who really are malnourished or infected with the disease in question divided by the sample population.

Quetelets index is an index of body mass— numerically weight/(height)^2 — said to be particularly suited for adults. It is less biased by height than other body mass indices and correlates with many health-related indices such as mortality risk. The numerical value of the index depends on the units used for height and weight.

Radioimmunoassay is based upon the binding-capacity of an antibody by the corresponding antigen. The degree to which the effective binding sites are saturated is determined by a radioactive tracer. The first step consists of adding radioactive antigen (*A) to the unlabelled antigen (Ag),

the latter being the compound to be assayed (i.e. ferritin). Specific antibody is then added to this mixture of Ag and *A in a proportion which allows part of the Ag pool to react with antibody (i.e. bound fraction) and the excess antigen to remain unaffected (i.e. free fraction). The final step consists of separating the bound fraction from the free fraction. The label commonly used is ^{125}I.

Random measurement errors may occur when the same examiner repeats the measurements (within- or intra-examiner error) or when several different examiners repeat the same measurement (between- or inter-examiner error). Such errors reduce the precision of a measurement by increasing the variability about the mean. They can be minimized by incorporating standardized measurement techniques and using trained personnel.

Reference limits are generally defined so that a stated fraction of the reference values is less than or equal to the limit, with a stated probability. Two reference limits are defined, the interval between and including them being termed the reference interval. For anthropometric indices, the 5th and 95th percentiles are frequently the two reference limits used to designate individuals with unusually low or unusually high anthropometric indices.

Respondent biases arise because the respondent may misunderstand what the interviewer has requested; receive nonverbal cues to the 'right answers' from the interviewer; or have a need to give 'socially desirable' answers.

Sensitivity of an index refers to the extent to which it reflects nutritional status, or predicts changes in nutriture. Sensitive indices show large changes as a result of only small changes in nutritional status, and, as a result have the ability to identify and classify those persons within a population who are genuinely malnourished.

Serum is obtained from blood which has been allowed to clot before centrifuging. It is similar to plasma except that it does not contain any fibrinogen. The latter was utilized to form the fibrin threads of the clot.

Single radial-immunodiffusion involves allowing an unknown amount of antigen to diffuse radially from a well in a uniformly thin layer of antibody-containing agar gel for a sufficient time to enable all the antigen to complex with the antibody, forming a precipitin zone around each well. The concentration of the unknown antigen varies directly with the area of the precipitin zone, which is proportional to the square of the diameter.

Skinfold thickness calipers measures quantitatively the compressed double fold of fat plus skin. Precision calipers are designed to exert a constant pressure of $10\,g/mm^2$ throughout the range of measured skinfolds and to have a standard 'pinch' area of 20 to $40\,mm^2$.

Social desirability response bias refers to the tendency to over-report the consumption of certain 'good' foods such as fresh fruits and vegetables, and to under-report the consumption of 'bad' items such as 'fast' and sweet foods, and alcohol.

Specificity of an index refers to the ability of the index to identify and classify those persons who are genuinely well-nourished. If an indicator has 100% specificity, all genuinely well-nourished individuals will be correctly identified: no well-nourished individuals will be classified as 'ill' (i.e. there are no false positives).

Spectrophotometry depends on the property of colored solutions to absorb light of specific wavelengths. Spectrophotometers have a continuously adjustable monochromator (prism) and can often measure the intensity of light from the near-ultraviolet region (180 or 200 nm) through the visible range (380–750 nm).

Stadiometer is a non-portable instrument that measures standing height of persons at least two years of age.

Standard deviation score is a measure of an individual's value with respect to the distribution of the reference population.

Static laboratory tests measure the level of a nutrient/metabolite in a biological tissue or fluid.

Stunting is the end result of a reduced rate of linear growth. Height for age is used as an index of stunting.

Systematic measurement errors may be present in any measurement process. Such errors reduce the accuracy by introducing a bias which alters the mean or median value. Such errors have no effect on the variance and hence do not alter the precision of the measurement.

Trigger levels are used in combination with cutoff points in population studies to set the level at which a predetermined intervention is initiated (or triggered). For example, an intervention may only be initiated if at least 10% of the population have a specific anthropometric index (e.g. weight for age) below the established cutoff point. In this case 10% is the 'trigger' level.

Validity describes the degree to which any measurement or index measures what it purports to measure.

Variance ratio is used in dietary assessment as a measure of the ratio of intra- to inter-subject variation in the true usual intake of a nutrient.

Volume/volume (v/v) is a term used for solutions composed of two liquids. A solution containing 5 mL glacial acetic acid diluted with water to a total volume of 100 mL is equivalent to 5% (v/v) acetic acid solution.

Wasting refers to gross deficits in both tissue and fat mass and is identified by a very low weight for height.

Abbreviations, conversion tables, and equipment suppliers

Measurement abbreviations

cm	centimeter
dL	deciliter (10^{-1}L)
fl oz	fluid ounces
g	gram
g	gravitational constant
hr	hour
in	inch
Kcal	kilocalorie
L	liter
lb	pound
MJ	megajoule (10^6 joules)
mL	milliliter (10^{-3}L)
mm	millimeter (10^{-3}m)
mmol	millimol (10^{-3}mol)
mg	milligram (10^{-3}m)
ng	nanogram (10^{-9}g)
nm	nanometer (10^{-9}m)
oz	ounce
pg	picogram (10^{-12}g)
sec	second
T	tablespoon
t	teaspoon
µg	microgram (10^{-6}g)
µL	microliter (10^{-6}L)
µmol	micromol (10^{-6}mol)
w/v	weight for volume

Other abbreviations

AFI	arm fat index
AMA	arm muscle area
ATP	adenosine triphosphate
BMI	body mass index
BMR	basal metabolic rate
BUN	body urea nitrogen
CAMA	corrected arm muscle area
CBC	complete blood count
CHD	coronary heart disease
CHI	creatinine height index
CPM	counts per minute
DHHS	Department of Health and Human Services
DNA	deoxyribonucleic acid
DNP	2,4-Dinitro-phenyl-hydrazine
DTT	dithiothreitol
EAA	essential amino acids
EDTA	ethylenediaminetetraacetic acid
EGR	erythrocyte glutathione reductase
EGTA	ethylene glycol-bis-(β-amino-ethyl-ether)-N,N^1-tetra-acetic acid
FAD	flavin adenine dinucleotide
FAO	Food and Agricultural Organization
HDL	high density lipoproteins
HES	Health Examination Survey (US)
HPLC	high performance (pressure) liquid chromatography

INQ	index of nutritional quality
LDL	low density lipoproteins
MAC	mid-arm circumference
MAMA	mid-arm muscle area
MAMC	mid-arm muscle circumference
MAR	mean adequacy ratio
MCH	mean cell (corpuscular) hemoglobin
MCHC	mean cell hemoglobin concentration
MCV	mean cell volume
NADPH	nicotinamide adenine dinucleotide phosphate
NAR	nutrient adequacy ratio
NCHS	National Center for Health Statistics
NEAA	non-essential amino acids
NHANES	National Health and Nutrition Examination Surveys
NIH	National Institutes of Health
NRC	National Research Council (US)
PCV	packed cell volume
PUFA	polyunsaturated fatty acids
RBC	red blood cell
RBP	retinol binding protein
RDA	recommended dietary allowance
RIA	radio-immunoassay
RNI	recommended nutrient intake
SD	standard deviation
SUN	serum urea nitrogen
TBPA	thyroxine-binding pre-albumin
TCA	trichloroacetic acid
TIBC	total iron-binding capacity
TSK	triceps skinfold
TTR	transthyretin
UIBC	unsaturated iron-binding capacity
UNU	United Nations University
UUN	urinary urea nitrogen
USDA	United States Department of Agriculture
WBC	white blood cell
WHO	World Health Organization

Small volume measures

Note: The American/Canadian standard measuring spoons used below are slightly smaller in capacity than the equivalent United Kingdom standard measuring spoons.

1 t	= 1/3 T	= 1/6 fl oz	= 4.9 mL
3 t	= 1 T	= 1/2 fl oz	= 14.8 mL
2 T	= 1/8 cup	= 1 fl oz	= 29.6 mL
4 T	= 1/4 cup	= 2 fl oz	= 59.1 mL
5 1/3 T	= 1/3 cup	= 2 2/3 fl oz	= 78.9 mL
8 T	= 1/2 cup	= 4 fl oz	= 118.3 mL
10 2/3 T	= 2/3 cup	= 5 1/3 fl oz	= 157.7 mL
12 T	= 3/4 cup	= 6 fl oz	= 177.4 mL
14 T	= 7/8 cup	= 7 fl oz	= 207.0 mL
16 T	= 1 cup	= 8 fl oz	= 236.6 mL
1 mL	= 0.034 fl oz	= 1 cc	= 0.001 liter
1 liter	= 34 fl oz	= 1000 mL	

Larger volume measures (North America)

1 pint	= 2 cups	= 16 fl oz	= 473 mL
1 quart	= 2 pints	= 0.946 liter	= 946 mL
1 gallon	= 4 quarts	= 3.785 liter	= 3785 mL
1 liter	= 1.06 quarts	= 0.26 gallons	= 1000 mL

Larger volume measures (United Kingdom)

1 pint	= 2 cups	= 20 fl oz	= 568 mL
1 quart	= 2 pints	= 1.137 liter	=1137 mL
1 gallon	= 4 quarts	= 4.546 liter	= 4546 mL
1 liter	= 1.76 pints	= 0.220 gallons	= 1000 mL

Weight measures

1000 mg	= 1 g	= 0.0352 oz	
100 g	= 3.52 oz		
1000 g	= 1 kg	= 35.2 oz	= 2.21 lb
1 oz	= 28.35 g		
16 oz	= 1 lb	= 453.59 g	= 0.454 kg

Suppliers of anthropometric equipment

Portable Length/Stature Measuring Board. Model: PE-A-1-M-101 Company: Perspective Enterprises, Inc., 7622 Sprinkle Rd., Kalamazoo, Michigan 49001. Tel: 616-327-0869. Description: Portable board, designed primarily for use in international surveys. Constructed of plywood and hardwood. Weight: approximately 20 pounds.

Recumbent Infant Length Board. Model: PE-RILB-122 (12 inches wide) Company: Perspective Enterprises 7622 Sprinkle Road, Kalamazoo, Michigan 49001. Tel: 616-327-0869. Description: This length board is constructed of plywood and has a clear plexiglass footboard. Calibration: $1/16$ th inch and 0.2 centimeters up to 39 inches and 100 centimeters. Dimension: $43 1/2$ inch long by 12 inches wide by 8 inches high. Weight: 12 pounds.

Infantometer. Model: 98-702 Company: Pfister Import-Export, Inc., 450 Barell Avenue Carlstadt, New Jersey 07072. Description: This infantometer is specifically designed for post-neonate growth studies. It has a measuring range of 300 mm to 940 mm.

Harpenden Portable Stadiometer. Model: 98-603 Company: Seritex, Inc., 450 Barell Avenue, Carlstadt, New Jersey 07072. Tel: 201-939-4606. Description: This instrument is a portable form of the 'Harpenden' standard Stadiometer. Range of 850 mm to 2060 mm. Easy to erect, free-standing unit. Measures to the nearest millimeter. Dimensions: Base 120 cm x 36 cm x 7.5 cm. Weight (including base): 20.5 kg.

Wall Mounted Measuring Board (Height). Model: PE-WM-103 Company: Perspective Enterprises 7622 Sprinkle Road, Kalamazoo, Michigan 49001 Tel: 616-327-0869. Description: This device permanently attaches to the wall and is constructed of $3/4$ inch laminated wood to prevent warping. Its clear plexiglass sliding head piece is spring-loaded to remain in place. Measures subjects up to 75 inches (190.5 cm). Dimensions: 48 inches by 10 inches wide by $3/4$ inch thick. Weight: 8 pounds.

'Handi-Stat' Measuring Device Kit. Model: PE-RA-108 Company: Perspective Enterprises, Inc., 7622 Sprinkle Road, Kalamazoo, Michigan 49001. Tel: 616-327-0869. Description: Right angle piece with tape. Calibration: $1/16$ th inch and millimeters. Weight: 10–12 oz. Suitable for those wishing to manufacture their own measuring equipment.

Microtoise Modified Tape Measure. Company: CMS Weighing Equipment Ltd., 18 Camden High Street, London, N.W.1 UK. Tel: 81-387-2060.

Portable Infant Weighing Scale. Model: MP 25: Infant weighing pack 800 Company: CMS Weighing Equipment Ltd., 18 Camden High Street, London, N.W.1. UK. Tel: 81-387-2060, or ITAC Corporation, P.O. Box 1742, Silver Springs, Maryland 20902. Tel: 301-593-8007. Weight: 1.5 kg net weight.

Pediatric Scale. Model No. 62449 (kg) Company: American Hospital Supply, 1250 Waukegan Road, McGaw Park, Illinois 60085. Tel: 800-322-6870; 708-689-8800. Calibration 20 gram increments.

Detector, Dual Reading Scale. Model No. 62408-WHI Company: American Hospital Supply, 1250 Waukegan Road, McGaw Park, Illinois 60085. Tel: 800-322-6870; 708-689-8800. Capacity 160 kilograms.

Standard Weights for Calibration. Company: Ricelake Bearing Co., 230 W. Coleman St., Ricelake, Wisconsin 54868. Tel: 800-472-6703; 715-234-9171. Weights 5, 10, 20, 25, 30, 50 pounds. (recommended to use two smaller weights rather than one large weight.)

Metropolitan Height and Weight Tables. Company: Metropolitan Life Insurance Company, Health and Safety Education Division, One Madison Ave., New York, N.Y., 10010.

Harpenden Skinfold Caliper. Company: Seritex, Inc., 450 Barell Avenue, Carlstadt, New Jersey 07072. Tel: 201-939-4606.

Lange Skinfold Caliper. Company: Seritex, Inc., 450 Barell Avenue, Carlstadt, New Jersey 07072. Tel: 201-939-4606.

Holtain Skinfold Caliper. Company: Seritex, Inc., 450 Barell Avenue, Carlstadt, New Jersey 07072. Tel: 201-939-4606.

McGaw Skinfold Caliper. Company: Ross Laboratories, Division of Abbott Laboratories, Columbus, Ohio 43216. Tel: 614-227-3706.

Elbow breadth Frame Gauge. Company: Seritex, Inc., 450 Barell Avenue, Carlstadt, New Jersey 07072. Tel: 201-939-4606.

Insertion Circumference Tape. Company: Ross Laboratories, Division of Abbott Laboratories, Columbus, Ohio 43216. Tel: 614-227-3706. Measures up to 22 inches (56 cm). Can be used for arm and head circumference.

Disclaimer: The information above is provided for the information of readers; it should not be taken as an endorsement by the author or publisher of the listed products, manufacturers, or suppliers. No significance should be attached to the absence from this list of any product, manufacturer, or supplier. A more extensive guide to equipment for nutritional assessment may be obtained from: Nutrition Services Section, Division of Health Assessment and Screening, Illinois Department of Public Health; and from: Dr. Catherine Geissler, Department of Food and Nutritional Sciences, Kings College, University of London, Campden Hill Rd., London W8 7AH, UK.

Index

Within the index, references to entries in the glossary are prefaced by the letter G.

Typeset in Adobe New Baskerville 11/13 and 9/11; figures are annotated in Adobe Helvetica.
Typeset at the University of Waterloo using a Linotronic-300, Professor Donald E. Knuth's program TeX,
and Dr. Leslie Lamport's package LaTeX. The diagrams were prepared using CorelDraw,
Harvard Graphics and Adobe Illustrator on a 386-PC. Book design by Ian L. Gibson
and Philip Taylor, with the assistance of Oxford University Press.